Maternal Mortality - Lessons Learnt from Autopsy

Kusum D. Jashnani
Editor

Maternal Mortality - Lessons Learnt from Autopsy

Springer

Editor
Kusum D. Jashnani
Department of Pathology
Topiwala National Medical College & B.Y.L. Nair Charitable Hospital
Mumbai, Maharashtra, India

ISBN 978-981-19-3419-3 ISBN 978-981-19-3420-9 (eBook)
https://doi.org/10.1007/978-981-19-3420-9

This Springer imprint is published by the registered company Springer Nature Singapore Pte Ltd.
The registered company address is: 152 Beach Road, #21-01/04 Gateway East, Singapore 189721, Singapore

To my Father Mr. Harkishindas Chhabaldas Nainaney

This compilation of case reports of the deceased patients' autopsies does not contain any identifiable information about any patient. The confidentiality and autonomy of each deceased patient is maintained throughout the manuscript and also in the images (both gross and microscopy) provided. All details that would enable any reader (including the individual or anyone else) to identify the deceased person are omitted. Principal author and all co-authors take full responsibility for this. This publication's benefits towards the society outweigh any potential harm.

Preface

Maternal mortality is an important public health problem with socioeconomic and clinical implications. Female death from any cause related to or aggravated by pregnancy or its management (excluding accidental or incidental causes) during pregnancy or within 42 days of childbirth or of an abortion, irrespective of the duration and site of the pregnancy, is defined as maternal mortality/death.

Direct maternal deaths are those "resulting from obstetric complications of the pregnant state (pregnancy, labour and puerperium), and from interventions, omissions, or incorrect treatment." Conditions like abruptio placentae, uterine rupture, and pulmonary thromboembolism are direct causes of maternal death. Indirect maternal deaths are those maternal deaths "resulting from previous existing disease or disease that developed during pregnancy and not due to direct obstetric causes but were aggravated by the physiologic effects of pregnancy." These include causes like chronic rheumatic heart disease, massive hepatic necrosis in HEV infection, severe anemia, and other infections like tuberculosis. Severe obstetric hemorrhage, puerperal sepsis, hypertensive disorders of pregnancy, and unsafe abortion constitute common causes of direct maternal deaths in developing countries. Accurate determination of causes of maternal deaths is critical for effective prevention, for which the gold standard evaluation for maternal deaths is autopsy or postmortem.

Maternal Death Review (MDR) process was started by the Government of India in the year 2010, to improve the quality of obstetric care & reduce maternal mortality by identifying gaps in existing health care. In our Institute of BYL Nair Ch. Hospital and TNMC, Mumbai, such meetings were already in place, being conducted by Dr Asha R Dalal, then HOD of Obstetrics & Gynecology Department, from the year 2003. It used to be a multidisciplinary meeting, with active participation of all concerned doctors, including presentation of autopsy findings by me. Maternal mortality ratio (MMR) in our Institute as well as in Mumbai city has shown a slight increase in trend over the years. The reason being late referrals of complicated cases from peripheral hospitals, nursing homes and hospitals from districts outside Mumbai. https://www.ncbi.nlm.nih.gov/p. More collaborative efforts are needed to bring down the MMR.

There are occasional cases, where even after complete gross and histopathologic examination after autopsy, I do not find a cause of death. I discuss these cases with the treating intensivists/obstetricians, and a consensus cause of death is then given. In this book, different cases of maternal death on autopsy—direct as well as indirect—are discussed with complete clinico-pathologic correlation, showing corresponding gross morphology and histo-pathology pictures. I am sure each of these cases will serve as a learning material to pathologists, obstetricians, intensivists, physicians, and all those involved in maternal care, and hospital administrators. What a better way to learn than getting to see authentic pictures of organs, pertaining to each case with complete clinicopathologic correlation. It has been rightly said that "Much can be learned about the living from the study of dead"—*Autopsy and Audit* (RC Path, RCP, RCS, 1991).

Thank You

Mumbai, Maharashtra, India Kusum D. Jashnani

Contents

About the Editor

Kusum D. Jashnani is currently Professor and Head of Department of Pathology, Topiwala National Medical College, Mumbai, India. She has done her undergraduation and postgraduation (MD Pathology) from Seth GS Medical College and KEM Hospital, Mumbai. She has a special interest in cytopathology, gynecologic pathology, placental pathology, and maternal autopsy and has participated as a faculty in various conferences and CMEs. Dr. Jashnani was the Organizing Secretary for CMEs on gynecologic pathology and cytopathology. She has several publications in various national and international journals and has been a postgraduate guide for MD Pathology students.

Part I

Direct Maternal Deaths

Catastrophic Abruptio Placentae: An Autopsy Case Series

1

Kusum D. Jashnani, Sumit Kumar Mandal, Lalita Yoganand Patil, and Vandana Rajesh Saravade

1.1 Case Series

1.1.1 Case 1

A 32-year-old pregnant woman (G2P1L1) was brought to the emergency room in a gasping state. Two hours prior, she had been taken to a local hospital with complaints of giddiness, vomiting and loss of consciousness. She had no previous antenatal check-up history. Her last menstrual period was also unknown. On examination, she was unconscious, not responding to deep painful stimuli. She had severe pallor, with bilateral pedal edema up to the knees. Her pulse and blood pressure were unrecordable. S1 and S2 were muffled with bilateral crepitations on auscultation. Per abdominal examination revealed a gravid uterus with 34 weeks of gestation and absent fetal heart sounds (FHS). The cervical os was closed on per-vaginal examination. Clinical impression was pre-eclampsia/eclampsia induced hypertensive cerebrovascular accident and aspiration pneumonitis. The patient died 1 h and 15 min later.

K. D. Jashnani (✉) · L. Y. Patil
Department of Pathology, Topiwala National Medical College & B.Y.L. Nair Charitable Hospital, Mumbai, Maharashtra, India

S. K. Mandal
SRL Diagnostics, Kolkata, West Bengal, India

V. R. Saravade
Department of Obstetrics and Gynecology, Topiwala National Medical College & B.Y.L. Nair Charitable Hospital, Mumbai, Maharashtra, India

1.1.2 Case 2

A 20-year-old female, primigravida with 8 months of amenorrhea, was admitted to a peripheral hospital with complaints of bleeding per vagina. She was referred to our tertiary care centre as a case of abruptio placenta with thrombocytopenia and intrauterine fetal death (IUFD). On examination, her general condition was poor. She had severe pallor (hemoglobin 6.4 g%). Her pulse and blood pressure were 120/min and 80/60 mmHg respectively. Per abdominal examination showed tonically contracted, 34–36 weeks uterus. The fetus was in cephalic presentation and FHS was not heard. On per-vaginal examination, cervical os was closed and 30% effaced. She was clinically diagnosed as having abruptio placentae with thrombocytopenia. She died 55 min after admission.

1.1.3 Case 3

A 36-year-old female (G5P5L3A1) was admitted with history of abdominal pain and severe anemia (hemoglobin 2.8 g%). There was no history of bleeding/leaking per vagina. On examination, she was unconscious and had severe pallor and cold

K. D. Jashnani (ed.), *Maternal Mortality - Lessons Learnt from Autopsy*,
https://doi.org/10.1007/978-981-19-3420-9_1

clammy extremities. Clinical impression was 9 months' amenorrhea with severe anemia and shock (hypovolemic) due to internal blood loss. She succumbed to death within 1 h of admission.

Complete autopsy was performed in all three cases.

1.2 Gross

1.2.1 Case 1

The uterus measured 35 × 27 × 11 cm. Placenta measuring 16 × 16 × 2 cm, was completely separated from the posterior uterine wall with the presence of a huge 700 g blood clot present behind the placenta (Fig. 1.1a).

1.2.2 Case 2

The uterus measured 31 × 24 × 5 cm. Placenta attached on the posterior wall measured 21 × 18 × 1.6 cm. The placenta was bulging into the uterine cavity over a thickness of 6 cm with a huge blood clot measuring 4 × 14 × 6 cm and weighing 600 g between the placenta and the uterine wall, causing almost complete placental separation from the uterine bed (Fig. 1.1b).

1.2.3 Case 3

The uterus enlarged in size (40 × 30 × 15 cm). The uterus was dusky on the external surface and was full of blood clots (total weighing 800 g) and liquid blood about 1.5 L on the cut surface. Gestational sac with the fetus was inside. The placenta was floating in the uterus, weighed 450 g and measured 15 × 15 × 2.5 cm (Fig. 1.2a, b).

In all three cases, there was no evidence of infarct in the placenta. The rest of the organs were very pale, otherwise unremarkable, except for case No. 2, where 60% of glomeruli showed the presence of fibrin thrombi within glomerular capillaries and patchy areas of acute tubular necrosis in the kidneys on histopathologic examination.

1.2.4 Final Cause of Death

Hemorrhagic shock following abruptio placentae with retroplacental hematoma and severe anemia

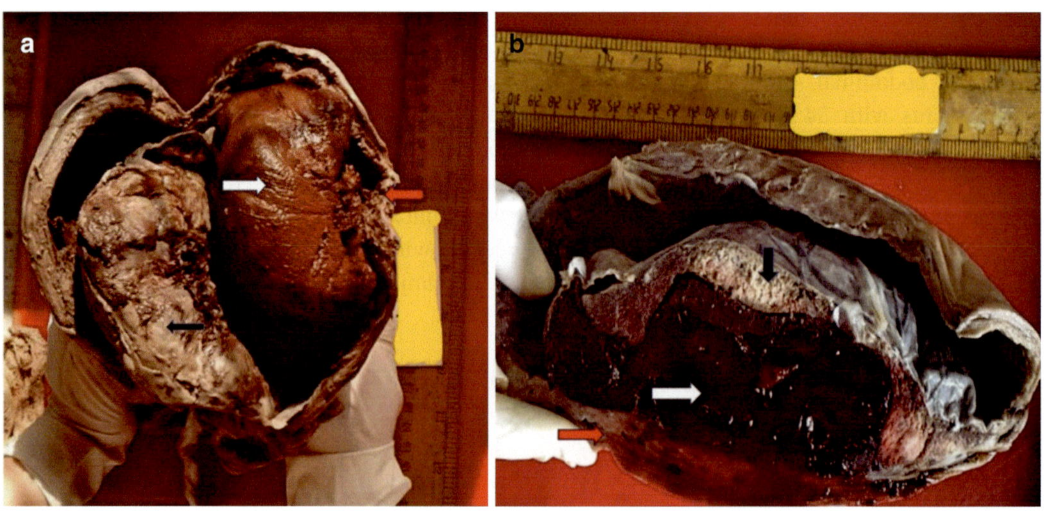

Fig. 1.1 (**a**) Case 1 Gross image—the placenta (black arrow) was completely separated from the posterior uterine wall (red arrow) with the presence of a huge blood clot (white arrow) present behind the placenta. No evidence of missing cotyledons or red or white area. (**b**) Case 2 Gross image—the placenta (black arrow) was bulging into the uterine cavity over a thickness of 6 cm with a huge blood clot (white arrow) between the placenta and the uterine wall (red arrow), causing almost complete placental separation from the uterine bed

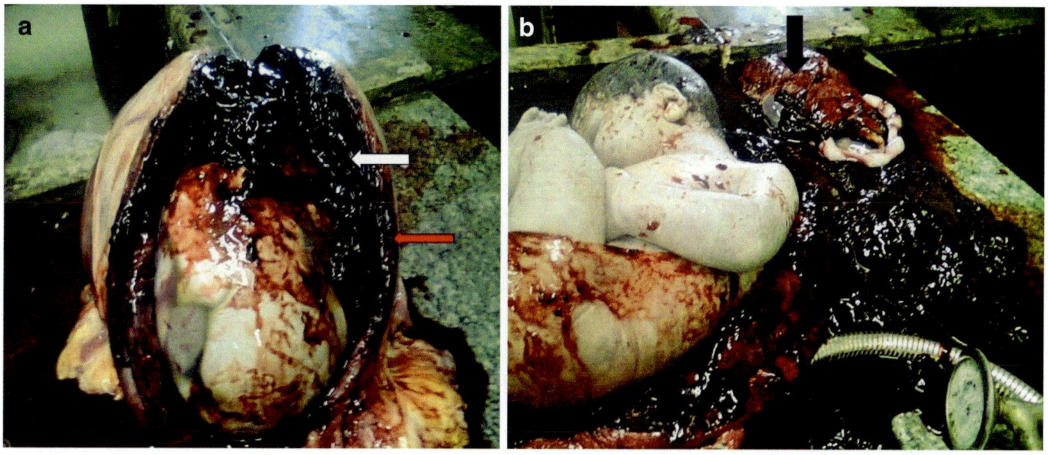

Fig. 1.2 Case 3 Gross image (**a**) the uterus was dusky and full of blood clots (white arrow) and liquid blood. The gestational sac with a fetus was seen inside, and the placenta was completely separated. (**b**) Flacid completely separated placenta (black arrow) from the uterus kept next to the fetus

(in all three cases) with the addition of coagulopathy in the cause of death in Case 2.

1.3 Clinicopathologic Discussion

Antepartum hemorrhage (APH) is an obstetric emergency responsible for maternal and fetal loss. It is defined as vaginal bleeding after 24 weeks of gestation. There are different causes of APH, commonest being placenta previa and abruptio placentae (AP), which account for almost 50% of cases of APH. Uterine rupture is a rare cause of APH. An AP is characterised by the partial or complete premature separation of the placenta, before the delivery of the fetus. Approximately 1% of births are complicated by placental abruption, which most often occurs in the third trimester. Risk factors for abruption are many, including advanced maternal age, increased parity, lack of prenatal care and low socio-economic status which were seen in our cases [1, 2]. Abruption in a previous pregnancy leads to 15- to 20-fold increased risk of recurrence in the following pregnancy [3]. The clinical hallmarks of AP are vaginal bleeding (in cases of a revealed type of AP), abdominal pain and uterine contractions/tenderness. In two of our patients, AP was of the concealed type with no symptoms of vaginal bleeding, and they had presented with signs of hypovolemic shock. Placental abruption may also be diagnosed based on pathologic findings including the presence of a significant retroplacental or marginal blood clot; a placenta with a large separately received blood clot and depression or indentation on the maternal surface of the placenta. Abruptio is associated with maternal complications like disseminated intravascular coagulation (DIC), shock, acute renal failure, post-partum hemorrhage (PPH) and anemia. Fetal complications include prematurity, hypoxia, growth restriction and fetal death [4]. In our case series, all the deceased had intrauterine fetal death. In cases with acute presentation and a live fetus, emergency cesarean section independent of gestational age is carried out, unless there is an indication of impending vaginal delivery. On the other hand, in acute symptoms and IUFD, either an induced vaginal delivery or an emergency cesarean section is done if there is risk of maternal death.

The key factor in the pathophysiology is hemorrhage at the decidual–placental interface which separates the decidua, leaving a thin layer attached to the placenta. The size of the hematoma increases gradually or suddenly, resulting in further separation and compression of the overlying intervillous space and local destruction of placental tissue [5]. Thrombin plays an important role in the clinical consequences and pathogenesis of placental abruption. It is formed via two pathways: (a) decidual bleeding leads to release of tissue factor (thromboplastin) from decidual cells, which leads to generation of thrombin, and (b) decidual hypoxia leads to production of vascular endothelial growth factor (VEGF). VEGF acts directly on decidual endothelial cells to induce expression of tissue factor, which subsequently generates thrombin [6]. Thrombin production accounts for various clinical sequelae:

1. As thrombin is a potent uterotonic agent, it leads to uterine tonicity and contractions [7].
2. There is increased expression of matrix metalloproteinases, upregulation of genes involved in apoptosis and enhanced expression of inflammatory cytokines (predominantly TNF, interleukin 1 and interleukin 8), resulting in tissue necrosis and extracellular matrix destruction. This results in the destruction of cellular connections that secure the placenta, ending in premature detachment [6].
3. Thrombin enters the maternal circulation instantaneously, inundates hemostatic control mechanisms. Consequently, there is widespread intravascular fibrin deposition, ischemic tissue injury and microangiopathic hemolytic anaemia, leading to severe systemic bleeding diathesis (DIC) [8].

Pre-eclampsia is strongly associated with abruptio placentae. Normally maternal spiral arteries are invaded by trophoblast cells, which maintains high flow and low resistance uteroplacental circulation. In case of pre-eclampsia, there is low pro-angiogenic placental growth factor (PlGF) and high anti-angiogenic soluble fms-like tyrosine kinase 1 (sFlt1). This leads to incomplete spiral artery remodelling and increased resistance to uterine artery blood flow. Subsequently, there is increased chance of vascular rupture and placental abruption [9].

Immunological rejection also plays an important role in placental abruption. Normally, human leukocyte antigen (HLA)-G defends the fetus (a semi-allograft) from maternal immune attack. It has been observed that placental abruption is associated with low maternal plasma levels of soluble HLA-G [10].

References

1. Sheiner E, Shoham-Vardi I, Hallak M, Hadar A, Gortzak-Uzan L, Katz M, et al. Placental abruption in term pregnancies: clinical significance and obstetric risk factors. J Matern Fetal Neonatal Med. 2003;13(1):45–9.
2. Salman M, Saraswathi K, Shyamala R, Ali SSA, Azam I, Khan MI. Placental Abruption An Obstetricians Nightmare-A Study of Risk Factors and Maternofoetal Outcomes at Two Tertiary Care Teaching Hospitals in South India. Asian Pacific J Heal Sci. 2017;4(1):220–30.
3. Ananth C V, Savitz DA, Williams MA. Placental abruption and its association with hypertension and prolonged rupture of membranes: A methodologic review and meta-analysis. Obstet Gynecol. 1996;88(2):309–18.
4. Sengodan SS, Dhanapal M. Abruptio placenta: a retrospective study on maternal and perinatal outcome. Int J Reprod Contraception, Obstet Gynecol. 2017;6(10):4389.
5. Hall DR. Abruptio Placentae and Disseminated Intravascular Coagulopathy. Semin Perinatol. 2009;33(3):189–95.
6. Krikun G, Huang STJ, Schatz F, Salafia C, Stocco C, Lockwood CJ. Thrombin activation of endometrial endothelial cells: A possible role in intrauterine growth restriction. Thromb Haemost. 2007;97(2):245–53.
7. Elovitz MA, Ascher-Landsberg J, Saunders T, Phillippe M. The mechanisms underlying the stimulatory effects of thrombin on myometrial smooth muscle. Am J Obstet Gynecol. 2000;183(3):674–81.
8. Thachil J, Toh CH. Disseminated intravascular coagulation in obstetric disorders and its acute haematological management. Blood Rev. 2009;23(4):167–76.
9. Powe CE, Levine RJ, Karumanchi SA. Preeclampsia, a disease of the maternal endothelium: the role of antiangiogenic factors and implications for later cardiovascular disease. Circulation. 2011;123(24):2856–69.
10. Steinborn A, Rebmann V, Scharf A, Sohn C, Grosse-Wilde H. Placental abruption is associated with decreased maternal plasma levels of soluble HLA-G. J Clin Immunol. 2003;23(4):307–14.

Liver Infarct in Pregnancy: A Complex, Rare and Dreadful Affair

2

Kanchan Dilip Trichal, Kusum D. Jashnani, and Vrinda Kiran Kulkarni

2.1 Clinical History

We present a case of 25-year-old multigravida with twin gestation who was referred from a local hospital with pain in abdomen at 37 weeks of pregnancy. In addition, she had history of yellow discoloration of the sclera, high-coloured urine and fever with chills in the last 3–4 days. She tested positive for HbsAg (hepatitis B surface antigen) in the first month of gestation. She had two previous pregnancies with a male and a female child at ages 5 years and 3 years, respectively (details of previous obstetric history were unavailable). Vaginal delivery was conducted and both babies were delivered safely. During delivery, blood clots were removed, and this was followed by massive bleeding per vaginum. On examination, she had severe pallor and drowsiness. She was transferred to MICU immediately with clinical impression of 'post-partum hemorrhage (PPH) with HbsAg positive status to rule out disseminated intravascular coagulation (DIC)'.

On the first examination in MICU, her general condition (GC) was moderate, BP 140/90, respiratory system was clear, pallor was present, and rashes were seen over her body. She was conscious, oriented but drowsy. Reports concluded severe anemia with hemoglobin 5 g/dL, thrombocytopenia (platelets reduced to 24,000), deranged values of LFT and raised INR (INR 3.9) and D dimer >10,000 ng/ml. Creatinine was also raised to 2.4 g/dL. Ultrasound reported the presence of bilateral mild pleural effusion, moderate ascites and minimal perihepatic free fluid and medical renal disease. She was started with immediate supportive treatment and multiple blood transfusions (4 units of PCV, 1 unit each of FFP and platelet). Despite all the measures, the patient's condition continued to deteriorate; she could not be revived and was declared dead on the fifth day of post-partum. A complete autopsy was performed after taking due permissions.

K. D. Trichal
Histopathology, University Hospital of North Durham, County Durham and Darlington NHS Foundation Trust, Durham, UK

K. D. Jashnani (✉)
Department of Pathology, Topiwala National Medical College & B.Y.L. Nair Charitable Hospital, Mumbai, Maharashtra, India

V. K. Kulkarni
Department of Medicine and Clinical Hematology, Topiwala National Medical College & B.Y.L. Nair Charitable Hospital, Mumbai, Maharashtra, India

K. D. Jashnani (ed.), *Maternal Mortality - Lessons Learnt from Autopsy*,
https://doi.org/10.1007/978-981-19-3420-9_2

2.2 Autopsy Findings

On gross examination, the liver weighed 1.7 kg, showing subcapsular hemorrhages. On cut section—chronic passive congestion (CPC) changes were noted with no evidence of cirrhosis. The caudate lobe showed necrosis involving almost the total lobe and necrosis extending up to the superior surface (Figs. 2.1 and 2.2). The pleural cavity was filled with blood and clots (about 500 g); the peritoneal cavity had around 1000 mL of dark yellow-coloured free fluid. The stomach mucosa and kidney capsule showed petechial haemorrhages. The lungs showed subplcural hemorrhage forming a clot measuring 3 × 3 × 1 cm. The uterus and cervix showed petechial hemorrhages on the serosa and blood clots in the cavity.

On microscopy, sections from the caudate lobe showed evidence of coagulative necrosis of hepatocytes involving large areas. Border of the infarct showed a dense mixed inflammatory infiltrate with loss of hepatocytes (Fig. 2.3). The subcapsular region showed proliferating capillaries and the deposition of fibrin. Portal tract vessels were dilated and markedly congested. Sections from the surrounding cholestatic liver showed preservation of normal lobular hepatic architecture with the presence of multiple focal areas of hepatocytic necrosis randomly scattered over the liver parenchyma. Impression: caudate lobe infarct of the liver.

Microscopy of the kidney showed cloudy change in tubules. Sections from the lung showed a large focus of subpleural hemorrhage with collapse of the underlying alveolar spaces. Similarly, areas of hemorrhagic necrosis were seen in the adrenals with fibrin thrombi in vessels. Areas of hemorrhage were also confirmed in the uterus, cervix and heart (subendocardial).

The rest of the organs were unremarkable on microscopy.

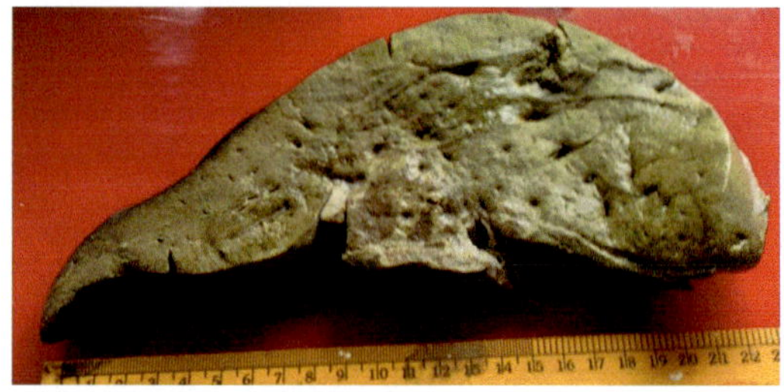

Fig. 2.1 Caudate lobe infarct. The weight was 1.7 kg. A large infarct involving almost the whole of the caudate lobe is seen

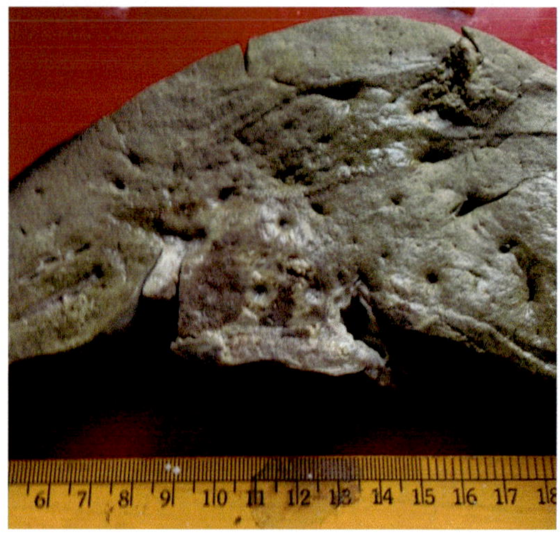

Fig. 2.2 Close-up view of the same caudate lobe infarct

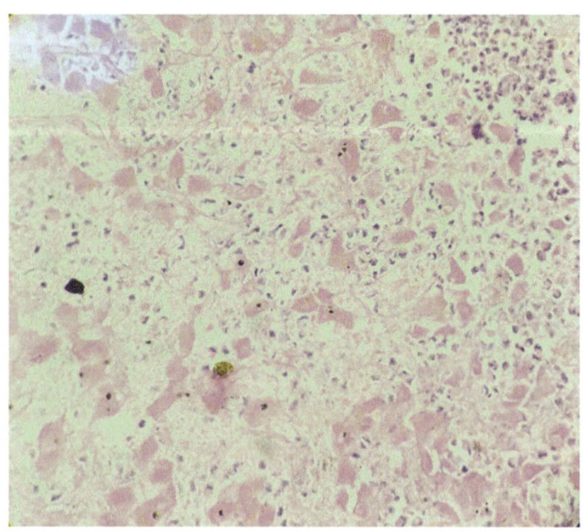

Fig. 2.3 Large areas of coagulative necrosis of hepatocytes. The border at right upper corner shows mixed inflammatory infiltrate (H&E, ×200)

2.3 Final Cause of Death

DIC with caudate lobe infarct following postpartum hemorrhage with known HbsAg positive status.

2.4 Clinicopathologic Discussion

Hepatic infarction is an extremely rare situation because the liver has a dual blood supply from the hepatic artery and portal vein. Liver infarction is usually reported at autopsy. Most cases are seen after liver transplantation or hepatobiliary surgery. There are two different mechanisms of vascular injury to the liver tissue, *ischemic hepatitis and hepatic infarction. Ischemic hepatitis* involves the whole liver. It is caused by systemic hypoperfusion, or it may be caused by decreased perfusion from the hepatic artery and/or portal vein. For example, it can occur in patients who undergo *liver transplantation* and have *hepatic artery thrombosis*. It is mostly self-limiting and removing the insult that caused the liver hypoperfusion is the only effective treatment [1]. In contrast, hepatic infarction represents a focal ischemic injury to the liver. This infarction can be caused by *occlusion of the hepatic artery due to arteriosclerosis, thrombosis or emboli*. Infarction without hepatic artery occlusion is mainly caused by *trauma during surgery*, *hypercoagulable state*, *pre-eclampsia*, *eclampsia* and *postpartum HELLP syndrome* (hemolysis, elevated liver function tests, and low platelets).

Clinical manifestations of liver infarction are non-specific; it can initially present as chest or upper right abdominal pain, fever, jaundice with or without associated nausea and vomiting [2, 3]. In addition, related laboratory studies for hematological and biochemical markers are not specific, which makes the diagnosis challenging. Hepatic encephalopathy, prolonged jaundice, and concomitant renal failure suggest poor prognosis [4]; two of these features were present in our case. In such circumstances, the short-term mortality rate is high.

Pregnancy is a hypercoagulable status. Obstetric complications include PPH (defined as haemorrhage above 500 mL after vaginal delivery or above 1000 mL after a cesarean section), pre-eclampsia, HELLP syndrome (hemolysis, elevated liver function tests, and low platelets), amniotic fluid embolism, and acute fatty liver are all conditions linked to high risk of developing DIC [1]. If we do not stop the bleeding at an early stage, severe consequences including DIC and organ failure can develop.

A literature search on hepatic infarction reveals previous reports which also presented cases of hepatic infarctions related to pregnancy. A report by Ting Peng et al. in Taiwan [1] presented a similar case of severe PPH complicated by DIC and hepatic infarction resulting in acute hepatic failure. In their case, they intervened with liver transplantation, but even then the patient couldn't survive and expired on the 36th day after the primary PPH episode. In their report, they discussed how the timing of effective hemostasis plays a substantial role in determining a woman's prognosis after PPH. Intervening earlier when the estimated blood loss is less seems to improve the outcome [5].

Another recent case report by Qinyue Guo et al. [6] discussed a pregnant woman with pre-eclampsia who was diagnosed with HELLP syndrome, following which 3 days later, they found a hepatic infarct on CT scan. However, with timely intervention through CRRT, plasma exchange, hormone therapy and supportive treatments, fortunately, further damage of the liver was prevented, and the patient recovered. R. Pauzner et al. describe four patients with pregnancy-associated hepatic infarctions. All four had APS and HELLP syndrome. They developed hepatic infarction despite anticoagulant treatment. All the fetuses were lost. Another rare case of severe PPH complicated by acute MI and ischemic hepatitis was reported by Meng-Han Chou et al. [7] AFLP (acute fatty liver of pregnancy) is a rare but significant cause of maternal morbidity and mortality. The initial presentation of AFLP mimics that of HELLP syndrome, making its diagnosis and management challenging. DIC and bleeding are the common complications in cases of AFLP. A recent case report of AFLP complicated by DIC discusses the long-complicated course of the disease in such cases [8].

In our case, autopsy showed the presence of a caudate lobe infarct; a similar interesting case of isolated caudate lobe infarct post-liver transplantation is described by C.F. Hung et al. [9] **Amongst all the references discussed, our study is the only one with autopsy evidence of caudate lobe infarct**. Our patient had tested *HbsAg positive*; hence, we tried to do a literature search to establish relation between hepatitis and hepatic infarction, but the data available is not plentiful. It is uncertain whether HBV and HCV themselves cause thrombosis. There is some evidence suggesting that chronic viral infection is a thrombotic risk factor, perhaps by infection-mediated inflammation and hemostatic impairment [9]. APL and the prothrombotic state associated with chronic liver disease seem to play an important role in virus-associated thrombosis [10]. The risk of developing other arterial and venous thromboembolic events in patients with chronic liver disease is not well defined. So, it is difficult to define the role of hepatitis B in the cascade of events that followed in our case.

In conclusion,

- The causes of liver infarction are complex with an outcome that can sometimes even be fatal. Since liver infarction is rare, we should be well aware of its imaging appearance, clinical characteristics and serum results for early suspicion and diagnosis. This is important for controlling further progression and improving prognosis.
- The management of PPH remains one of the significant challenges to obstetricians; the timing of intervention plays a substantial role in determining a woman's prognosis after PPH [1].
- Finally, although the case that we presented of PPH leading to DIC and hepatic infarction is rare in an uncomplicated pregnant woman, we have to be well prepared to detect and manage these uncommon but serious complications closely and timely.

References

1. Peng I-T, Chung M-T, Lin C-C. Severe postpartum hemorrhage complicated with liver infarction resulting in hepatic failure necessitating liver transplantation. Case Rep Obstet Gynecol. 2018;2018:1–5.
2. Mor F, Beigel Y, Inbal A, Goren M, Wysenbeek AJ. Hepatic infarction in a patient with the lupus anticoagulant. Arthritis Rheum. 1989;32(4):491–5. https://pubmed.ncbi.nlm.nih.gov/2495803/. Accessed 11 Jan 2021.
3. Wang F-H, Yang N-N, Liu F, Tian H. Unexplained huge liver infarction presenting as a tumor with bleeding: a case report. World J Clin Cases. 2020;8(10):2016–22. https://www.wjgnet.com/2307-8960/full/v8/i10/2016.htm. Accessed 11 Jan 2021.
4. Yantorno SE, Kremers WK, Ruf AE, Trentadue JJ, Podestá LG, Villamil FG. MELD is superior to King's college and Clichy's criteria to assess prognosis in fulminant hepatic failure. Liver Transpl. 2007;13(6):822–8. https://aasldpubs.onlinelibrary.wiley.com/doi/full/10.1002/lt.21104. Accessed 11 Jan 2021.
5. Howard TF, Grobman WA. The relationship between timing of postpartum hemorrhage interventions and adverse outcomes. Am J Obstet Gynecol. 2015;213(2):239.e1–3. http://www.ajog.org/article/S0002937815003816/fulltext. Accessed 11 Jan 2021.
6. Guo Q, Yang Z, Guo J, Zhang L, Gao L, Zhou B, et al. Hepatic infarction induced by HELLP syndrome: a case report and review of the literature. BMC Pregn Childb. 2018;18(1):191. https://bmcpregnancychildbirth.biomedcentral.com/articles/10.1186/s12884-018-1799-9. Accessed 7 Jan 2021.
7. Chou MH, Chen YC, Hwang KS, Yu MH, Su HY. Myocardial infarction and ischemic hepatitis complicated by postpartum hemorrhage. Taiwan J Obstet Gynecol. 2016;55(3):437–40.
8. Chalifoux M, Blank H. Acute fatty liver of pregnancy and disseminated intravascular coagulation: a case report. J Obstet Anaesth Crit Care. 2020;10(1):42.
9. Hung CF, Tseng JH, Jeng LB, Lee WC, Ng KK, Wan YL. Isolated caudate lobe infarct after orthoptic liver transplantation. Transplant Proc. 2000;32(7):2223–4. https://pubmed.ncbi.nlm.nih.gov/11120142/. Accessed 12 Jan 2021.
10. Tripodi A, Mannucci PM. The coagulopathy of chronic liver disease. N Engl J Med. 2011;365(2):147–56. https://pubmed.ncbi.nlm.nih.gov/21751907/. Accessed 12 Jan 2021.

Cerebral Venous Sinus Thrombosis: An Avertable Catastrophe

3

Asha Shenoy

3.1 Clinical History

A 24-year-old woman presented with a severe throbbing headache since 1 day. She later on developed generalized tonic and clonic convulsions and weakness of left-sided extremities, for which she was admitted to our hospital. She had a history of normal vaginal delivery 16 days ago and no history of gestational diabetes mellitus, pregnancy induced hypertension, or abnormal thyroid function. There was no history of fever, epilepsy, or any other complaint.

On examination She was afebrile with a pulse rate of 84/min and a blood pressure of 110/70 mmHg. Systemic examination of the central nervous system revealed she was drowsy, with decreased movements on the left side of her body, with ipsilateral decreased tone, and exaggerated reflexes. Subsequently, the patient developed two more episodes of convulsions. The routine hematological investigations showed leucocytosis and biochemical investigations were normal.

Imaging Thrombosis of the superior sagittal sinus and bilateral transverse sinuses. Venous infarct with hemorrhagic transformation.

The patient was treated with anticonvulsants and anticerebral edema measures. She expired within 18 hours of admission.

3.2 Autopsy Findings

Brain The brain along with the dura was suspended and fixed in 10% formalin for 2 weeks. The brain weighed 1.2 kg and the dura showed thrombosis of the superior sagittal sinus along its entire length and thrombosis of draining veins. The basal dura showed thrombosis of bilateral transverse sinuses. The cerebral hemispheres were asymmetrical, and bilaterally cortical veins were prominent, congested, tortuous, and cord-like. The right parietal cortex showed a hemorrhagic infarct measuring 4 × 3 × 3 cm, reaching superficially up to the thrombosed veins. Surrounding white matter edema with a shift of midline structures to the opposite side was seen.

A. Shenoy (✉)
Neuropathology Laboratory, Department of Pathology, Seth G.S. Medical College & K.E.M Hospital, Mumbai, Maharashtra, India

K. D. Jashnani (ed.), *Maternal Mortality - Lessons Learnt from Autopsy*,
https://doi.org/10.1007/978-981-19-3420-9_3

Cerebellar tonsillar herniation was present more on the right side (Fig. 3.1).

All the other organs were unremarkable on gross examination. No foci of infection seen in any organ including pelvic cavity.

On histology Brain with dura: Sections from the dura showed recent thrombi within the sinus lumina and draining veins. Sections from the infarct showed typical ball and ring hemorrhages, which were confluent in areas forming lakes of hemorrhages. Capillaries showed recent fibrin thrombi and a few vessels were plugged with neutrophils. No significant inflammation was seen in any section (Fig. 3.2).

Sections from other organs also did not show any inflammation.

3.3 Final Cause of Death

Cerebral venous sinus thrombosis, hemorrhagic cerebral infarction, and raised intracranial pressure.

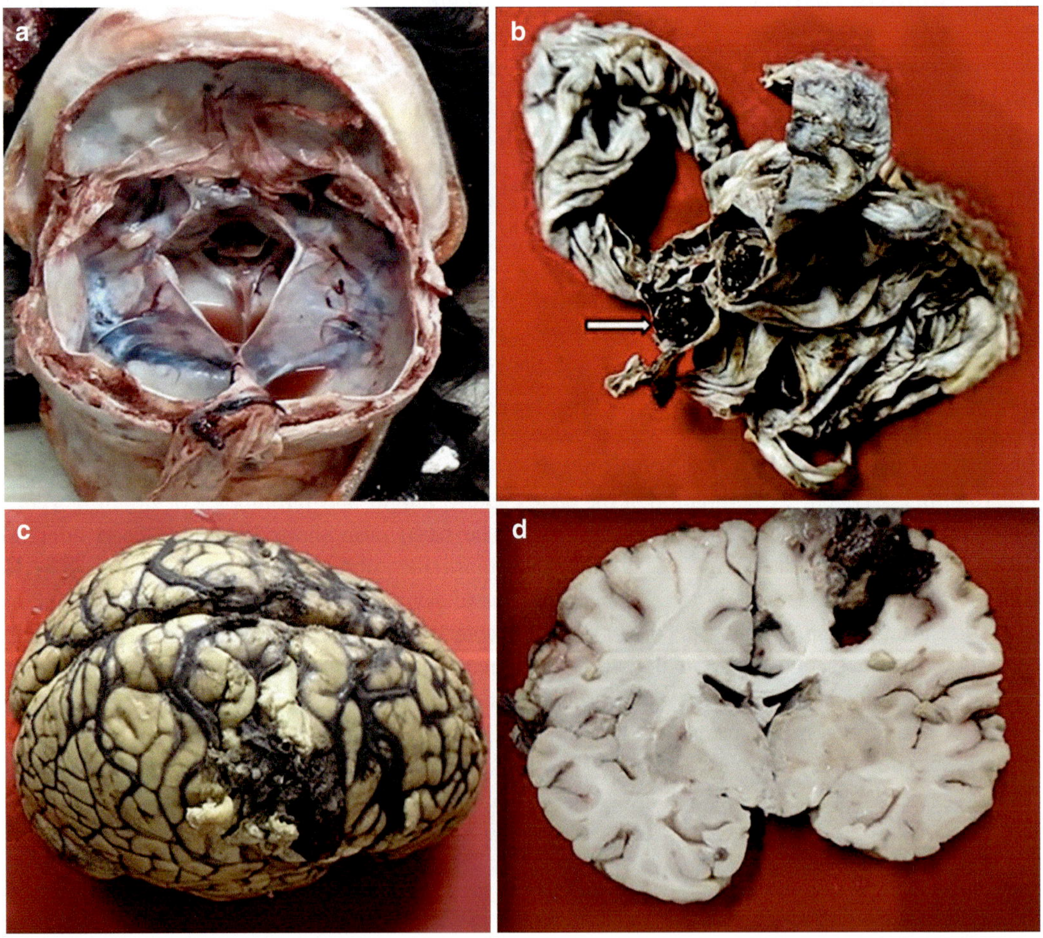

Fig. 3.1 (**a**) The basal dura showing thrombosis of bilateral transverse sinuses. (**b**) Dural sinus occluded by recent thrombus (arrow). (**c**) The brain showing edema and prominent cord-like tortuous thrombosed cortical veins. (**d**) Coronal slice showing hemorrhagic infarct in the parietal region reaching the surface

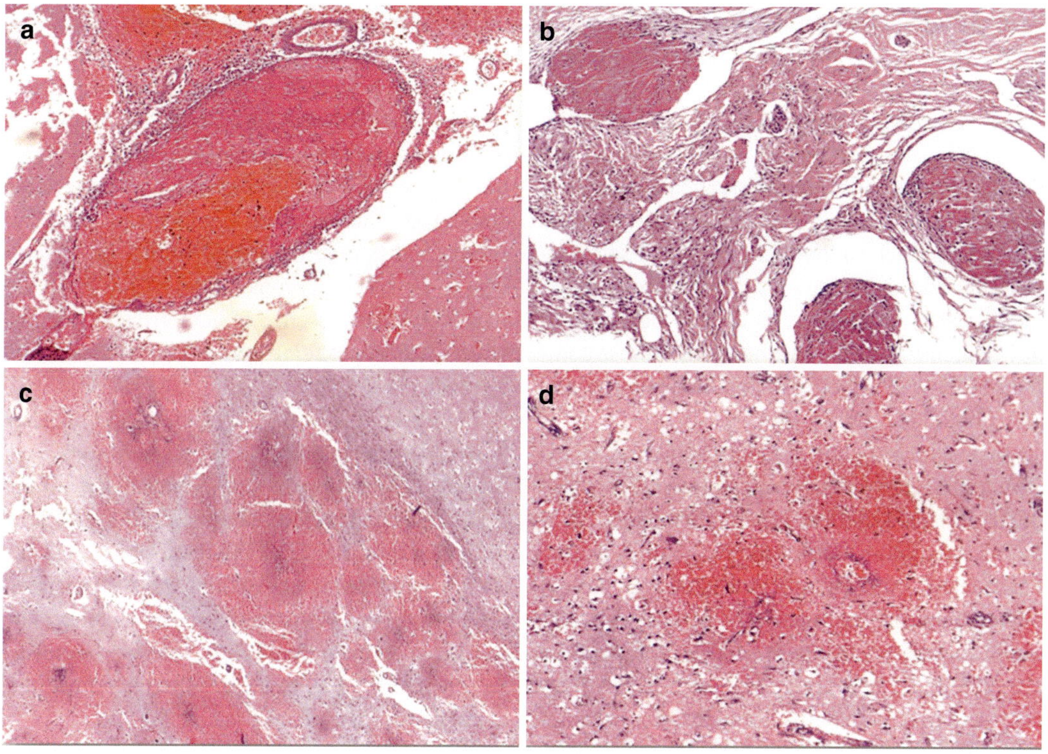

Fig. 3.2 (**a**) The cortical vein showing recent thrombus H&E ×400. (**b**) The dura showing recent thrombi in draining veins H&E ×400. (**c**) Hemorrhagic infarct showing ball and ring hemorrhages H&E ×100. (**d**) Hemorrhagic infarct showing ring hemorrhages H&E ×400

3.4 Clinicopathologic Discussion

Cerebral venous sinus thrombosis (CVST) accounts for 0.5–1% of all cases of strokes [1]. Women outnumbered men in a ratio of 3:1, especially in the young (20–35 years) [2]. This increased incidence is due to gender specific risk factors like pregnancy, puerperium, use of oral contraceptives, and hormone replacement therapy. In addition, other factors predisposing to (CVST) are infections, systemic diseases, malignancy, trauma to the head and neck, severe dehydration, and hereditary thrombophilia [2].

Pregnancy is known to cause several changes in the coagulation system including increased pro-coagulant factors, an impaired physiological anticoagulant system, and decreased fibrinolysis. Additional risk factors in puerperium include infection, cesarian section, dehydration, increased maternal age, hypertension, etc. Most cases of CVST during this period present in the last trimester of pregnancy and up to the first 2 weeks of puerperium. Additional risk factors like genetic thrombophilia may play a synergistic role, and screening for the same is recommended in all patients as this has been reported in as many as half the patients in this group [3].

The case highlighted was that of a 24-year-old woman who presented on Day 16 postpartum. She had no predisposing risk factors in the antenatal and intranatal period. There was no fever and no symptoms to suggest infection in the postnatal period. Her short ward stay precluded ancillary tests for thrombophilia. Her routine hemogram showed neutrophilia (but autopsy examination did not reveal any source of infection). Imaging studies (MRI/MRVenography) were performed and showed SSS and transverse sinus thrombosis and hemorrhagic cerebral infarction.

The clinical and neuroradiological appearance of CVST are identical whatever the etiology and depend on the location and extent of thrombus/thrombi. The highly variable clinical presentation makes early diagnosis difficult and delays therapy. Patients present with headache (most common), followed by seizures, motor weakness, and coma/obtunded status [4–6].

Headache is a clinical manifestation of raised intracranial pressure which follows extensive dural sinus and cortical venous thrombosis. It is an early symptom, but in the post-partum period, headache is often wrongly attributed to postdural puncture headache, especially in cases of epidural anesthesia/caesarean section. Patients are prescribed analgesics and there is a delay in diagnosis and treatment until significant clinical deterioration is seen. In our patient, despite severe throbbing-generalized headache, medical aid was sought only after multiple episodes of convulsions and motor weakness. This delay in seeking medical assistance possibly resulted in fatal outcome.

In pregnancy induced hypertension, seizures are treated initially as part of eclampsia, and imaging studies are often carried out after the failure of anticonvulsant therapy. This delay worsens the survival and prognosis [4]. A high index of clinical suspicion is therefore necessary and imaging studies like MRI and MR Venography (MRV) are required for clinching the diagnosis.

In a clinically suspected/diagnosed case of CVST at autopsy, the dural sinuses are examined for recent/recanalizing thrombi. The extent of involvement of the sinus and draining veins is noted. The basal dura is examined after the brain is removed and the basal sinuses are opened and inspected for thrombi. This step has to be performed during autopsy as these sinuses lie at the base of the skull. The basal dura can be stripped off the skull base and also examined later. The brain is suspended and fixed in 10% formalin for a minimum period of 2 weeks. The thrombosed cortical veins on the surface of the brain look prominent, tortuous, congested and feel cord-like. They may be accompanied by a variable amount of subarachnoid hemorrhage. Cerebral edema and herniation are additional gross findings to be noted. Coronal slices of the brain are studied for the presence of hemorrhagic infarcts, which are superficial and often bilateral and symmetrical.

In our case, besides extensive SSS, bilateral transverse sinus and cortical venous thrombosis, autopsy also confirmed the hemorrhagic infarct in the right parietal cortex which had produced a left-sided motor deficit. The hemorrhagic venous infarct was superficial, reaching the surface, up to the thrombosed veins, resulting in seizures. The resultant cerebral edema and consequent cerebellar tonsillar herniation had resulted in a fatal outcome in our case.

The management of a patient with CVST in pregnancy and puerperium is challenging due to restrictions of pharmacological and procedural management. Administration of anticoagulant therapy, thrombolysis, and thrombectomy are the therapeutic modalities used. Decompression surgery/craniotomy is carried out if herniation is imminent. Our patient was however only administered anticonvulsants and anti-edema measures due to short ward stay.

CVST has generally a favorable prognosis though severe sequelae and death can occur in few cases. Patients with headache alone at the time of treatment have a better outcome than those with obtunded status. A deteriorating clinical picture, delay in diagnosis and treatment leads to a guarded prognosis. Brain herniation due to large hemorrhagic venous infarcts is the most common cause of death in the acute setting of CVST. In survivors, the recurrence of CVST is 1–3% with the highest risk in the first year after diagnosis [7]. Investigation for thrombophilic diseases should be carried out as they are associated with recurrent thrombotic episodes. Tests for hereditary thrombophilias (protein-C/S deficiency, anti-thrombin III deficiency, factor V Leiden mutation, prothrombin mutation, etc.), antiphospholipid/anticardiolipin antibodies, and homocysteine levels are few important investigations [6].

References

1. Saposnik G, Barrinagarrementaria F, Brown RD Jr, Bushnell CD, Cucchiara B, Cushman, et al. Diagnosis and management of cerebral venous thrombosis: a statement for healthcare professionals from the American Heart Association/American Stroke Association. Stroke. 2011;42(4):1158–92.
2. Bousser MG, Crassard I. Cerebral venous thrombosis, pregnancy and oral contraceptives. Thromb Res. 2012;130(Suppl 1):S19–22.
3. Coutinho JM, Ferro JM, Canhao P, Barrinagarrementaria F, Cantu C, Bousser MG, et al. Cerebral venous and sinus thrombosis in women. Stroke. 2009;40(7):2356–61.
4. Kashkoush AI, Ma H, Agarwal N, Panczykowski D, Tonetti D, Weiner GM, et al. Cerebral venous sinus thrombosis in pregnancy and puerperium: a pooled, systematic review. J Clin Neurosci. 2017;39:9–15.
5. Sharma N, Sharma SR, Hussain M. An audit of cerebral venous thrombosis associated with pregnancy and puerperium in teaching hospital in North Eastern India. J Fam Med Prim Care. 2019;8(3):1054–7.
6. Gazioglu S, Dinc G. Cerebral venous sinus thrombosis in pregnancy and puerperium. Acta Neurol Belg. 2020;6:1–6.
7. Hiltunen S, Putaala J, Haapaniemi E, Tatlisumak T. Long-term outcome after cerebral venous thrombosis: analysis of functional and vocational outcome, residual symptoms, and adverse events in 161 patients. J Neurol. 2016;263(3):477–84.

4 Fatty Liver: More Likely To Be Fatal in Pregnancy!

Kusum D. Jashnani, Lalita Yoganand Patil, Shruti Lande, and Rosemarie de Souza

4.1 Clinical History

A 22-year-old primigravida, with 38 weeks of gestation, came with complaints of vomiting and pain in her abdomen, for 4 days for which she was treated at a primary health care center. Same-day ultrasound was done, and it was suggestive of intrauterine fetal death. Labor was induced, and the fetus delivered vaginally. In view of excessive and prolonged vaginal bleeding and blood oozing out from the mouth and gums, the patient was referred to our tertiary care hospital for further management. She did not have any comorbidities or any major medical and surgical illnesses. Her general condition was poor, she was unconscious and not responding to deep painful stimuli, with dilated pupils. On per abdomen examination, it was soft and non-tender. She was in the hospital for almost one and a half days during which her clinical condition remained the same as at the time of admission. The bleeding continued for which she received two units of packed red blood cells, eight units of fresh frozen plasma, and seven units of platelet concentrate. The patient was anemic with markedly low hemoglobin level (3.3 g/dL) with leukocytosis (19,500/μL) and thrombocytopenia (90,000/μL). There was mild derangement of the coagulation profile, which showed raised prothrombin time (20.2 s with control of 12 s), INR (1.52), and APTT (37 s with control of 30 s). Liver function test showed raised total and direct bilirubin (5.6 mg/dL and 3.4 mg/dL, respectively), SGOT and SGPT were within normal limits (61 and 31 IU), and alkaline phosphatase was raised (340 IU). Serum albumin was slightly low (2.1 g/dL), with raised serum creatinine (2.8) and a raised serum uric acid level (10 mg/dL). Hepatitis viral markers were negative.

Patient's condition deteriorated with a systolic blood pressure of 60 mmHg, and she was intubated in view of respiratory distress and falling saturation. Despite all measures, the patient could not be revived and succumbed to death after one and half days of hospital stay. A complete autopsy was performed after taking adequate permission.

K. D. Jashnani (✉) · L. Y. Patil · S. Lande
Department of Pathology, Topiwala National Medical College & B.Y.L. Nair Charitable Hospital, Mumbai, Maharashtra, India

R. de Souza
Department of Medicine, MICU, Topiwala National Medical College & B.Y.L. Nair Charitable Hospital, Mumbai, Maharashtra, India

K. D. Jashnani (ed.), *Maternal Mortality - Lessons Learnt from Autopsy*, https://doi.org/10.1007/978-981-19-3420-9_4

4.2 Autopsy Findings

The liver was enlarged weighing 1.3 kg, yellow in color with rounded margins on gross examination (Fig. 4.1). Histopathologic examination showed normal hepatic lobular architecture with zone 2 and 3 hepatocytes showing extensive microvesicular fatty change with normal periportal hepatocytes (Figs. 4.2 and 4.3). There was some degree of intrahepatocytic cholestasis also. In microvesicular fatty change, the hepatocytes retain their polygonal shape and also the central position of nuclei; show multiple tiny vacuoles in the cytoplasm which are due to dissolved fat during the paraffin embedding process, which is a characteristic feature of acute fatty liver of pregnancy. The kidneys showed few patchy areas of acute tubular necrosis, and uterine myometrium showed physiologic changes of hypertrophy and preischemia. The rest of the organs were very pale on gross examination. There was no evidence of any internal organ hemorrhage.

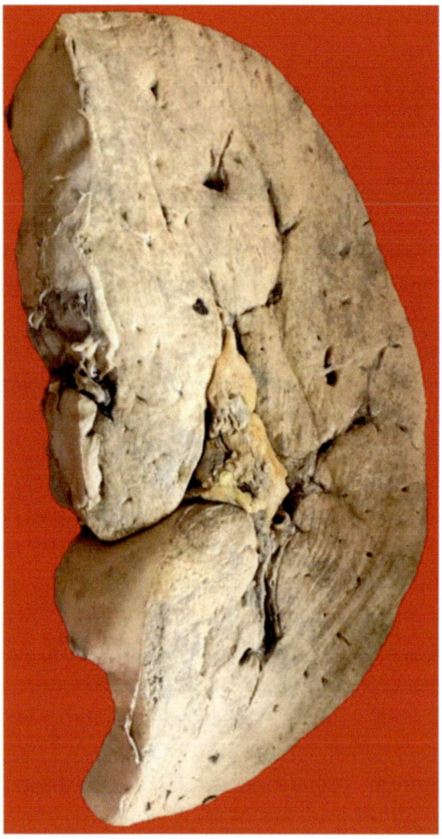

Fig. 4.1 Gross photograph of the liver showing an enlarged liver with yellow color, greasy to touch and rounded margins on the cut surface

4.3 Final Cause of Death

Acute fatty liver of pregnancy with hepatic encephalopathy, coagulopathy and severe anemia in a postpartum female.

4.4 Clinicopathologic Discussion

Acute fatty liver of pregnancy (AFLP) is a rare, life-threatening condition which usually occurs in the third trimester of pregnancy [1]. Defects in the genes encoding for the transport and oxidation pathways of fatty acids are inherited as autosomal recessive traits and are known as fatty acid

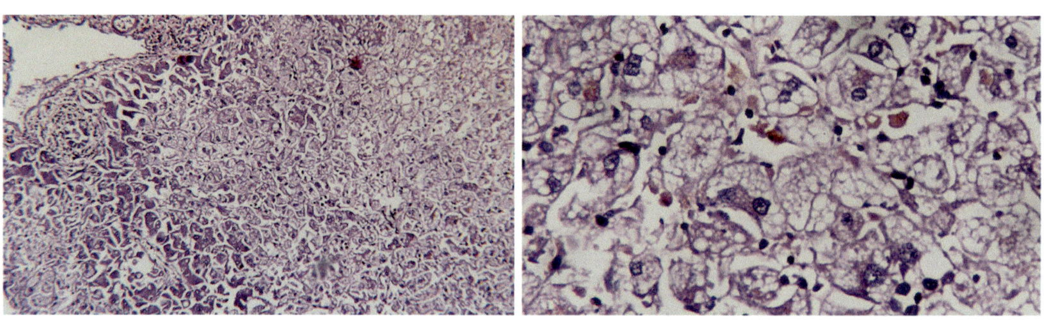

Figs. 4.2 and 4.3 (H&E ×100 and ×400) The microphotograph shows extensive microvesicular fatty changes with focal intrahepatocytic cholestasis

oxidation disorders. The most common disorder of fatty acid oxidation disorder in AFLP is a deficiency of long-chain 3-hydroxylacyl-CoA dehydrogenase (LCHAD) [2]. These have been shown to be associated with maternal, placental, and fetal complications. In this case, it resulted in both fetal and maternal death.

During the last trimester, the metabolic demands of the fetus increase. Mothers heterozygous for a fatty acid oxidation disorder and pregnant with an affected fetus can develop AFLP because of their inability to metabolize fatty acids for energy production and fetal growth. Fatty acids are then deposited in the liver. Delivery of the fetus unloads the excess of fatty acid delivery to the liver and can lead to fast recovery without sequelae of chronic liver disease [2].

Early diagnosis and prompt delivery are known to greatly improve the prognosis in such cases. The offspring of mothers affected by AFLP should also be screened and monitored for fatty acid oxidation disorders.

Swansea criteria is used to make the diagnosis of AFLP. Presence of six or more features included in the Swansea criteria, in the absence of any other explanation/cause, makes the diagnosis of AFLP [3]. These include vomiting, abdominal pain, polydipsia/polyuria, encephalopathy, elevated bilirubin, hypoglycemia, elevated urate, leukocytosis, ascites or bright liver on ultrasound, elevated transaminases, elevated ammonia, renal impairment, coagulopathy, and microvesicular steatosis on liver biopsy/autopsy. Liver biopsies are not routinely performed during pregnancy, knowing the procedural risks. We, as pathologists, usually get to see the classic histopathologic hepatic features of microvesicular steatosis on a postmortem liver specimen, as seen in the present case. Microvesicular steatosis is in contrast to macrovesicular steatosis, wherein the hepatocyte becomes oval in shape with an eccentrically placed nucleus and cytoplasm occupied by a single large vacuole. It is possible to demonstrate fat within the hepatocytes, whether microvesicular or macrovesicular, by carrying out a frozen section of the fresh, non-formalin-fixed liver tissue followed by staining with special stains for fat—Oil Red O, Sudan black, or Sudan III. In the case being discussed, the patient presented with nine of the above-mentioned features, thus fulfilling the Swansea criteria. If this disease is not intervened early, major life-threatening complications like upper gastrointestinal bleeding due to altered coagulation profile, acute kidney injury, sepsis, pancreatitis, and hypoglycemia follow it.

Maternal mortality in AFLP ranges from 7% to 18% and fetal mortality from 9% to 23%. Varied maternal complications which could eventually be the cause of death are coagulopathy, hemorrhage, acute renal failure, hepatorenal syndrome, acute liver failure, encephalopathy, etc. The common causes of icterus during pregnancy are intrahepatic cholestasis of pregnancy, viral hepatitis, HELLP syndrome, and AFLP. These conditions share a lot of similarities in clinical features and investigation findings, and hence, the diagnosis of AFLP may be difficult. In acute viral hepatitis, serum transaminase values are above 1000 IU/L and uric acid levels are rarely elevated. Intrahepatic cholestasis distinctly presents with intense pruritus and elevated serum bile acid levels (>10 μmol/L) confirms the diagnosis. This is not a fatal condition, as it usually resolves after delivery, though it can recur in the next pregnancy. In HELLP syndrome, jaundice is not so prominent, as also the development of encephalopathy with rapid progressive acute liver failure is not so often. Here, neurological symptoms like severe headache and visual disturbances are more common along with history of hypertension [4]. Incorporation of an important diagnostic test of AT—antithrombin activity <65% into the diagnostic criteria for AFLP may facilitate prompt diagnosis of AFLP and contribute to better differentiation from other causes of icterus during pregnancy [5]. However, most patients affected by AFLP have no known risk factors, and it may not be possible to do routine antithrombin III screening. Thus a high level of clinical suspicion with timely diagnosis followed by delivery/early termination of pregnancy can lead to a favourable outcome in AFLP [6].

References

1. Liu J, Ghaziani TT, Wolf JL. Acute fatty liver disease of pregnancy: updates in pathogenesis, diagnosis, and management a review. Am J Gastroenterol. 2017;112(6):838–46.
2. Italian Association for the Study of the Liver (AISF). AISF position paper on liver disease and pregnancy. Dig Liver Dis. 2016;48:120–37.
3. Morton A, Laurie J. Physiological changes of pregnancy and the Swansea criteria in diagnosing acute fatty liver of pregnancy. Obstetric Med. 2018;11(3):126–31.
4. Rath W, Tsikouras P, Stelzl P. HELLP syndrome or acute fatty liver of pregnancy: a differential diagnostic challenge: common features and differences. Gebertshilfe Frauenheilkd. 2020;80(5):499–507. https://doi.org/10.1055/9-1091-8630.
5. Minakami H, Morikawa M, Yamada T, Yamada T, Akaishi R, Nishida R. Differentiation of acute fatty liver of pregnancy from syndrome of hemolysis, elevated liver enzymes and low platelet counts. J Obstet Gynaecol Res. 2014;40(3):641–9. https://doi.org/10.1111/jog.12282. PMID: 24428400.
6. Perera, et al. A case of fatal acute fatty liver of pregnancy and literature review. Int J Reprod Contrac Obstet Gynaecol. 2018;7:2026–30.

5 Eclampsia: A Risk Factor for Intracranial Hemorrhage

Sakshi Agrawal, Kusum D. Jashnani,
Lalita Yoganand Patil,
and Vandana Rajesh Saravade

5.1 Clinical History

A 21-year-old female, unregistered, P1L1, had history of one episode of generalized tonic clonic convulsions (GTCS) in the morning and was taken to primary health care center in a drowsy state. A single live male child was delivered by forceps delivery on the same day. Injection labetalol and injection magnesium sulfate were given. Convulsions stopped after delivery, but the patient noticed left-sided weakness. The CT brain performed on Day 3 postpartum was suggestive of a 4.5 × 3.5 cm intraparenchymal hemorrhage in the bilateral parietooccipital region with a midline shift to the left side. Her BP was 200/100 mmHg. Hematological investigations were suggestive of anemia (Hb—7.3 g/dL). The rest of the biochemical investigations were within normal limits. The patient was then referred to our tertiary care hospital in view of intracerebral hemorrhage with complaints of headache, vomiting, left-sided weakness, and one episode of convulsion followed by unconsciousness. Her general condition was poor. She was intubated and started on mechanical ventilation. The patient's condition further deteriorated, and she succumbed to death within 2 hours of hospital stay. A complete autopsy was performed.

5.2 Autopsy Findings

On in situ examination, there was no evidence of any external injury or fracture. On opening the cranial cavity, there was no evidence of extradural hematoma, subdural hematoma, or superior sagittal sinus thrombosis. The brain weighed 1.4 kg, had congested meningeal vessels. There were a few foci of SAH with marked cerebral edema (Fig. 5.1a). On the cut surface, intracerebral hematoma was seen in the right parietooccipital region measuring 6 × 5 × 3 cm (Fig. 5.1b)

S. Agrawal
Histopathology Laboratory, Lilavati Hospital and Research Centre, Mumbai, Maharashtra, India

K. D. Jashnani (✉) · L. Y. Patil
Department of Pathology, Topiwala National Medical College & B.Y.L. Nair Charitable Hospital, Mumbai, Maharashtra, India

V. R. Saravade
Department of Obstetrics and Gynecology, Topiwala National Medical College & B.Y.L. Nair Charitable Hospital, Mumbai, Maharashtra, India

K. D. Jashnani (ed.), *Maternal Mortality - Lessons Learnt from Autopsy*,
https://doi.org/10.1007/978-981-19-3420-9_5

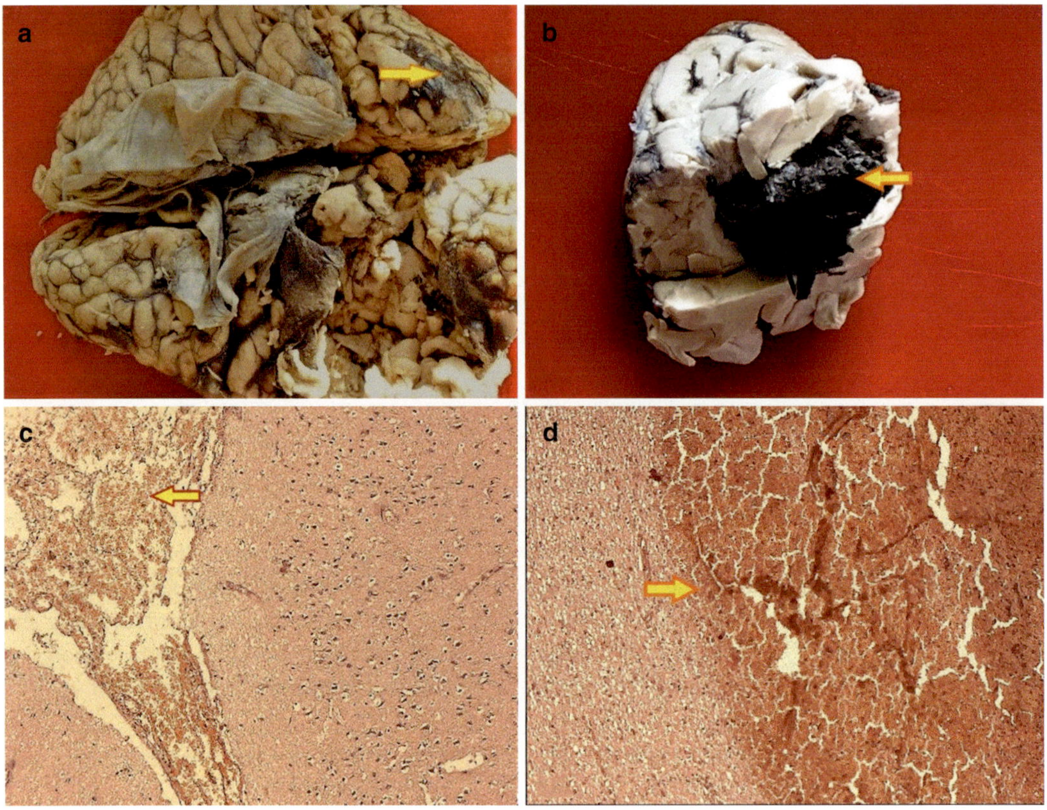

Fig. 5.1 (**a**) Gross specimen of cerebrum showing few foci of subarachnoid hemorrhage (yellow arrow) and cerebral edema. (**b**) Gross specimen of intracerebral hematoma (yellow arrow). (**c**) Subarachnoid hemorrhage (yellow arrow) of (**a**) (H&E, ×400). (**d**) large area of hemorrhage (yellow arrow) in the cerebral parenchyma (H&E, ×400)

and at the left parietooccipital region measuring 2 × 2 × 2 cm. Ventricles were unremarkable. The cerebellum showed tonsillar and uncal herniation. On microscopy, multiple sections from the cerebrum showed subarachnoid hemorrhage (Fig. 5.1c) along with congested and dilated meningeal blood vessels. A large area of intracerebral hemorrhage (Fig. 5.1d) with the presence of few hypoxic ischemic red neurons was seen.

Lungs weighed 380 g each, rubbery to firm in consistency and on cut surface showed scanty reddish frothy fluid oozing out on pressure, which was confirmed on histopathologic examination as intra alveolar hemorrhage (Fig. 5.2a). Rest of the organs were unremarkable.

5.3 Final Cause of Death

Intracerebral and subarachnoid hemorrhage with raised intracranial tension in a postpartum eclamptic female.

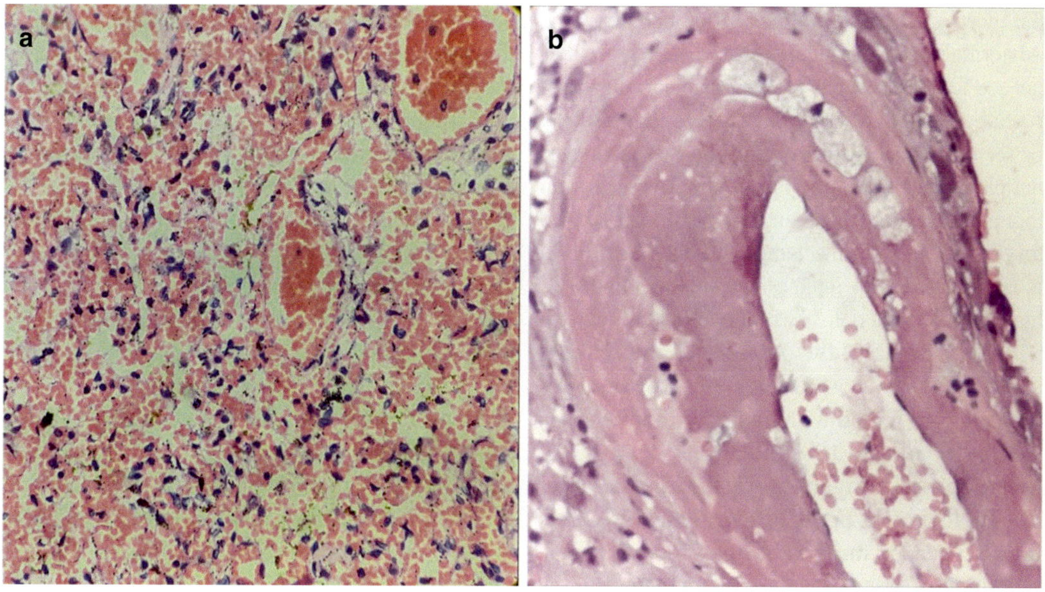

Fig. 5.2 (**a**) Intraalveolar hemorrhage showing alveolar spaces filled with RBCs admixed with few alveolar macrophages (H&E, ×400). (**b**) Decidual artery showing fibrinoid deposition in the wall and the presence of few foamy macrophages-acute atherosis (H&E, ×400)

5.4 Clinicopathologic Discussion

Pregnancy-associated ICH is an uncommon but potentially life-threatening event that markedly contributes to maternal mortality. Pre-eclampsia complicates 3–5% of pregnancies and, according to ACOG guidelines, is defined as the new development of hypertension (blood pressure >140/90 mmHg) on two occasions, at least 4 h apart, and proteinuria arising after 20 weeks of gestation in previously normotensive women [1]. Preeclampsia is associated with risk factors like advanced maternal age, obesity, multifetal gestation, previous history of preeclampsia, and family history of hypertension in first-degree relatives [2]. Eclampsia includes preeclampsia with the presence of convulsions not attributable to other neurologic disease [3]. The seizures are generalized and can appear at any time before, during, or after labor.

Nonvillous intermediate trophoblast has the physiological function of invading the walls of uterine spiral arteries, causing replacement of their muscular walls by fibrinoid material deposition, resulting in their conversion from small-caliber high-resistance arteries into large-caliber low-resistance uteroplacental arteries (remodeling). These changes permit a greatly increased blood flow into the intervillous space, which takes care of increasing oxygen demands of the growing fetus. In preeclamptic-eclamptic pregnancies, there is inhibition of this secondary endovascular trophoblast migration in the second trimester, so that the myometrial segments of the uteroplacental arteries remain as musculoelastic arteries, i.e., failure of physiological remodeling. This leads to ischemia/hypoxia-mediated increases in sFlt-1, AT1-AA, and inflammatory cytokines, resulting in subsequent detrimental effects on several downstream targets. The decrease in pro-angiogenic factors such as VEGF and PlGF and the increased production of reactive oxygen species lead to maternal endothelial dysfunction. As a result, increased endothelin (ET-1) production and the decreased bioavailability of NO lead to the characteristic widespread vascular abnormalities in various organs such as the kidneys and brain [1].

Acute atherosis, a necrotizing arteriopathy, affects small muscular arteries in the placental bed, a term coined to describe the maternal-fetal interface (the area in which the placenta attaches itself to the uterus) [4], and arterioles in the decidua vera. Abnormal immunological response between maternal and fetal tissues may be responsible for this arteriopathy. Sometimes, by chance, these changes may be seen in the vessels present just outside the maternal plate of the placenta (Fig. 5.2b). This was seen in a placenta sent to our surgical pathology laboratory from a case of an eclamptic mother. Eclampsia is best treated with magnesium sulfate, control of hypertension, and delivery of the infant.

In present case, the patient had intracranial bleed on Day 3 postpartum. She was unregistered and presented with history of convulsions with a BP of 200/100 mmHg at 34 weeks of gestation and diagnosed to have eclampsia. The incidence of pregnancy-associated ICH is highest during the postpartum period [5] as seen in the present case also. Other neurological symptoms that can be seen in patients with eclampsia include headaches, blurred vision, nausea, and drowsiness, which were not reported in our patient. Rapid hormonal and hemodynamic changes during the postpartum period may promote the development of ICH due to effects on coagulation and blood vessel walls [3]. Patients with pregnancy-associated ICH have poorer prognosis for both the mother and fetus [5]. In present case, newborn was alive and healthy.

Intracerebral hemorrhage has been found in up to 40% of patients with eclampsia in autopsy series. Hypertension, obesity, age >30 years, and multiple pregnancy-induced hypertension (PIH) occurrences are independent risk factors for ICH in PIH patients. Hemorrhages may be extensive or petechial with an intraparenchymal type of ICH typically seen with preeclampsia-eclampsia, however subdural hematomas and SAH have also been described in association with PIH. Possible effects of preeclampsia or eclampsia on cerebral vessels include endothelial dysfunction, microangiopathy, vasospasm, increased cerebral perfusion pressure, and brain capillary permeability, with subsequent vasodilation and cerebral edema. Additionally, high blood pressure with increased cerebrovascular resistance and loss of autoregulation, persistently damages vessel walls and leads to rupture and bleeding. Treatment options include surgical evacuation of intracerebral clots in cases of a declining conscious state or worsening neurological deficit. A non-operative approach is appropriate in cases of devastating hemorrhage that is non-recoverable.

While performing an autopsy in such cases, we should start with an external examination to look for any external injury which might suggest trauma as a cause of intracranial hemorrhage. After opening the cranium, a thorough examination is a must to look for the exact location of the hemorrhage [3]. Apart from confirming the clinical diagnosis of intracranial hemorrhage, autopsy also helps in examining other organs for any complications caused by preeclampsia or eclampsia like placental abruption, disseminated intravascular coagulation, HELLP syndrome, heart failure, postpartum hemorrhage, etc. Though the incidence of preeclampsia and eclampsia is on the decline, still it remains the major contributor to poor maternal and fetal outcome. Regular antenatal checkups, early diagnosis, prompt multidisciplinary treatment, and optimum timing of delivery reduce the incidence of complications and maternal mortality.

References

1. Warrington JP, George EM, Palei AC, Spardley FT, Granger JP. Recent advances in the understanding of the pathophysiology of preeclampsia. Hypertension. 2013;62(4):666–73.
2. Kongwattanakul K, Saksiriwuttho P, Chaiyarach S, Thepsuthammarat K. Incidence, characteristics, maternal complications, and perinatal outcomes associated with preeclampsia with severe features and HELLP syndrome. Int J Women's Health. 2018;10:371–7.
3. Lin LT, Tsui KH, Cheng JT, Cheng JS, Huang WC, Liou WS, Tang PL. Increased risk of intracranial hemorrhage in patients with pregnancy-induced hypertension: a nationwide population-based retrospective cohort study. Medicine (Baltimore). 2016;95(20):e3732.
4. Brosens I, Puttemans P, Benagiano G. Placental bed research: I. The placental bed: from spiral arteries remodeling to the great obstetrical syndromes. Am J Obstet Gynecol. 2019;221(5):437–45.
5. Liang ZW, Lin L, Gao WL, Feng LM. A clinical characteristic analysis of pregnancy-associated intracranial hemorrhage in China. Sci Rep. 2015;5:9509.

6 Cervical Trauma: Clinical Conundrum and Correlation

Kusum D. Jashnani and Reena J. Wani

6.1 Case A

6.1.1 Clinical History

A 25-year-old female, G4P3L3, ANC registered in a private maternity hospital, referred in view of jaundice with labor pain, was admitted to the gynecology ward with history of pain in the abdomen (labor pain) for 1 day, history of high-colored urine, and yellow discoloration of sclera since the past 10 days. History of left leg swelling since 3–4 years, details of any treatment taken not known. Obstetric history: married for 10 years, G1-FTND F 9-year-old, G2-FTND F 8-year-old, and G3-FTNDF 3-year-old.

On examination, she was afebrile, icterus +++ with pulse 100/min and BP 100/70 mmHg. On per abdomen examination, she was at 38 weeks gestation, with cardiovascular system and central nervous system examinations being normal.

Investigations done on admission revealed hemoglobin of 16.4 g/dL, T WBC of 20, 4000/mm^3, and a platelet count of 132,000/mm^3. SGOT/SGPT were 212/159 U/L, total bilirubin was 19.15 mg/dl, and creatinine was 0.90 mg/dl. Prothrombin time was >60 s (control 12.5 s). The investigations done 25 days back revealed Hemoglobin of 8.9 g/dL, T WBC of 8300/mm^3, platelet count of 192,000/mm^3. SGOT/SGPT were 15/21 U/L. She was transfused with two pints of whole blood 1 month ago, details of which were not available.

The patient delivered 3 h after admission with outlet forceps delivery in view of shoulder dystocia++. The cork screw method was attempted, and the baby was fresh still birth. After delivery, the patient was disoriented and conscious, with pulse 104/min and BP 100/70 mmHg. One hour later, the patient had altered sensorium with labored breathing. She was intubated for the same and transferred to MICU. There was bleeding per vaginum noted. Clinical impression: was postpartum state with acute fulminant hepatitis? viral with encephalopathy? hypotensive shock. Her condition continued to be precarious, and in spite of all resuscitative measures, the patient could not be survived and was declared dead 7 h after admission. A complete autopsy was performed after taking due permission.

K. D. Jashnani (✉)
Department of Pathology, Topiwala National Medical College & B.Y.L. Nair Charitable Hospital, Mumbai, Maharashtra, India

R. J. Wani
Department of Obstetrics & Gynecology, Hindu Hridaysamrat Balasaheb Thackeray Medical College & Dr R N Cooper Municipal Hospital, Mumbai, Maharashtra, India

K. D. Jashnani (ed.), *Maternal Mortality - Lessons Learnt from Autopsy*,
https://doi.org/10.1007/978-981-19-3420-9_6

6.1.2 Autopsy Findings

The deceased was averagely built and nourished with evidence of icterus ++ all over and edema over the lower limbs. The peritoneal cavity showed a clot of 100 g over the Gerota's fascia on the left kidney. Anterior extraperitoneal utero-vesical space showed blood clots weighing 200–300 g (Fig. 6.3b). Mesentery of the small and large intestines showed hemorrhages. The urinary bladder showed serosal hemorrhages. The liver weighing 600 g (Fig. 6.1a) showed wrinkled capsule, it was soft and foldable on cut surface.

The weight of the uterus, the cervix along with broad ligament hematoma, was 1.7 kg. The uterus measured 20 × 15 × 9 cm; the cervix measured 8 × 7 × 6 cm. There was a left lateral cervical wall tear measuring 8 cm long with ragged borders and hemorrhages, extending to the lower uterine segment (Fig. 6.1b). This tear led to a broad ligament hematoma measuring 10 × 9 × 1 cm. The uterus on opening showed a raw posterior wall suggestive of placental bed, with no evidence of retained products of conception. Sections from the site of the tear showed large areas of hemorrhage in the wall of the cervix as well as the lower uterine wall along with neutrophils. The endometrium showed decidual change and the myometrium showed physiologic changes of hypertrophy and preischemia. The kidneys (icteric on external surface), the brain (extremely pale), the heart, the lungs, the spleen, the bilateral ovaries and the fallopian tubes, and the rest of the organs were unremarkable.

6.1.3 Final Cause of Death

Hypovolemic shock due to a lateral cervical wall tear extending into the lower uterine segment with broad ligament hematoma and massive hepatic necrosis.

6.2 Case B

6.2.1 Clinical History

A 26-year-old female G4P3L2D1 with 39 weeks of gestation was admitted with pain in the abdomen. During the course of the next 6 days in the hospital, her general condition was fair, she was afebrile, with a pulse of 80–90/min and a BP of 110/70 mmHg. P/A-Uterine Palpation-Fetus was cephalic with

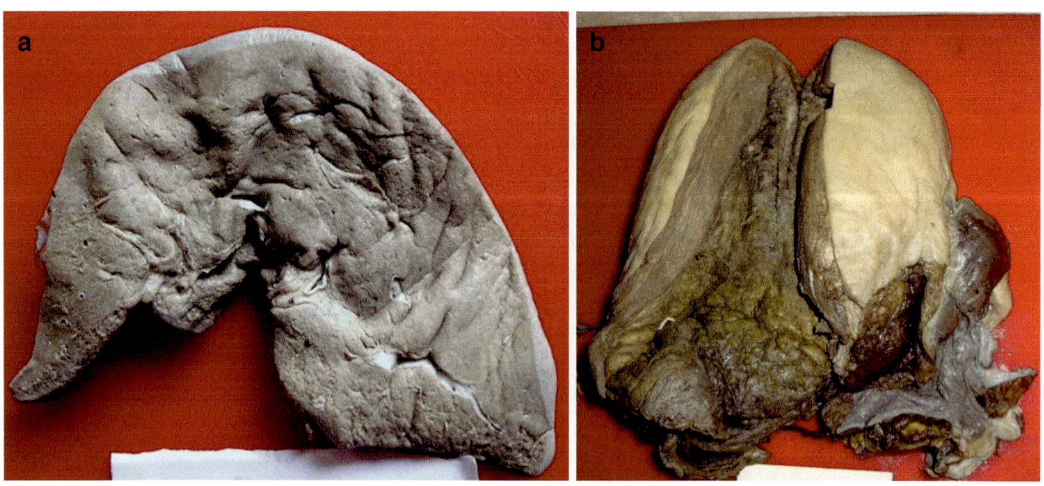

Fig. 6.1 Case A—Gross specimen of a liver slice showing a soft foldable liver with a wrinkled capsule (**a**). Gross specimen of the uterus with the cervix showing a tear in the lateral wall of the cervix extending to the lower uterine wall (**b**)

FHS+, regular. The course was uneventful for the next 6 days. On the seventh day, early morning, she complained of PV leak, was given Inj Pitocin at 4:00 am. After one and a half hours, she delivered a female child (2.93 kg in weight) by vaginal delivery with lateral episiotomy. Baby CIAB had APGAR score of 8,9,9. The placenta was expelled completely and spontaneously. However, she continued to bleed following vaginal delivery; the uterus was well contracted, for which she was given oxytocin and methergine. Exploration of the episiotomy wound and the cervix was done, which revealed cervical tears at both angles-which were sutured; a blood clot of 500 g was removed. Her BP was 90/60 with P—110 min, the patient continued to bleed even after the sutures, she was given T Misoprostol per rectum with inj oxytocin, and atonic PPH was suspected. Her condition continued to deteriorate in view of persistent bleeding PV, hypotension, and shock with gasping respiration and arterial blood gas (ABG) suggestive of severe metabolic acidosis. The patient was intubated, resuscitated, systolic 70 mmHg, but could not be revived, so she was declared dead after 12 h of exploration and cervical suturing. A complete autopsy was performed after taking due permission.

6.2.2 Autopsy Findings

The lungs bilateral weighed 350 g each, the pleura was smooth and shiny, and the cut surface was subcrepitant. Almost 30 cm in length of the mesocolon of the transverse and descending colon showed extensive areas of hemorrhages corresponding to the site of tear. The enlarged postpartum uterus showed a raw area on the posterior surface corresponding to placental attachment, with no evidence of retained products of conception, there were four sutures seen on each right and left side of the cervix. In addition, there was one cervical tear 6 cm long in the left lateral wall, close to the area of sutures, extending to the lower uterine segment (Figs. 6.2a, b and 6.3a). The broad ligament corresponding to the cervical tear showed a large area of hemorrhage of 25 × 10 cm and one blood clot of 20 g was seen close to it. The uterus on microscopy showed endometrial decidual change and physio-

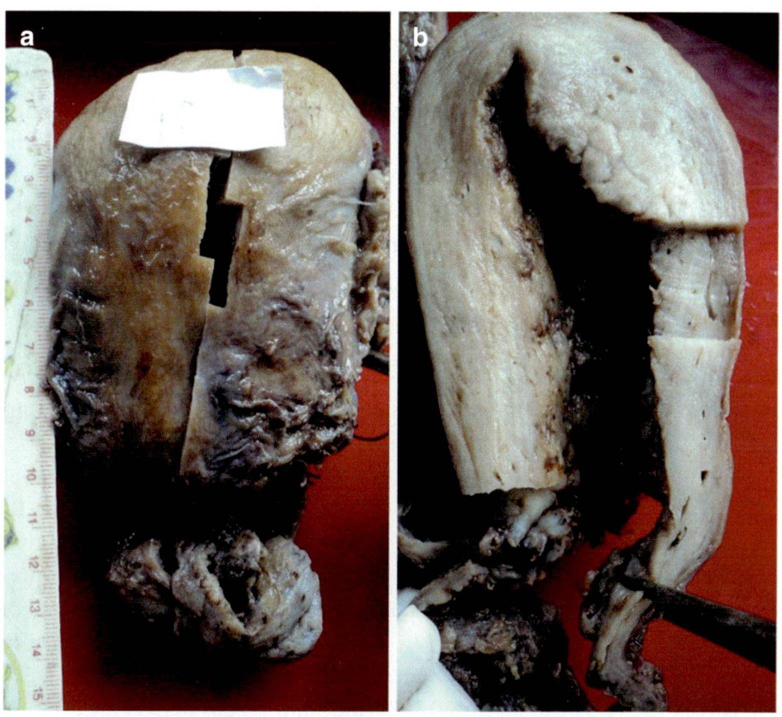

Fig. 6.2 Case B—Gross specimen of uterus with cervix showing a cervical tear with the presence of sutures at the periphery on external (**a**) and cut (**b**) surface

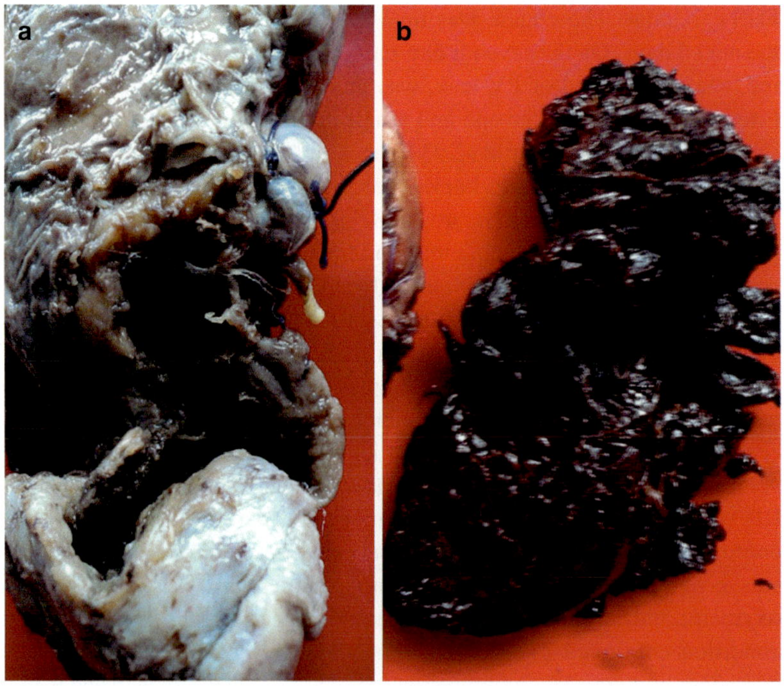

Fig. 6.3 Case B—Close-up of cervical wall tear with the presence of sutures of previous repair (**a**). Blood clot in Case A (**b**)

logic changes of myometrial hypertrophy and pre-ischemia along with the presence of intermediate trophoblasts in the myometrium and in the vessel wall. The right kidney showed chronic pyelonephritis with hydronephrosis and hydroureter with no evidence of calculus or stricture, while the left kidney was unremarkable. A section from the cervical tear showed epithelial ulceration, with neutrophils and fibrin, and hemorrhage. The underlying wall showed large areas of hemorrhage. Sections from blood clots showed red blood cells, with no evidence of retained products of conception.

6.2.3 Final Cause of Death

Hypovolemic shock following a left-sided lateral cervical wall tear extending into the lower uterine segment in a postpartum female with cervical tear repair.

6.3 Clinicopathologic Discussion

Labor is considered obstructed when the presenting part of the fetus cannot progress further into the birth canal, in spite of strong uterine contractions. The most frequent cause of obstructed labor is cephalopelvic disproportion—usually being a large fetal head and a smaller pelvic brim of the mother. More causes of obstructed labor may be malpresentation or malposition of the fetus (shoulder, brow, or occipito-posterior positions). Occasionally, locked twins or pelvic tumors can be the cause of obstruction. The obstruction can only be relieved by means of an operative delivery, either cesarean section or other instrumental delivery (forceps, vacuum extraction or symphysiotomy), or by manual maneuvers carried out like in cases of shoulder dystocia [1]. In the present case no. A, forceps delivery was carried out in view of shoulder dystocia. The incidence of clinically diagnosed shoulder dystocia range cited by the American College of Obstetricians and Gynecologists (ACOG) and the Royal College of Obstetricians and Gynecologists (RCOG) are 0.6–1.4% and 0.58–0.70%, respectively [2].

Clinically, significant lesions of the cervix occur in 0.2–1.7% of vaginal deliveries [3]. Cervical tears have been frequently reported with instrumental delivery, particularly with forceps delivery. Cervical tears are one of the causes of postpartum hemorrhage. Other causes of postpartum hemorrhage are uterine atony (tone); laceration, hematoma, inversion, rupture (trauma); retained placental tissue or invasive placenta (tissue); and coagulopathy (thrombin)—the four Ts are helpful to remember. A cervical tear should be suspected in cases of postpartum hemorrhage where there is good uterine retraction and the uterine rupture has been ruled out. The tear can also be felt during vaginal examination, and the source of the bleeding is discovered during inspection of the birth canal, with careful examination of the vagina and the cervix using two vaginal retractors. Other causes of cervical lacerations include manual dilatation of the cervix; improper use of oxytocins and precipitate labor. Predisposing factors are cervical rigidity, scarring of the cervix, edema as in prolonged labor, and placenta praevia due to increased vascularity. Apart from postpartum hemorrhage, other complications of cervical tear being ruptured uterus due to upward extension; local infection; cervical incompetence leading to future recurrent abortion or preterm labor and ureteric injury from the extension of the tear or during its repair. Types of cervical tears are unilateral: more common on the left side due to dextro-rotation of the uterus; lateral; stellate: multiple tears extending radially from the external os like a star or annular detachment. Management of cervical tear consists of immediate repair under general anesthesia. Annular detachment usually doesn't need any sutures as there is usually no bleeding due to ischemia at the edges of detachment [4].

In a study by Biru S et al., overall maternal complications related to instrumental delivery were 12.1%. Mothers who had forceps delivery were 3.4 times more likely to develop maternal complications than those mothers who had vacuum delivery. Mothers who had episiotomy had about 86% less risk of maternal complication from instrumental delivery than those who had no episiotomy [5]. Other complications due to instrumental delivery can be minor complications like laceration of the vagina and perineum and major complications associated with traumatic hemorrhage, bladder injury, and pelvic muscle injury.

The patient in case A also suffered from massive hepatic necrosis with encephalopathy. The cervical wall tear was therefore not considered or missed under the cover of this hepatic necrosis. Since she was in the hospital for less than a total of 7 h, a complete serology workup had not been done. So, the exact cause of massive hepatic necrosis in the present case was not known. Fulminant liver failure (FLF) is clinically characterized by an abrupt onset of jaundice with subsequent development of encephalopathy and coagulopathy in patients with or without preexisting liver disease. Viral hepatitis, autoimmune hepatitis, and drug induced liver injury (DILI) are some of the common etiologies for fulminant liver failure. Other precipitating events comprise alcoholic liver disease, ischemia, portal vein thrombosis, and infection. In some cases, a precipitating factor is never identified. Whatever the etiology, FLF is typically associated with high morbidity and mortality [6]. In the present case A, both conditions massive hepatic necrosis with encephalopathy and cervical wall tear with hypovolemic shock if present as solitary condition were also enough to cause death. In case B, bilateral cervical tears were identified and sutured, however the PV bleeding continued, and subsequently, within 12 h, the patient died. Autopsy showed one more cervical lateral wall tear, which had been the cause of her continued bleeding with hypovolemic shock and death. She had received oxytocin, which could have been one of the risk factors for her cervical tear.

References

1. The Royal Women's Hospital. n.d.. https://thewomens.r.worldssl.net/images/uploads/downloadable-records/clinical-guidelines/shoulder-dystocia-guideline_280720.pdf.
2. Garland J, Little D. Maternal death and its investigation. Acad Foren Pathol. 2018;8(4):894–911.
3. Djokovic D, Costa C, Martins A, Abushad S. Spontaneous delivery through a cervical tear without cervical os dilatation. Clin Case Rep. 2015;3(1):3–6. PMCID: PMC4317200, PMID: 25678963.
4. Geneva Foundation for Medical Education & Research GFMER Cervical Lacerations. n.d.. https://www.

gfmer.ch/Obstetrics_simplified/maternal_obstetric_injuries.htm.
5. Biru S, Addisu D, Kassa S, Animen S. Maternal complication related to instrumental delivery at Felege Hiwot Specialized Hospital, Northwest Ethiopia: a retrospective cross-sectional study. BMC Res Notes. 2019;12:482.
6. Ndekwe P, Ghabril MS, Zang Y, Mann SA, Cummings OW, Lin J. Substantial hepatic necrosis is prognostic in fulminant liver failure. World J Gastroenterol. 2017;23(23):4303–10. https://doi.org/10.3748/wjg.v23.i23.4303. PMID: 28694671.

7 Amniotic Fluid Embolism Syndrome: A Rare, Unpredictable, and Catastrophic Complication of Pregnancy

Kusum D. Jashnani, Sakshi Agrawal, and Asha R. Dalal

7.1 Clinical History

A 31-year-old asymptomatic primigravida came to our hospital at 41 weeks of gestation. She was posted for LSCS on the seventh day of admission in view of a lower uterine fibroid. During LSCS, vertical upper segment incision was given due to a lower uterine fibroid and the baby was delivered by breech extraction. The patient suddenly developed bradycardia (pulse 34/min) and hypotension (systolic BP-70 mmhg). Cardiopulmonary resuscitation was started, she was intubated and put on mechanical ventilation. The uterus was closed and around 650 ml of blood loss occurred during the operation. Complete blood count done post-operative was suggestive of fall in Hb (1.5 gmsg/dL) and platelet count (13,000/cmm), and TLC raised to 38,680/cmm. One packed cell volume, 25 units of FFP, 22 units of cryoprecipitate, and 12 units of platelets were transfused over 2 days. Hb increased to 4.8 gmg/dL, and the platelet count rose to 34,000/cmm. SGOT/SGPT was 715/339, serum creatinine 2 mg/dl, fibrinogen 55 mg/dl, d-dimer 3.6 μg/ml, and LDH 2460 U/L. On examination, she was pale, her BP was 94/58 mmHg, pedal edema was present, and petechial hemorrhages were seen on the shoulder, thighs, and lower abdomen. Clinically acute renal injury and disseminated intravascular coagulation secondary to amniotic fluid embolism were suspected. USG performed showed free fluid in the pelvic cavity suggestive of hemoperitoneum, which was confirmed by USG guided tapping. Despite all efforts, the patient's condition deteriorated, and the patient succumbed on day 3 post-LSCS. Complete autopsy was performed.

K. D. Jashnani (✉)
Department of Pathology, Topiwala National Medical College and BYL Nair Charitable Hospital, Mumbai, Maharashtra, India

S. Agrawal
Histopathology Laboratory, Lilavati Hospital and Research Centre, Mumbai, Maharashtra, India

A. R. Dalal
Department of Obstetrics and Gynecology, Sir H N Reliance Foundation Hospital, Mumbai, Maharashtra, India

K. D. Jashnani (ed.), *Maternal Mortality - Lessons Learnt from Autopsy*,
https://doi.org/10.1007/978-981-19-3420-9_7

7.2 Autopsy Findings

On external examination, petechial hemorrhages were present on the shoulder, thighs, and lower abdomen. LSCS incision of 11 cm with 9 sutures was noted. The abdominal cavity showed the presence of 300 cc of blood-mixed fluid which on microscopic examination showed plenty of red blood cells with a few lymphocytes and neutrophils. The lungs weighed 350 gms each, firm in consistency with petechial hemorrhages on the pleura. Microscopy showed a slightly thickened pleura with patchy areas of intra-alveolar edema, pleural and intra-alveolar hemorrhages. There was the presence of fetal squames and bile pigment of meconium in multiple small vessels of lung (Fig. 7.1), and some vessels also showed fibrin thrombi (Fig. 7.2). Petechial hemorrhages were seen on the epicardial surface of the heart and on the capsular and cut surfaces of the liver and bilateral kidneys. The stomach contained 30 cc of blood-stained fluid with markedly congested mucosa. The uterus showed vertical incision with a small hematoma and a lower uterine fibroid. The rest of the organs were unremarkable on gross and microscopy.

7.3 Final Cause of Death

Amniotic fluid embolism with disseminated intravascular coagulation.

7.4 Clinicopathologic Correlation

Amniotic fluid embolism (AFE) is an obstetric emergency which occurs in 1 in 8000 to 1 in 80,000 deliveries [1]. The true incidence is unknown because of inaccurate diagnosis and inconsistent reporting of nonfatal cases. Currently, no definitive diagnostic test exists for AFE. The following four criteria are recom-

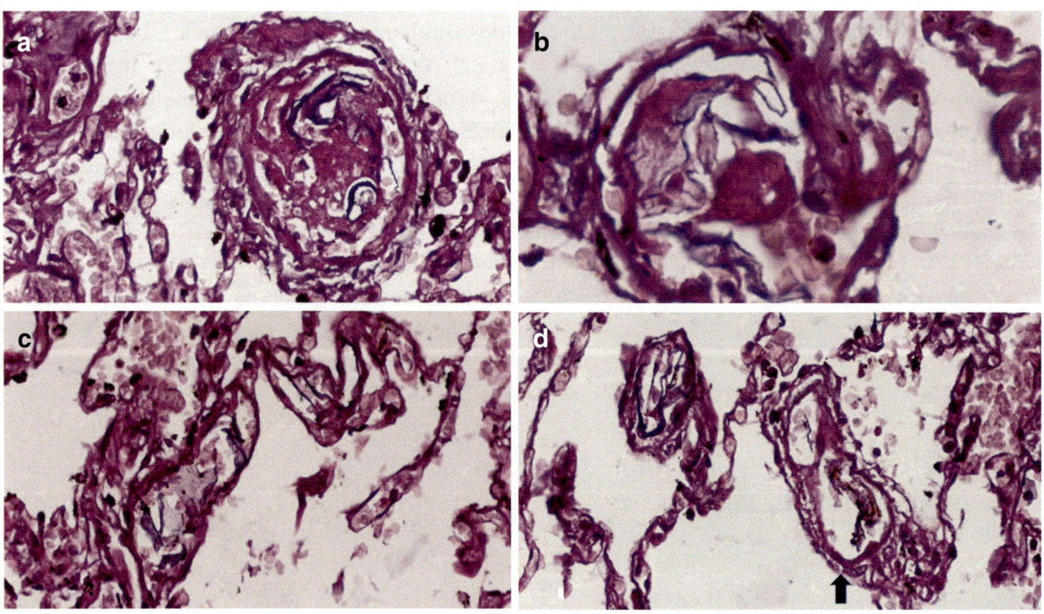

Fig. 7.1 Small-sized pulmonary arteries showing the presence of anucleate squames, bile pigment of meconium within their lumina. H&E, (**a**, **c**, **d**) all 400×. (**b**) 1000×

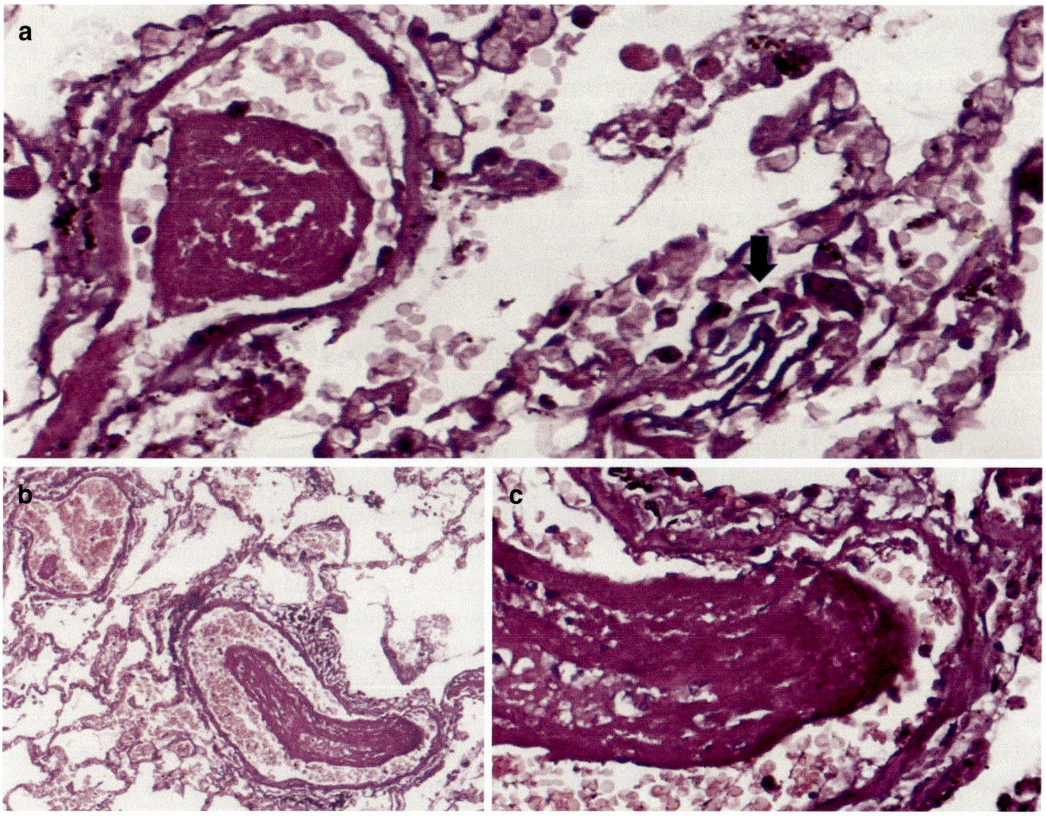

Fig. 7.2 Small- and medium-sized pulmonary arteries showing the presence of fibrin thrombus within their lumina (**b**, **c** H&E, 200× and 400×, respectively). (**a**) shows the presence of thrombus and squames (black arrow) and bile pigment in two different arteries, side by side, H&E, 400×

mended, all of which must be present to make the diagnosis of AFE: [2]

1. Acute hypotension or cardiac arrest.
2. Coagulopathy or severe hemorrhage in the absence of other explanations.
3. All of these occurring during labor, cesarean section, dilatation and evacuation, or within 30 min postpartum with no other explanation of findings.
4. No fever (38.0 ° C) during labor.

All the above features were seen in the present case. Here, the patient had a sudden onset of hypotension and bradycardia during a cesarean section after delivery of baby and the patient was put on ventilatory support for 2 days. Other symptoms that can be seen in cases of AFE are altered mental status due to encephalopathy, cough, cyanosis, and postpartum hemorrhage due to uterine atony. In view of clinical presentation and coagulation investigations, diagnosis of disseminated intravascular coagulation secondary to amniotic fluid embolism was suspected clinically. The syndrome typically occurs during labor in 70% cases, 19% during cesarean delivery, or 11% soon after vaginal delivery [1]. All the cases noted during cesarean section had their onset soon after the delivery of the fetus which was also seen in the present case.

Steiner and Lushbaugh described AFE for the first time in 1941 after they found fetal debris in the pulmonary circulation of women who died during labor at postmortem. It was postulated that amniotic fluid with fetal cells, hair, or other debris enters the maternal pulmonary circulation, causing cardiovascular collapse. Usually, there is a tear in the fetal membranes, permitting exposure of the fetal tissue to the maternal vasculature, thereby increasing the risk of AFE. Recent advances suggest that the occurrence of death in AFE is not a consequence of mechanical respiratory obstruction, but a humoral effect causing anaphylactoid reaction or complement activation. Progression occurs in two phases [1]. Phase I, which may last up to 30 min, consists of pulmonary artery vasospasm with pulmonary hypertension and increased right ventricular pressure causing hypoxia. This hypoxia causes myocardial and pulmonary capillary damage, left heart failure, and acute respiratory distress syndrome. Women who survive these events may enter phase II which is the hemorrhagic phase wherein fatal consumptive coagulopathy may be the initial presentation. This is characterized by massive hemorrhage with uterine atony and DIC. Amniotic fluid contains vasoactive and procoagulant products. The endothelin of amniotic fluid causes bronchoconstriction as well as pulmonary and coronary arterial vasoconstriction, which contributes to cardiovascular collapse. The direct procoagulant property of amniotic fluid may explain the prevalence of DIC in AFE. Thus, the process of AFE is similar to anaphylaxis than to embolism, hence the term anaphylactoid syndrome of pregnancy is now given, because fetal tissue or amniotic fluid components are not always found in all women who present with signs and symptoms similar to AFE. In the present case, the patient succumbed to death 3 days post-symptoms onset. On autopsy, we found squames and bile stain meconium as well as fibrin thrombi in small vessels of the lungs on histopathological examination. Apart from fetal squames and bile stain meconium, other components of amniotic fluid that can enter into maternal circulation include lanugo hair, fetal gut mucin, vernix caseosa, and trophoblast. Also seen were petechial hemorrhages in multiple organs and blood-tinged fluid in the peritoneal cavity and stomach. These features confirmed the clinical diagnosis of DIC secondary to AFE.

Previous studies revealed mortality rates as high as 61–86%, but recent estimates suggest a case fatality of 13–26% [3]. This decrease in mortality from AFE may be because of early diagnosis and better resuscitative care. The most important goal of therapy is to prevent additional hypoxia and multi-organ failure by giving oxygen expeditiously. However, though the mortality has come down, both the maternal and fetal morbidity are still very high, and 85% of those who survive have permanent neurological deficit. Amniotic fluid embolism is therefore considered an unpredictable and unpreventable event with an unknown cause. Pulmonary thromboembolism, air embolism, aspiration of gastric contents into the lungs, and hemorrhagic shock are some of the differential diagnoses of AFE clinically [4].

References

1. Viswanathan M, Viswanathan KV, Daniel S. Amniotic fluid embolism: a comprehensive review. Int J Reprod Contracept Obstet Gynecol. 2014;3:304–9.
2. Clark SL, Romero R, Dildy GA, et al. Proposed diagnostic criteria for the case definition of amniotic fluid embolism in research studies. Am J Obstet Gynecol. 2016;215:408–12.
3. Kaur K, Bhardwaj M, Kumar P, Singhal S, Singh T, Hooda S. Amniotic fluid embolism. J Anaesthesiol Clin Pharmacol. 2016;32:153–9.
4. Rudra A, Chatterjee S, Sengupta S, Nandi B, Mitra J. Amniotic fluid embolism. Indian. J Crit Care Med. 2009;12(3):129–35.

Systemic Thromboembolism and Giant Gastric Mucormycotic Ulcer

8

Kusum D. Jashnani, Pratibha Suryakant Shete, and Vandana Rajesh Saravade

8.1 Clinical History

A 22-year-old G3P2L1 23 weeks pregnant woman was referred to the hospital with episodes of heavy bleeding per vaginum. She had history of previous two lower segment cesarean sections (LSCS). Her BP on admission was 100/70 mm Hg, pulse rate 100/min, pallor ++, and no pedal edema. USG showed SLIUF 23 weeks + 2 days, liquor adequate, lower border of placenta 1.8 cm away from internal os s/o placenta previa type 1. Retro placental clot measuring 3.2 × 2.1 cm noted in the right lower part of the placenta suggestive of abruptio placenta. After few hours, a live female child (preterm) was delivered spontaneously (weight: 492 g); the baby cried immediately after birth. Placenta and membrane expelled out completely and spontaneously. Fresh bleeding ++ continued, per abdomen uterus was not well contracted. As the pulse was feeble, BP—not recordable, per abdomen—uterus flabby, bleeding++, patient was shifted to operation theatre.

During the operation, 1000 cc of blood was present in the abdomen suggestive of hemoperitoneum. Uterus—16 weeks size, flabby with rupture of anterior wall of lower segment with peritoneum over it intact. Rent identified on the left side. 343 g of blood clot was removed. A chest tube was inserted into the peritoneal cavity. Exploratory laparotomy with obstetric subtotal hysterectomy with bilateral internal iliac artery ligation with repair of rupture site of the uterus as well as repair of bladder wall injury was done.

On day 12, in view of the deranged creatinine level, the patient was put on hemodialysis for few days. One day later, she was not following simple oral commands and had twitching movements of her left upper limb intermittently. The patient had a large ecchymosis on her right lower limb with a 6 × 8 cm blister on her left lower limb. Clinical impression was hypoxic encephalopathy, disseminated intravascular coagulation (DIC), septic shock, and acute renal

K. D. Jashnani (✉)
Department of Pathology, Topiwala National Medical College and BYL Nair Charitable Hospital, Mumbai, Maharashtra, India

P. S. Shete
PH Diagnostic Center, Pune, Maharashtra, India

V. R. Saravade
Department of Obstetrics and Gynecology, Topiwala National Medical College and BYL Nair Charitable Hospital, Mumbai, Maharashtra, India

K. D. Jashnani (ed.), *Maternal Mortality - Lessons Learnt from Autopsy*,
https://doi.org/10.1007/978-981-19-3420-9_8

failure (ARF). The drain out continued to be hemorrhagic, gradually decreasing in amount. The baby expired on day 7, and the patient was declared dead on day 17 of admission. A complete autopsy was performed.

Investigations: D dimer—positive >10,000 ng/mL, fibrinogen level—590 mg/dl, fibrinogen degradation products—20 mcg/mg. Rapid Malaria Antigen Test (RMAT), rapid test for Leptospira IgM antibodies, rapid test for dengue IgM/IgG antibodies, and dengue NS1 antigen test were all negative. There was no growth in the blood culture. Total transfusions given were 15 units PCV, 27 units FFP, 5 units cryoprecipitate, and 24 units platelet concentrate.

8.2 Autopsy Findings

General examination: Pallor++, bilateral lower limbs showed blackening of skin and eroded skin surface of size 15 × 5 cm on the medial aspect in addition to surgical wound of obstetric hysterectomy on the anterior abdominal wall. A large ulcer measuring 5 × 4 × 1.5 cm with a greenish necrotic floor and elevated edges was seen in the body of

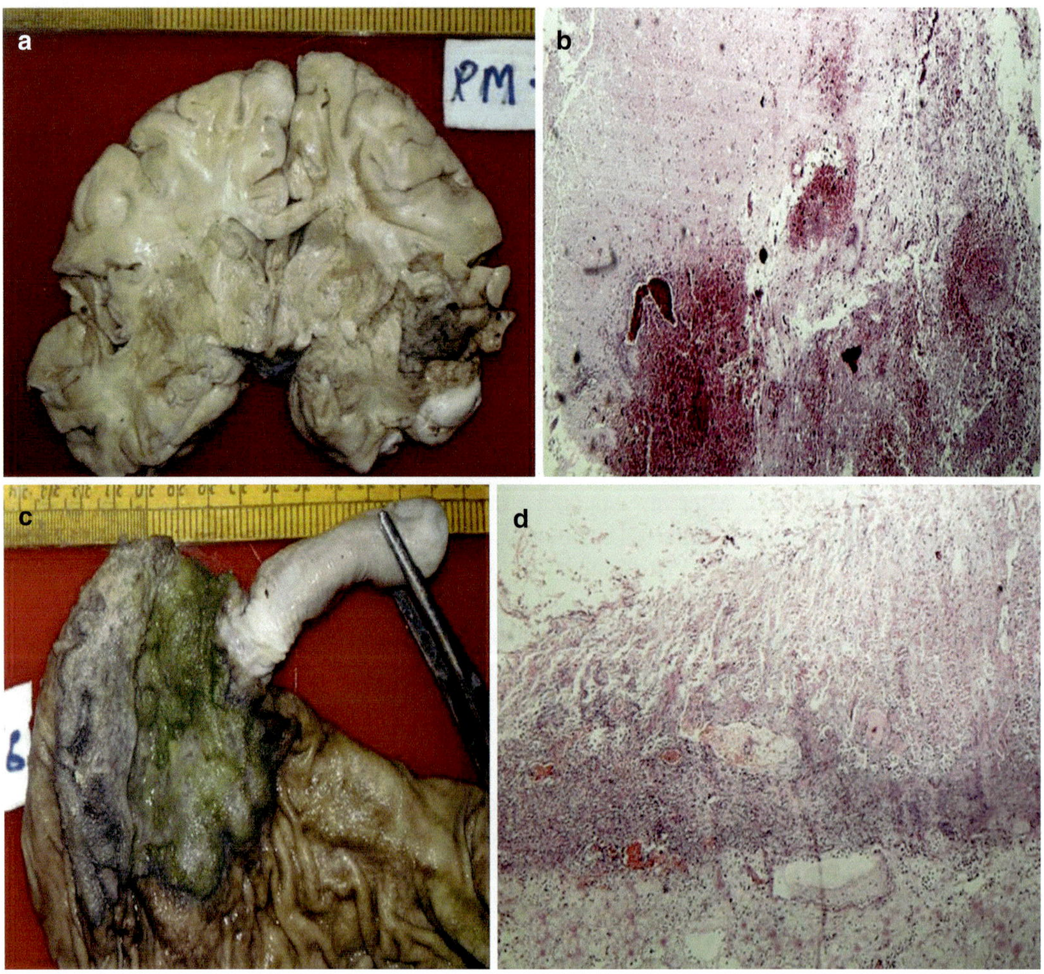

Fig. 8.1 (**a**) Brain showed a hemorrhagic lesion of 2.5 × 2.0 × 2.0 cm in the right temporoparietal lobe. (**b**) Microscopy showed a hemorrhagic infarct with the presence of few thrombosed small vessels in the surrounding viable parenchyma, H&E, 100x. (**c**) Large ulcer measuring 5 × 4 × 1.5 cm with a greenish necrotic floor and elevated edges was seen in the body of the stomach. (**d**) Ischemic ulcer with the presence of fibrin thrombi in the submucosal blood vessels, H&E, 100x

the stomach (Fig. 8.1c). Microscopy revealed an ischemic ulcer with the presence of fibrin thrombi in the submucosal blood vessels (Fig. 8.1d). On higher magnification, broad, obtuse-angled, non-septate fungal hyphae were seen in the ischemic mucosa as well as in the thrombi and in the walls of thrombosed vessels (Fig. 8.3a, c). Special stains of periodic acid-Schiff (PAS) (Fig. 8.3d) and Gomori's methenamine silver (GMS) confirmed the fungi to be mucormycosis. Brain showed a hemorrhagic lesion of 2.5 × 2.0 × 2.0 cm in the right temporoparietal lobe. Microscopy showed a hemorrhagic infarct with the presence of few thrombosed small vessels in the surrounding viable parenchyma (Fig. 8.1a, b). Both lungs showed multiple patchy elevated firm areas, gray-yellow in color, varying from 1.5 × 2.0 × 1.0 cm to larger 3.5 × 2.0 × 1.5 cm in size, suggestive of bronchopneumonia. Microscopy showed ulceration of the bronchial mucosa with the presence of neutrophils in the ulcerated area as well as within the bronchial lumen. A similar neutrophilic infiltrate was seen within the alveolar spaces (Fig. 8.2a, b). Few small- and medium-sized arteries showed fibrin thrombi; however, fungal hyphae were not seen (Fig. 8.3b). The urinary bladder and cervix appeared grossly as an irregular hemorrhagic soft tissue mass with few sutures seen (Fig. 8.2c). A cordlike thrombosed blood vessel was also seen over the surface. Multiple sections from this hemorrhagic mass identified them by their respective lining epithelium with ischemic hemorrhagic necrosis of both the cervix and urinary bladder walls and the presence of thrombosed blood vessels in their walls, without fungal hyphae. The cervix in addition showed the presence of retained placental tissue in the form of chorionic villi. A part of the uterine wall identified by hypertrophied myometrial fibers was also seen. Kidneys showed focal areas of acute

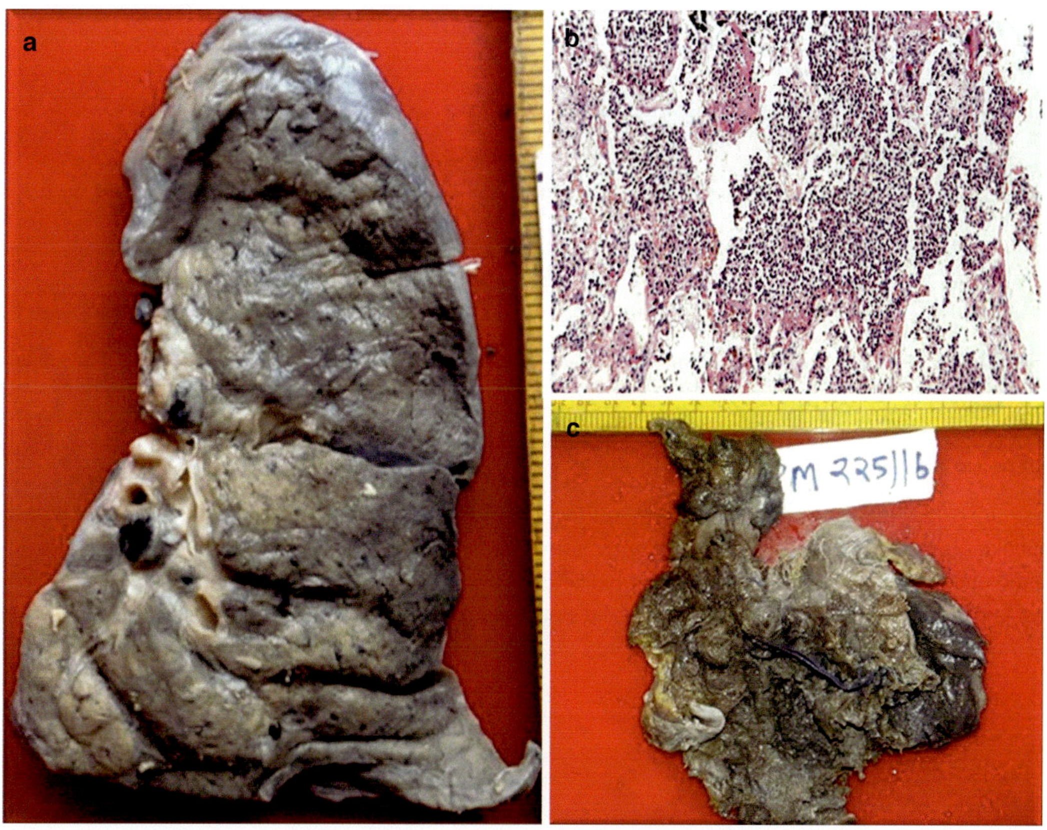

Fig. 8.2 (**a**) Lung shows multiple patchy elevated firm areas, gray-yellow in color, varying from 1.5 × 2.0 × 1.0 cm to larger 3.5 × 2.0 × 1.5 cm in size, suggestive of bronchopneumonia. (**b**) Neutrophilic infiltrate seen within alveolar spaces, H&E, 100x. (**c**) The urinary bladder and cervix appeared grossly as an irregular hemorrhagic soft tissue mass

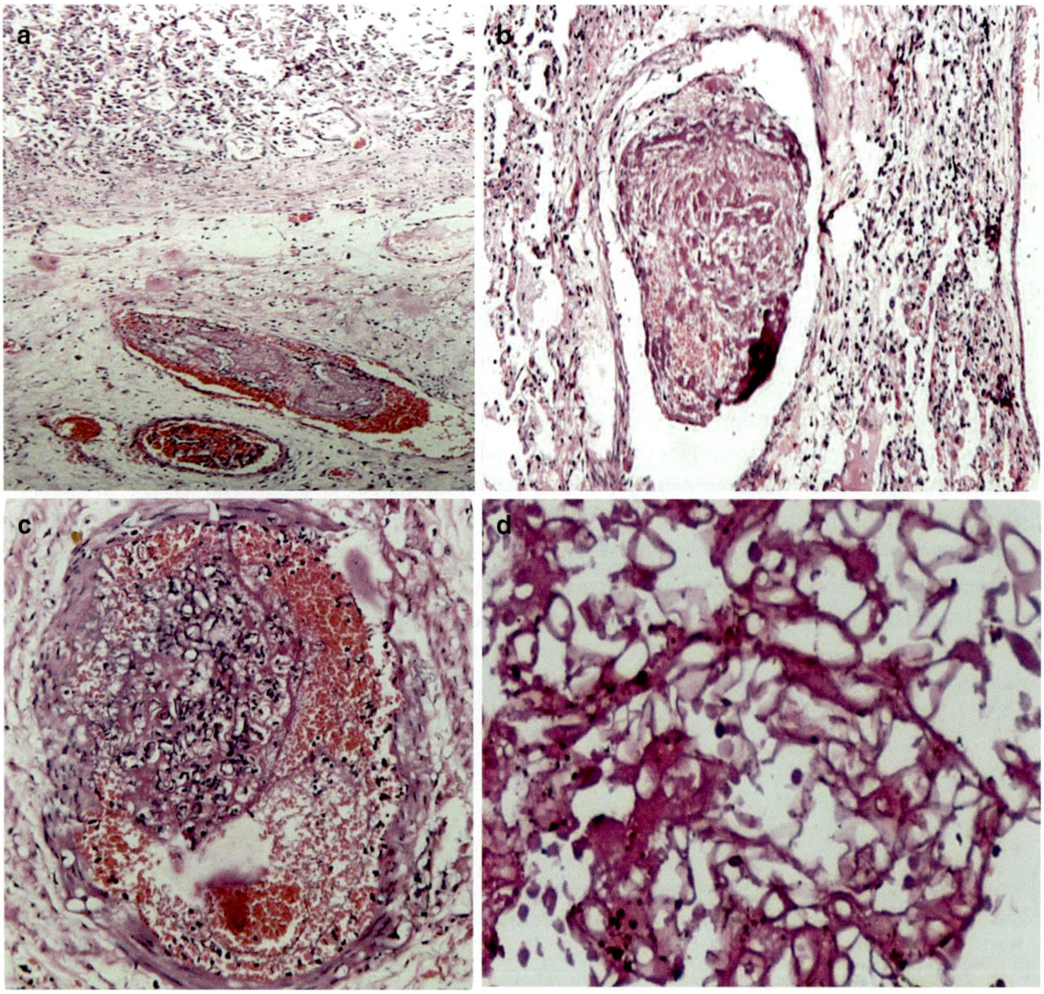

Fig. 8.3 (**a**) Fibrin thrombi with fungal filaments in gastric submucosal blood vessels, H&E, 200x. (**b**) Few small and medium sized arteries showed fibrin thrombi; however, fungal hyphae were not seen, H&E, 400x. (**c**) Broad, obtuse-angled, non-septate fungal hyphae were seen in the ischemic mucosa as well as in the thrombi and in the walls of thrombosed vessels, H&E, 400x. (**d**) Special stain periodic acid-Schiff (PAS) confirmed the fungi to be mucormycosis, 1000x

tubular necrosis. Rest of the organs were unremarkable on gross and microscopy. Histopathologic examination of the subtotal hysterectomy did not show any evidence of rent nor any sutured area.

8.3 Final Cause of Death

Systemic thromboembolism, bronchopneumonia, and septicemia in a case of obstetric subtotal hysterectomy (unnatural).

8.4 Clinicopathologic Discussion

Venous thromboembolism (VTE) is a collective term that describes deep vein thrombosis (DVT) and pulmonary embolism (PE). Pregnancy, being a hypercoagulable state, is a risk factor for both arterial and venous thromboembolism (TE). Approximately 20% of these events are arterial, and the rest 80% are venous. The pelvic and lower limb veins have increased stasis due to physical obstruction from the gravid uterus. Also, the coagulation factor levels are increased in pregnancy in preparation for the hemostatic challenge of delivery as well as the injury to pelvic vessels occurring during delivery. Thus, all three components of "Virchow's triad" of venous stasis, hypercoagulability, and vascular damage occur in the course of pregnancy and delivery. The risk for TE is present in the antenatal as well as until at least 12 weeks postnatal, although most thromboembolic events occur in the first 3 weeks after delivery. Postnatal risk factors include cesarean section, particularly if this was associated with a prolonged hospital stay or emergency delivery, and complicated by other factors such as postpartum hemorrhage and/or sepsis. Pre-existing factors such as parity >3, varicose veins, smoking, and medical comorbidities (e.g., cancer) are some of the risk factors for VTE. All women should be assessed for their risk of VTE early in the pregnancy. This assessment should be repeated in the intrapartum and postnatal periods. It is not so easy to diagnose pulmonary thromboembolism clinically as the physiologic signs and symptoms of pregnancy very often mimic it [1–3].

There was no evidence of rent identified in the uterine wall of subtotal hysterectomy (reported by the first author in the surgical pathology laboratory), and products of conception (POCs) in the form of chorionic villi were seen in the cervical wall on autopsy. So, with subtotal hysterectomy, the rent as well as POCs remained inside the body. Total obstetric hysterectomy should have been the procedure carried out in this case of uterine rent and placenta previa. This retained POCs as well as the surgery acted as the stimulus for continuing bleeding (postpartum hemorrhage), systemic thromboembolism (cervix, urinary bladder, brain, stomach, lung) in addition to the already existing hypercoagulable state of pregnancy, and mucormycotic infection followed by death.

Mucormycosis is a life-threatening infection caused by fungi of the subphylum Mucoromycotina, order Mucorales. Traditional risk factors for the development of invasive mucormycosis include diabetes, defects in host phagocytes, cancer, corticosteroid use, and organ or stem cell transplantation. The common factor acting in all these risk factors is immunosuppression status. In recent years, the disease has also increasingly been described in patients without these risk factors. Mucormycosis can affect any organ system, but the most common presentations involve either the nasal sinuses, orbit, and brain (rhino-orbital-cerebral) or the lungs. Gastrointestinal mucormycosis is very rare, with the stomach being the most common site, followed by the colon and ileum [4].

There are two possibilities for giant gastric ulcer with mucormycosis: the first is ischemic gastric ulcer due to systemic thromboembolism with superadded mucor infection. The second possibility is primary mucor infection causing a giant gastric ulcer due to vascular invasion.

Ingestion of infected sputum or pathogens in food such as fermented milk or dried bread products or ingestion of spore contaminated herbal or homeopathic medicines or during intubation are the pathways of entry of mucor into the stomach. Hallmark features of mucormycosis infection are angioinvasion, vascular thrombosis, and tissue necrosis. Because this infection is acute and rapidly fatal, it is often diagnosed on postmortem. Affected patients may present with fever, nonspecific abdominal pain, nausea, vomiting to hematemesis, melaena, hematochezia or gastrointestinal perforation. The diagnosis is by biopsy of the suspected area at surgery/endoscopy. Treatment is usually with intravenous amphotericin B or oral posaconazole; however, surgical intervention may be considered for uncontrollable gastrointestinal hemorrhage or perforation [5, 6].

References

1. Alsheef MA, Alabbad AM, Albassam RA, Alarfaj RM, Zaidi ARZ, Al-Arfaj O, Abu-Shaheen A. Pregnancy and venous thromboembolism: risk factors, trends, management, and mortality. BioMed Int Res. 2020;2020:4071892. https://doi.org/10.1155/2020/4071892.
2. Unger HW, Bhaskar S, Mahmood T. Venous thromboembolism in pregnancy. Obstetr Gynaecol Reprod Med. 2018; https://doi.org/10.1016/j.ogrm.2018.11.002.
3. Friel L. Thromboembolic disorders in pregnancy. Gynecology and obstetrics, MSD manual professional version. 2020.

4. Adhikari S, Gautam AR, Paudyal B, Sigdel KR, Basnyat B. Case report: gastric Mucormycosis-a rare but important differential diagnosis of upper gastrointestinal bleeding in an area of Helicobacter pylori endemicity. Wellcome Open Res. 2019;4:5. https://doi.org/10.12688/wellcomeopenres.15026.2.
5. Sehmbey G, Malik R, Kosa D, Srinivasan I, Chuang K-Y, Bellapravalu S. Case Report: Gastric ulcer and perforation due to mucormycosis in an immunocompetent patient. ACG Case Rep J. 2019;6(8):e00154. https://doi.org/10.14309/crj.0000000000000154.
6. Chhaya V, Gupta S, Arnaout A. Mucormycosis causing giant gastric ulcers. Endoscopy. 2011;43:E289–90.

9 Puerperal Sepsis: A Preventable Cause of Maternal Death

Kusum D. Jashnani, Sakshi Agrawal, Lalita Yoganand Patil, and Vandana Rajesh Saravade

9.1 Clinical History

A 20-year-old primigravida, 33 weeks of gestation, came with complaints of abdominal pain with history of gestational hypertension and twin gestation, with non-availability of NICU. There was no other significant history (leaking per vagina, absence of fetal movements, bladder/bowel disturbance, headache, epigastric pain, blurring of vision and vomiting). She was afebrile with a blood pressure of 130/100 mmHg and abdominal wall edema with bilateral pedal edema. On abdominal examination, fetal heart sounds were present. Ultrasound of the abdomen and pelvis was suggestive of diamniotic monochorionic twins. Emergency LSCS was carried out with IUCD insertion within 24 h of admission. On post-operative day 1, the patient's vitals were stable. Then from day 2 to day 5, the patient started complaining of loose motions, fever with chills, vomiting, abdominal distension and abdominal pain. So, augmentin was stepped up to ceftriaxone, artesunate and piperacillin. Tazobactum was also given. She was also given one cycle of peritoneal dialysis in view of acute renal failure and a packed red blood cell transfusion in view of low Hb. Her symptoms however progressively worsened, and she suddenly collapsed in ward on day 8. The patient was revived after CPR and intubated. Clinical examination showed abdominal distension and tenderness, and clinical impression was anemia with hypokalemia, severe metabolic acidosis with sepsis secondary to abdominal cause. USG pelvis done showed bulky uterus with collection in the lower uterine segment and mild ascites. Her condition deteriorated, with poor general condition and BP

K. D. Jashnani (✉) · L. Y. Patil
Department of Pathology, Topiwala National Medical College and BYL Nair Charitable Hospital, Mumbai, Maharashtra, India

S. Agrawal
Histopathology Laboratory, Lilavati Hospital and Research Centre, Mumbai, Maharashtra, India

V. R. Saravade
Department of Obstetrics and Gynecology, Topiwala National Medical College and BYL Nair Charitable Hospital, Mumbai, Maharashtra, India

K. D. Jashnani (ed.), *Maternal Mortality - Lessons Learnt from Autopsy*,
https://doi.org/10.1007/978-981-19-3420-9_9

varying from 90 to 60 systolic and 60 to 33 diastolic, finally she expired on day 12.

9.2 Investigations

Hemoglobin varied from 8.8 to 9.5 g/dL, total WBC counts were in the range of 8000 to 8800/cmm, serum creatinine varied from 2.73 to 4 mg/dl, and D-dimer was raised to 9297 ng/ml. Ascitic fluid showed plenty of degenerated white blood cells on microscopic examination. Complete autopsy was performed.

9.3 Autopsy Findings

The abdominal cavity showed 800 ml of yellow with red tinge fluid. Microscopic examination of this fluid showed 3000 cells/cmm with 80% polymorphs and 20% lymphocytes against a background of reactive mesothelial cells and RBCs. The uterus weighed 700 g and measured 24 × 17 × 7 cm. The external surface showed yellowish white granular exudate with the presence of a 6 × 1.5 cm incision of the lower uterine cesarean segment with sutures in place (Fig. 9.1a). Margins of the incision showed the

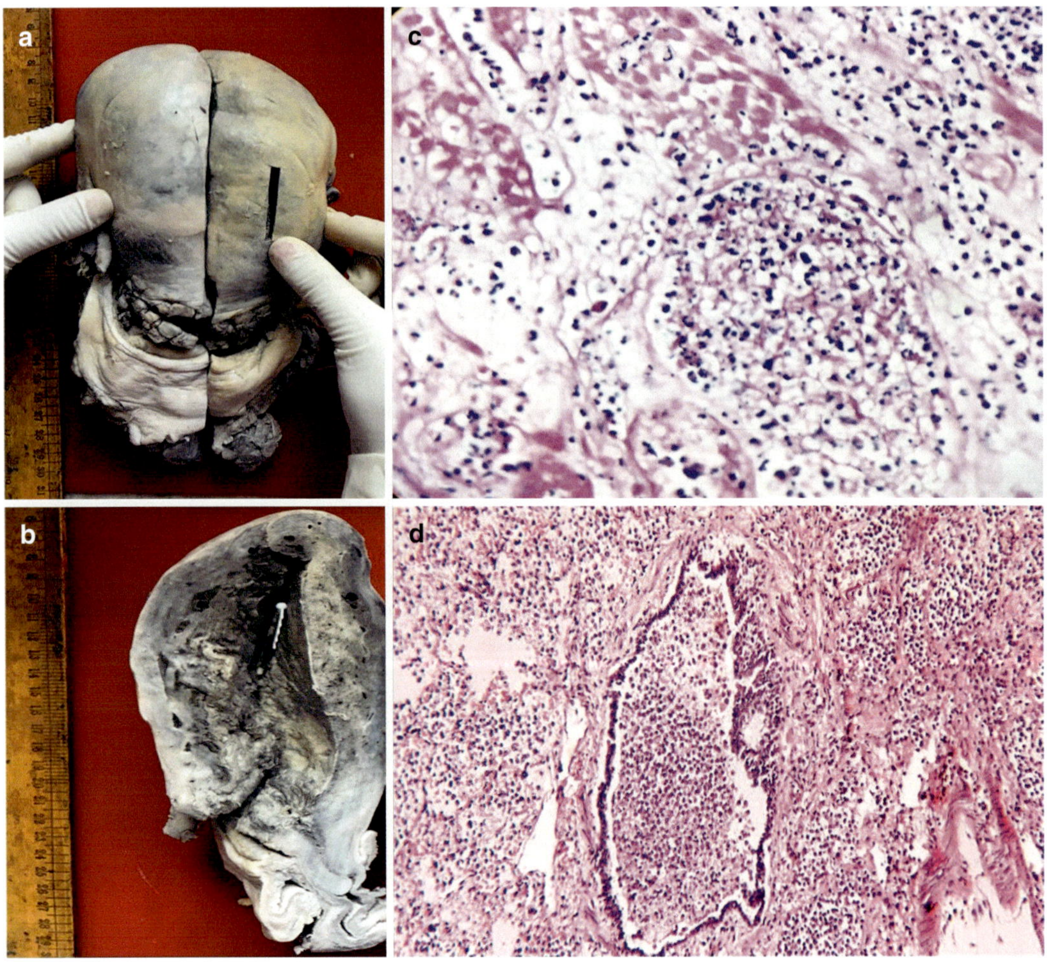

Fig. 9.1 (**a**) Gross specimen of the uterus with the cervix showing granular, thick exudate over the external surface of the uterine fundus. (**b**) Cut surface of the uterus showing copper T and yellowish exudate over the entire endometrial surface. (**c**) Necrosis of the myometrial fibres with multiple aggregates of neutrophils (H & E, 400×). (**d**) Bronchopneumonia showing alveolar spaces and a bronchiole packed with neutrophilic inflammatory infiltrate (H & E, 100×)

presence of thick yellow exudate. The cut surface of the uterus showed granular exudate on the endometrial surface and copper T noted in the endometrial cavity (Fig. 9.1b). The cervix, fallopian tubes and ovaries were unremarkable. On microscopic examination, the uterine serosa showed dense fibrino-neutrophilic exudate which at places was extending into the underlying deep myometrium with abscess formation (Fig. 9.1c). The endometrium showed decidual change with a dense neutrophilic inflammatory infiltrate which was extending into the underlying superficial myometrium. Few bacterial colonies were also seen in this inflammation. At places, the endometrium and inner half of myometrium showed infarction with a few decidual vessels showing fibrin thrombi.

Small and large intestines showed edematous mucosa and a yellowish white granular fibrino-neutrophilic exudate on the serosal surface on gross and microscopic examination (Fig. 9.2a, b).

The liver was enlarged and showed thick yellowish white exudate on the capsule (Fig. 9.2c), cut surface showed alternating light and dark areas suggestive of chronic passive congestion (CPC). On microscopic examination, the capsule was thick with the presence of a band of fibrino-neutrophilic exudate (Fig. 9.2d) and features of CPC. Sinusoids were dilated and showed the presence of neutrophils.

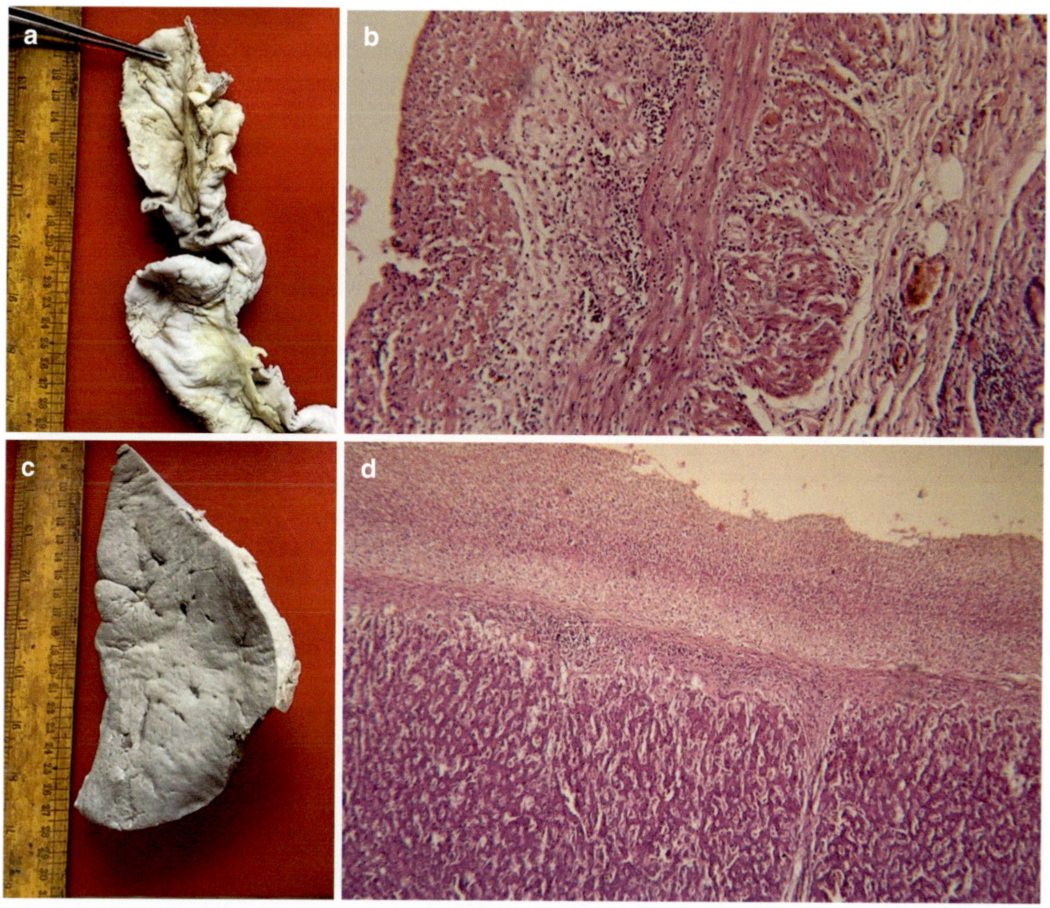

Fig. 9.2 (**a**) Gross specimen of the small intestine showing a greyish white granular, thick exudate over the serosal surface. (**b**) The serosal surface of small intestine showing band of fibrino-neutrophilic exudate (H & E, 100×). (**c**) Gross specimen of the liver showing a greyish white granular, thick exudate over the capsule. (**d**) The liver in (**c**) showing a band of fibrino-neutrophilic exudate on the capsule (H & E, 100×)

The lungs weighed 450 g each. The pleura showed focal areas of opacity. The cut surface of the lungs showed patchy firm raised areas suggestive of bronchopneumonia. On microscopic examination, the pleura showed fibrous thickening with patchy areas of alveolar spaces packed with neutrophilic inflammatory infiltrate. Some bronchioles showed ulcerated epithelium with presence of neutrophils in their lumina. Few alveolar septae were focally lined by eosinophilic hyaline membranes. Features were suggestive of bronchopneumonia with early acute respiratory distress syndrome. The kidneys on microscopic examination showed multiple patchy areas of acute tubular necrosis. No evidence of thrombi in the glomerular capillaries. Rest of the organs were unremarkable.

9.4 Final Cause of Death

Septic shock due to puerperal sepsis and peritonitis in a case operated for lower segment cesarean section with wound dehiscence (unnatural).

9.5 Clinicopathologic Discussion

Puerperal sepsis is one of the preventable causes of maternal mortality occurring in developing countries like India. It is one of the five leading causes of maternal mortality worldwide, the others being hypertension, hemorrhage, obstructed labour and unsafe abortion [1]. According to the World Health Organization (WHO), puerperal sepsis is defined as the infection of the genital tract occurring at labour or within 42 days of the post-partum period [2]. WHO report estimated 3,58,000 maternal deaths yearly due to child birth problems, and out of these up to 15% are associated with puerperal sepsis [3]. Patients with puerperal sepsis present with complaints of persistent fever, malodorous vaginal discharge, abdominal pain with distension and a delay in the rate of reduction of the size of the uterus. Cesarean section is found to be the single most important risk factor for puerperal sepsis. Puerperal sepsis has been observed in 1% to 3% of normal vaginal deliveries, 5–15% in scheduled cesarean deliveries performed before labour begins, and 15–20% in non-scheduled cesarean deliveries performed after labour begins. Other risk factors being retained products of conception, prolonged rupture of membranes, multiple gestation, multiple vaginal examinations during labour, amniocentesis or other invasive procedure, etc. In developing countries like India, especially in rural areas, home delivery by an unskilled attendant using unsterile/unhygienic methods for delivery is also an important cause of puerperal sepsis. Relevant clinical examination findings are elevated body temperatures, abdominal distention, foul smelling lochia and supportive investigations are leucocytosis or leukopenia, thrombocytopenia, deranged coagulation profile and altered serum electrolytes. Ultrasound examination may show intraperitoneal collection, uterine collection or retained products of conception, etc. Detailed history along with clinical examination and specific investigations helps in early diagnosis of puerperal sepsis, and its prompt treatment can be initiated, which can reduce mortality. Detailed history should also include presence of predisposing factors if any, such as poor hygiene, poverty, illiteracy, frequent vaginal examinations (>5), delivery/abortion by untrained persons, home delivery, prolonged labour, prolonged rupture of membrane, postpartum hemorrhage and comorbidities like diabetes, tuberculosis, anemia [4]. Delayed diagnosis or improper treatment can lead to complications of puerperal sepsis which include disseminated intravascular coagulation, septicemia and maternal death [4].

The case discussed here presented with abdominal pain and gestational hypertension with twin gestation and was afebrile at the time of admission. Post second day of LSCS with IUCD insertion, she started complaining of fever and abdominal distension with pain. So, the source of infection was related to LSCS and/or IUCD insertion or it was following wound dehiscence (this looks more likely). Due to altered physiology during pregnancy and puerperium, the signs and symptoms of sepsis may be obscured, leading to rapid deterioration and death. If sepsis is suspected, current guidelines support the initiation of emperic antibiotic treatment as early as possible. In the present case, antibiotic treatment had been started as a protocol following LSCS. Findings of granular exudate on the serosal and endometrial surfaces of the uterus and other organs during autopsy with histopathological examination, in the background of clinical correlation confirmed the diagnosis of puerperal sepsis. Microbiological studies like blood for culture can be sent during autopsy of suspected cases of puerperal sepsis. Puerperal sepsis is often a polymicrobial infection. Escherichia coli is a common cause of severe maternal sepsis with origin from the genital tract. Group A *Streptococcus*, *S. aureus*, *Streptococcus* spp., *Klebsiella* spp., *Pseudomonas* spp. and anaerobes are other types of bacteria involved [5]. In addition to assisting in determining the cause of death, autopsy also helps in identifying comorbidities that could have affected recovery and also identification of any complication caused by puerperal sepsis or its management, e.g. presence of hemorrhage and fibrin thrombi in the kidney or other organs indicative of the presence of disseminated intravascular coagulation which is one of the complications of puerperal sepsis.

References

1. Buddeberg BS, Aveling W. Puerperal sepsis in the 21st century: progress, new challenges and the situation worldwide. Postgrad Med J. 2015; https://doi.org/10.1136/postgradmedj-2015-133475.
2. Khaskheli MN, Baloch S, Sheeba A. Risk factors and complications of puerperal sepsis at a tertiary healthcare centre. Pak J Med Sci. 2013;29(4):972–6.
3. World Health Organization: Trends in maternal mortality 1990–2008. Estimates developed by WHO, UNICEF, UNFPA and World Bank, Geneva; 2010.
4. Marwah S, Topden SR, Sharma M, Mohindra R, Mittal P. Severe puerperal sepsis-a simmering menace. J Clin Diagn Res. 2017;11(5):QC04–8.
5. Majangara R, Gidiri MF, Chirenje ZM. Microbiology and clinical outcomes of puerperal sepsis: a prospective cohort study. J Obstet Gynaecol. 2018;38(5):635–41.

Peripartum Cardiomyopathy: Failed Cardiac Physiology

10

Rushabh Shah, Pranita Zare, and Pradeep Vaideeswar

10.1 Clinical History

A diagnosis of pregnancy-induced hypertension (160/100 mm Hg) was made in the second trimester of a 35-year-old primigravida. She, at 34 weeks of pregnancy, developed shortness of breath for the past 1 month. It had progressed to affect her routine activities and later persisted even at rest in the past 1 week. Subsequently, she had an episode of tonic-clonic convulsions and was admitted to a private nursing home. Elective cesarean section was deferred due to dyspnea and she was transferred to our center. Her general condition was poor with a heart rate of 140 per min and a blood pressure of 200/110 mm Hg. There were bilateral coarse crepitations. The routine hematological (including coagulation profile) and biochemical investigations were within normal limits. A two-dimensional transthoracic echocardiography revealed sinus tachycardia, generalized left ventricular hypokinesia with an ejection fraction of 40%, moderate mitral regurgitation, and mild tricuspid regurgitation. No fetal cardiac activity was noted on ultrasonography. She expired within 2 days of admission, despite anti-failure and anti-hypertensive therapy.

10.2 Autopsy Findings

The heart was mildly enlarged in size (270 g) and globular in shape due to mild biventricular dilatation and hypertrophy (Fig. 10.1a, b). The myocardium appeared a little pale brown. Foci of congestion or fibrosis were not seen. Valves and other chambers appeared to be normal. On histology, there was mild hypertrophy of the cardiomyocytes (Fig. 10.1c) of the right and left ventricles with fine interstitial and interfiber increase in connective tissue (Fig. 10.1d). Small foci of necroses with lymphocytic infiltrate, larger subendocardial foci of scarring and focal myocytolysis were also present. The lungs showed diffuse alveolar damage and pulmonary edema. Lymphocytic thyroiditis was also present. The uterus showed a male fetus with normal placentation. Other organs were normal.

R. Shah
SRL Dr Avinash Phadke Labs,
Mumbai, Maharashtra, India

P. Zare · P. Vaideeswar (✉)
Department of Pathology (Cardiovascular and Thoracic Division), Seth GS Medical College and KEM Hospital, Mumbai, Maharashtra, India

K. D. Jashnani (ed.), *Maternal Mortality - Lessons Learnt from Autopsy*,
https://doi.org/10.1007/978-981-19-3420-9_10

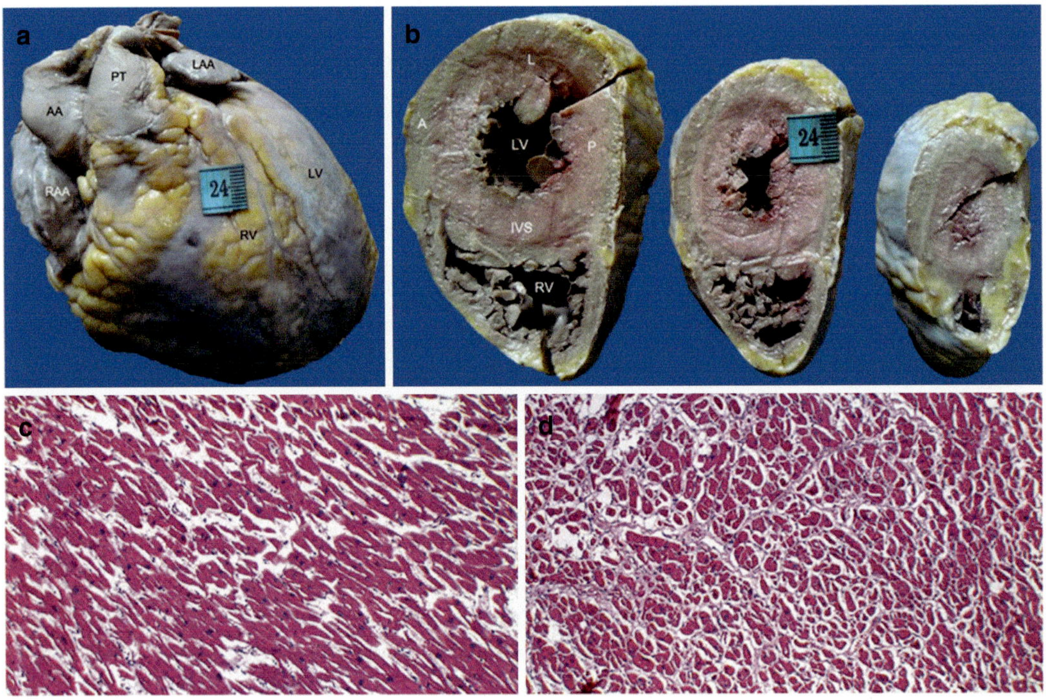

Fig. 10.1 (**a**) Mild cardiomegaly due to enlargement of the right RV and left LV ventricles. Note that the apex is formed by both ventricles. (**b**) Serial transverse sections reveal mild hypertrophy with pale myocardium (*A* anterior wall, *AA* ascending aorta, *IVS* inter-ventricular septum, *L* lateral wall, *LAA* left atrial appendage, *P* posterior wall, *PT* pulmonary trunk, RAA right atrial appendage). (**c**) Cardiomyocyte hypertrophy (H&E ×200). (**d**) Prominent interfiber increase in connective tissue (H&E ×200)

10.3 Final Cause of Death

PPCM with diffuse alveolar damage.

10.4 Clinicopathologic Discussion

The case depicts the development of heart failure during the third trimester of pregnancy in a woman in her third decade of life. She had gestational hypertension, but no other evidence of toxemia of pregnancy despite an episode of tonic-clonic convulsion. Heart failure is an important cause of morbidity and mortality in pregnancy (about 9% of all maternal deaths), particularly in the postpartum period [1]. It occurs when the physiological changes overwhelm the compensatory mechanisms in a pre-existing CVD or the changes unmask a subclinical but significant CVD. Such disorders mainly include valvular, ischemic, and certain congenital heart diseases and pulmonary hypertension [2]. Apart from the more common pregnancy-induced hypertensive disorders, an uncommon manifestation that culminates in heart failure is PPCM, which was the diagnosis made in this patient after autopsy evaluation. PPCM is an idiopathic cardiomyopathy characterized by signs and symptoms of heart failure that develop in the last month of pregnancy or within 5 months of the postpartum period without any identifiable or known cause; the left ventricular ejection fraction is less than 45% [3]. The cardiomyopathy can sometimes occur after a miscarriage, and the systolic dysfunction can also occur with ejection fractions between 45% and 50% [4]. In this context, it is also interesting to note that left ventricular dysfunction can also be documented in asymptomatic pregnant women [5]. The approximate world-wide incidence of PPCM is 1 in 1000 pregnancies [6]. The incidence, however, varies widely depending upon the geographic location, race (especially African descent), and ethnicity [6]. A recent study had a figure of 1 in 1541 live births [7]. Despite the variation, the risk factors are common and include advanced maternal age, multiparity, multifetal gestation, hypertensive disorders of pregnancy, use of tocolytic agents, diabetes mellitus, obesity, and history of smoking [3].

PPCM basically has a DCM phenotype but is a diagnosis of exclusion. In most cases, on gross examination, the heart is enlarged with biventricular dilatation and flabby consistency of the myocardium. It may be associated with pericardial effusions or mural thrombi within the chambers. On histopathology, the appearance is varied, and owing to the heterogeneity of the pathogenesis, it shows a myocarditic or a non-myocarditic picture. Some cases show features of a lymphohistiocytic myocarditis with elevated levels of pro-inflammatory cytokines, which is explained on the basis of reactivation of latent viruses or dysregulated immune responses with the generation of autoantibodies [8]. Apart from myocarditis, features of DCM (non-specific characteristics of increased interfiber or interstitial fibrosis, myocyte attenuation, degeneration, or hypertrophy) can be observed. These changes in some patients are directly associated with gene mutations, which are otherwise responsible for DCM and/or hypertrophic cardiomyopathy in other individuals [9]. Hemodynamic and unbalanced oxidative stress induce an angiogenic imbalance through pregnancy-related hormones (particularly prolactin and its metabolite) and cause endothelial dysfunction, thwarted angiogenesis, apoptosis, and impaired cardiomyocyte contractility [10]. Such effects can be enhanced by a genetic predisposition as well ("two-hit" model) [10]. These mechanisms can also produce a DCM phenotype or sometimes may be associated with almost normal histomorphology (barring the hypertrophy). Other potential mechanisms to explain the cardiac dysfunction are nutritional deficiencies, defective antioxidant defenses, or coronary artery spasm. Our case had shown features similar to DCM.

Though PPCM is a diagnosis of exclusion, heightened clinical suspicion and timely evaluation would ensure prompt therapy to alleviate the cardiac failure and to prevent thrombo-embolic episodes or arrhythmias, which are often associated with this condition. However, there would still be a non-salvageable group of patients (such as ours) or women who may not completely regain optimal cardiac function.

References

1. Mogos MF, Piano MR, McFarlin BL, Salemi JL, Liese KL, Briller JE. Heart failure in pregnant women: a concern across the pregnancy continuum. Circ Heart Fail. 2018;11:e004005.
2. Guimarães T, Magalhães A, Veiga A, Fiuza M, Ávila W, Pinto FJ. Heart disease and pregnancy: state of the art. Rev Port Cardiol. 2019;38:373–83.
3. Davis MB, Arany Z, McNamara DM, Goland S, Elkayam U. Peripartum cardiomyopathy. JACC state-of-the-art review. J Am Coll Cardiol. 2020;75:207–21.
4. Bauersachs J, König T, van der Meer P, Petrie MC, Hilfiker-Kleiner D, Mbakwem A. Pathophysiology, diagnosis and management of peripartum cardiomyopathy: a position statement from the heart failure Association of the European Society of cardiology study group on peripartum cardiomyopathy. Eur J Heart Fail. 2019;21:827–43.
5. Vettori DV, Rohde LE, Clausell N. Asymptomatic left ventricular dysfunction in puerperal women: an echocardiographic-based study. Int J Cardiol. 2011;149:353–7.
6. Isogai T, Kamiya CA. Worldwide incidence of peripartum cardiomyopathy and overall maternal mortality. Int Heart J. 2019;60:503–11.
7. Binu AJ, Rajan SJ, Rathore S, Beck M, Regi A, Thomson VS, et al. Perpartum cardiomyopathy: an analysis of clinical profiles and outcomes from a tertiary care Centre in southern India. Obstet Med. 2020;13:179–84.
8. Gupta D, Wenger NK. Peripartum cardiomyopathy: status 2018. Clin Cardiol. 2018;41:217–9.
9. Kamiya CA, Yoshimatsu J, Ikeda T. Peripartum cardiomyopathy from a genetic perspective. Circ J. 2016;80:1684–8.
10. Ricke-Hoch M, Pfeffer TJ, Hilfiker-Kleiner D. Peripartum cardiomyopathy: basic mechanisms and hope for new therapies. Cardiovasc Res. 2020;116:520–31.

HELLP Syndrome: The Snowball Effect 11

Shilpa Kapil Lad, Kusum D. Jashnani, and Shekhar T. Nabar

11.1 Clinical History

A 25-year-old primigravida at 38 weeks of gestation had a total hospital stay of 7 days. She was admitted with epigastric pain, fever, and episodes of blackout which were present for the last 5 days. Her blood pressure at the time of admission was 140/100 mmHg, and she was diagnosed with pregnancy-induced hypertension (PIH). For the last 15 days, she had started to develop pedal edema. She had jaundice one and a half months ago due to hepatitis E infection. On day 2 of admission, a forceps delivery was conducted in view of intrauterine fetal death (IUFD), following which she developed hypotension and was dyspneic. She was unconscious but was responding to deep painful stimuli and was shifted to ICU, put on a ventilator, and started with dopamine and antibiotics (Monocef and meterogyl). On day 2 postpartum, she developed sudden per vaginal bleeding and also developed a right labial hematoma with a gaping episiotomy wound. She remained unconscious during her postpartum state with a complete renal shutdown in her last 2 days. Her hemoglobin at the time of admission was 9.6 g/dL, which dropped to 3.6 g/dL in the immediate postpartum period. She was given 8 pints of packed cells, which helped to increase her hemoglobin levels to 8 g/dL terminally. Her total WBC count showed a steady rise from 24,400/cmm on day 2 postpartum to 32,800/cmm with neutrophilia and a left shift suggestive of sepsis. In view of her platelet counts of 69,000/cmm in the antenatal period, she was given 10 units of platelets, which helped to maintain the platelet count in the normal range with counts of 169,000/cmm terminally. Her serum bilirubin levels were 9.2 mg/dl with direct bilirubin of 6.8 mg/dl on the day of admission which rose steadily from 12.8 mg/dl on day 2 postpartum to 27.5 mg/dl with direct hyperbilirubinemia in the terminal stages. Her liver enzyme levels continued to be deranged with SGOT/SGPT levels of 1064/421 U/L in the immediate postpartum period with slight improvement at day 6 postpartum to 204/93 U/L, respectively. During her ward stay of 7 days, she underwent hemodialysis daily in view of her creatinine levels of 4.3 mg/dl; her BUN level was 41 mg/dl with serum creatinine of 3.1 mg/dl on the last day. Clinical impression was hepatic encephalopathy with HELLP syndrome with PIH to rule out disseminated intravascular coagulation (DIC). Terminally her coagulation profile showed serum fibrinogen level <150 mg %, prothrombin time (PT) was 2.2 min (control was 13 s), and FDP (fibrin degradation products) level was >1400 mcg/ml in spite of 12 units of FFP. She was HIV,

S. K. Lad · K. D. Jashnani (✉)
Department of Pathology, Topiwala National Medical College and BYL Nair Charitable Hospital, Mumbai, Maharashtra, India

S. T. Nabar
Ex Head, Department of Medicine, Topiwala National Medical College and BYL Nair Charitable Hospital, Mumbai, India

K. D. Jashnani (ed.), *Maternal Mortality - Lessons Learnt from Autopsy*,
https://doi.org/10.1007/978-981-19-3420-9_11

HBsAg, and HCV nonreactive. She succumbed on day 7 of delivery in spite of all resuscitative measures. A complete autopsy was performed.

11.2 Autopsy Findings

At autopsy, she was averagely built and nourished. A blood-soaked vaginal pad was removed from the vagina. A right labial hematoma and a gaping episiotomy wound were noted. Her skin showed yellow discoloration and was pale. Her abdomen was distended due to 2.5 liters of blood in the peritoneal cavity. Hemorrhages were seen on the pleural surfaces and in the uterine adnexae. All the organs were severely pale.

The brain weighed 1200 g and showed cerebral edema. The cerebellum showed multiple tiny petechial hemorrhages. The heart was normal in size and shape, weighed 350 g, and showed multiple roughened pale patches of 1 cm^2 on the epicardium. The heart was opened along the flow of blood and showed multiple pale lesions with hyperemic borders ranging from 0.5 to 1.5 cm in the ventricular myocardium, suggestive of multiple myocardial abscesses. (Fig. 11.1a).

Lungs weighed 350 g each and showed focal patches of consolidation with sinking test positive. Bilateral kidneys weighed 130 g each and showed wedge shaped pale areas in the cortex with hyperemic borders in the cortex. The liver weighed 1.4 kg and was soft, yellow, and foldable with a wrinkled capsule suggestive of hepatic necrosis. The uterus with bilateral adnexa weighed 250 g; serosa showed multiple hemorrhages with 200 g of clot in the uterine cavity. All the other organs were unremarkable.

Histopathological Examination Sections from the myocardial lesions showed focal areas of myocyte necrosis with septate fungal hyphae with acute branching suggestive of aspergillus along with neutrophilic infiltrate around it suggestive of

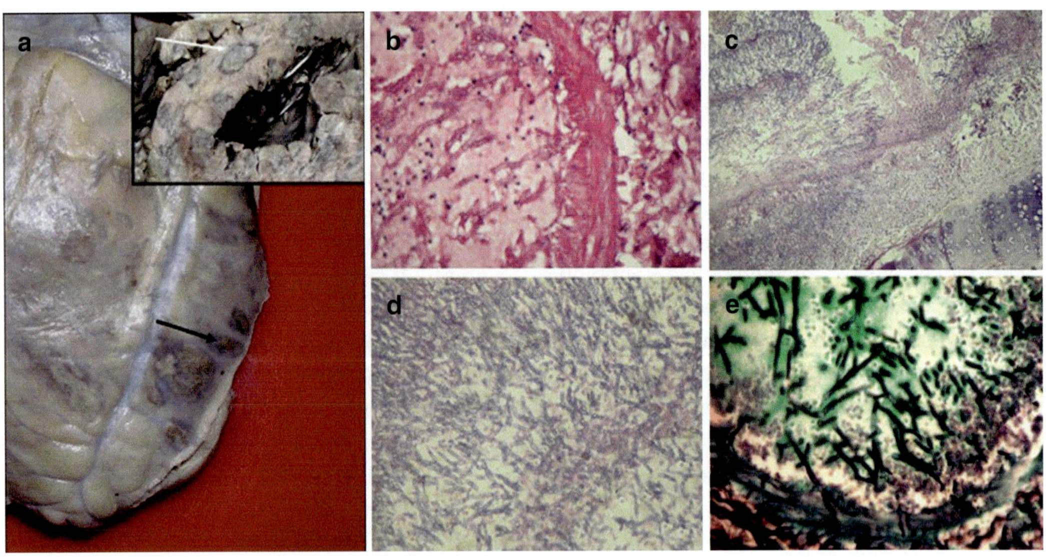

Fig. 11.1 (**a**) Anterior surface of heart shows roughened pericardium showing pale areas with hyperemic borders. (Black arrow) Inset—Myocardium shows similar 1 cm^2 pale areas with hyperemic borders suggestive of multiple myocardial abscesses shown by white arrow. (**b**) Heart showing necrosed tissue with septate dichotomously branching hyphae of aspergillus, 100× H&E. (**c**) Lung showing septate, branching hyphae of aspergillus in peribronchial tissue, 100× H&E. (**d**) Lung showing hyphae of aspergillus, 400× H&E. (**e**) Septate dichotomously branching hyphae of aspergillus seen invading a vessel wall, 400× GMS (Grocott-Gomori's methenamine silver stain)

fungal myocardial abscesses (Fig. 11.1b). Sections from the lung showed microabscesses with aspergillus hyphae (Fig. 11.1c, d). Special stains PAS and GMS were performed which confirmed aspergillosis (Fig. 11.1e). Sections from the pale areas in the renal cortex showed coagulative necrosis with the presence of neutrophils, nuclear debris, and fibrin suggestive of septic infarctions. Fungal filaments were not seen. Sections taken from the hemorrhagic areas in the cerebellum showed the presence of aspergillosis along with parenchymal hemorrhage. Histopathology of the liver showed loss of normal architecture due to submassive hepatic necrosis. There was no evidence of any fungal filaments. There was canalicular and intrahepatocytic cholestasis in preserved areas. A section from the uterus showed changes related to the postpartum state; however no fungal hyphae were seen in the uterus.

11.3 Final Cause of Death

Sepsis with coagulopathy and submassive hepatic necrosis in a postpartum female with HELLP syndrome.

11.4 Clinicopathologic Discussion

HELLP syndrome is a life-threatening, rapidly progressive pregnancy-associated disorder with significant maternal morbidity and mortality. A study conducted by Kongwattanakul K et al. on a total of 11,199 deliveries identified 213 preeclamptic women, of which 16 (1.4 per 1000 deliveries) had HELLP syndrome. [1] It is considered a severe form of preeclampsia by some while others think that it is a disease entity on its own. In the early twentieth century, HELLP was known as "edema-proteinuria-hypertension gestosis type B." It was later renamed by Louis Weinstein in 1982. It is usually seen in pregnant women at 26–40 weeks of gestation but can be seen even in the postpartum state. The disease usually has a rapid onset, and patients present with subtle and nonspecific symptoms like right upper quadrant abdominal or epigastric fluctuating or colicky pain, headache, visual disturbances, and nausea or vomiting. Rimaitis K et al. in their study of 64 patients with HELLP syndrome over a 10-year period suggest that the symptoms do not vary with the severity of HELLP syndrome but should be noted down as they act as "red flags" in the diagnosis of HELLP syndrome [2].

Hemolysis seen in HELLP is due to microangiopathic hemolytic anemia with the presence of schistocytes and burr cells in the peripheral smear. Hemolysis causes a rise in LDH, unconjugated bilirubin, and a fall in hemoglobin levels. Our patient had a low platelet count and low hemoglobin levels at admission; however, she showed direct hyperbilirubinemia due to hepatic parenchymal necrosis. The histology of the liver in HELLP syndrome usually shows characteristic sinusoidal fibrin deposition, periportal changes with hemorrhage, and hepatocyte necrosis. As the disease progresses, more extensive areas of necrosis may lead to hematomas and eventually to hepatic rupture. Elevation of liver transaminases and direct hyperbilirubinemia are seen due to liver injury. Disseminated intravascular coagulation (DIC) can occur in HELLP syndrome, which causes elevation of fibrin degradation products, low fibrinogen levels, and a secondary increase in the prothrombin time. Thrombocytopenia is mandatory for the diagnosis of HELLP syndrome.

There are two classification systems for HELLP syndrome (Table 11.1).

Kaur AP et al. in a study conducted on 71 patients with preeclampsia complicated by

Table 11.1 Classification of HELLP syndrome

HELLP class	Tennessee classification	Mississippi classification
1	Platelets $\leq 100 \times 10^9/L$ AST ≥ 70 IU/L LDH ≥ 600 IU/L	Platelets $\leq 50 \times 10^9/L$ AST or ALT ≥ 70 IU/L LDH ≥ 600 IU/L
2		Platelets $\leq 100 \times 10^9/L$ $\geq 50 \times 10^9/L$ AST or ALT ≥ 70 IU/L LDH ≥ 600 IU/L
3		Platelets $\leq 150 \times 10^9/L$ $\geq 100 \times 10^9/L$ AST or ALT ≥ 40 IU/L LDH ≥ 600 IU/L

HELLP syndrome reported severe maternal complications like postpartum hemorrhage, abruptio placentae, pulmonary edema, renal failure, and DIC and perinatal complications like prematurity, respiratory distress, intrauterine demise, intrauterine growth retardation, NICU admission, and early neonatal death [3]. It can also lead to life-threatening complications in the mother, like wound hematoma and infection, cerebral or brain stem hemorrhage, thrombosis, and infarction.

HELLP syndrome is known to cause generalized immunosuppression and also a profound decrease in monocyte phagocytic and bactericidal activity, thus predisposing the patient to bacterial infection. Our patient had microabscesses in the lungs, myocardium, and a septic infarct in the kidney, causing sepsis. A study conducted on 1199 deliveries had 16 (1.4 per 1000 deliveries) with HELLP syndrome, of which 10 (9.4%) had postpartum hemorrhage, placental abruption was seen in three patients, and neonatal complications were in the form of still birth, low birth weight, birth asphyxia, neonatal intensive care unit admission, and neonatal resuscitation. [1] However, the neonatal outcome largely depends on the gestational age, birth weight, and the available neonatal care facilities. The etiology of HELLP syndrome is unknown. A study by Arthur et al. showed that HELLP syndrome is characterized by both activation of the APC and frequent germline mutations in adenomatous polyposis coli (APC) genes [4]. Management consists of early delivery when HELLP syndrome develops after 34 weeks of pregnancy. If HELLP syndrome develops prior to 34 weeks, then there is controversy regarding follow-up expectant management and the use of cesarean section.

A case published in the literature is of a 31-year-old pregnant woman at 33 weeks of gestation with HELLP syndrome who underwent hysterectomy for postpartum hemorrhage; autopsy showed multiple cerebral and pontine hemorrhages and disseminated aspergillosis in the lungs, trachea, brain, esophagus, stomach, heart, and thyroid gland. [5] In our patient, HELLP syndrome and IUFD both could have acted as independent risk factors for the development of coagulopathy and DIC. She had complications due to HELLP syndrome in the form of overwhelming sepsis and coagulopathy, leading to massive blood loss along with hepatic failure. DIC and microangiopathy contributed to her renal failure and raised serum creatinine levels. Her weakened host immune responses have led to disseminated aspergillosis involving the heart, lungs, and cerebellum. The portal of entry of aspergillus is usually the lung with hematogenous dissemination.

This is a case of complicated HELLP syndrome leading to maternal mortality and adverse perinatal outcome.

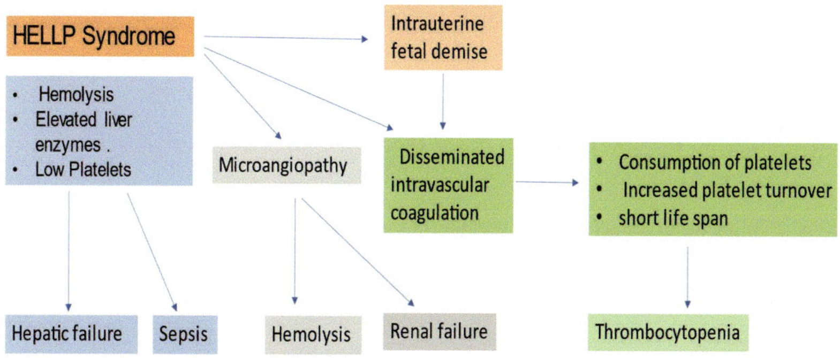

Flowchart: Pathophysiology of HELLP syndrome

References

1. Kongwattanakul K, Saksiriwuttho P, Chaiyarach S, Thepsuthammarat K. Incidence, characteristics, maternal complications, and perinatal outcomes associated with preeclampsia with severe features and HELLP syndrome. Int J Wome's Health. 2018;10:371–7. https://doi.org/10.2147/IJWH.S168569.
2. Rimaitis K, Grauslyte L, Zavackiene A, Baliuliene V, Nadisauskiene R, Macas A. Diagnosis of HELLP syndrome: a 10-year survey in a perinatology centre. Int J Environ Res Public Health. 2019;16(1):109. https://doi.org/10.3390/ijerph16010109.
3. Kaur AP, Kaur N, Dhillon SPS. HELLP syndrome and its implications on maternal and perinatal outcome. Int J Reprod Contracept Obstet Gynecol. 2018;7:1007–11.
4. Vaught AJ, Braunstein EM, Jasem J, Yuan X, Makhlin I, Eloundou S, Baines AC, Merrill SA, Chaturvedi S, Blakemore K, Sperati CJ, Brodsky RA. Germline mutations in the alternative pathway of complement predispose to HELLP syndrome. JCI Insight. 2018;3(6):e99128. https://doi.org/10.1172/jci.insight.99128.
5. Kobayashi M, Ito M, Hotchi M. An autopsy case of HELLP syndrome with disseminated aspergillosis. Nippon Ishinkin Gakkai Zasshi. 2000;41(2):103–7. Japanese. https://doi.org/10.3314/jjmm.41.103.

12 Uterine Anomalies: Less Common but Lethal if Not Detected!

Kusum D. Jashnani, Sushama A. Chandekar, and Reena J. Wani

12.1 Clinical History

A 19-year-old primigravida was brought with complaints of amenorrhea for 5 months, P/V spotting, and abdominal pain for 2 days. The patient was unconscious and gasping on admission. She was referred from a PHC in view of declining vitals with suspicion of abruptio placentae. On examination, pallor +++, abdominal distension present, uterus not felt separately. PV—cervix closed, show+, BP not recordable, pupils dilated. Patient was intubated, given AMBU support with O2, P 140/min with very low volume, and was unconscious with minimal response to DPS.

Hemoglobin reports available showed reduction from 10 to 6.8 g/dl, HIV nonreactive, blood group A+ve. USG revealed an intraabdominal pregnancy with no evidence of gestation in the uterus and moderate ascites. Over the next 55 min, her condition deteriorated; she succumbed in spite of resuscitative measures. A complete autopsy was performed after taking proper consent.

12.2 Autopsy Findings

The deceased was averagely built and nourished with pallor 3+, distended abdomen, and no pedal edema. The abdominal cavity was filled with 1500 cc of blood and 950 g of blood clots. The rudimentary horn with left-sided fallopian tube and ovary with attached placenta was seen ruptured at the lower end with extensive areas of hemorrhage (Fig. 12.1). The umbilical cord with a fetus was seen hanging out into the abdominal cavity from the lower ruptured part of the horn. It was a male fetus of 36 cm in length. This rudimentary horn was lying away from the main uterus and cervix with the right fallopian tube and ovary and did not seem to have any communication with the main uterus. Histology showed thin endometrium with focal decidual change and normal myometrium in the main uterus. The rudimentary horn showed placental tissue in the form of chorionic villi overlying decidualized endometrium, with a mild degree of myometrial hypertrophy (Fig. 12.2). The rest of the organs were very pale, otherwise unremarkable on gross as well as microscopy.

K. D. Jashnani (✉) · S. A. Chandekar
Department of Pathology, Topiwala National Medical College and BYL Nair Charitable Hospital, Mumbai, Maharashtra, India

R. J. Wani
Department of Obstetrics and Gynecology, Hindu Hriday Samrat Balasaheb Thackeray Medical College and Dr R N Cooper Municipal Hospital, Mumbai, Maharashtra, India

K. D. Jashnani (ed.), *Maternal Mortality - Lessons Learnt from Autopsy*,
https://doi.org/10.1007/978-981-19-3420-9_12

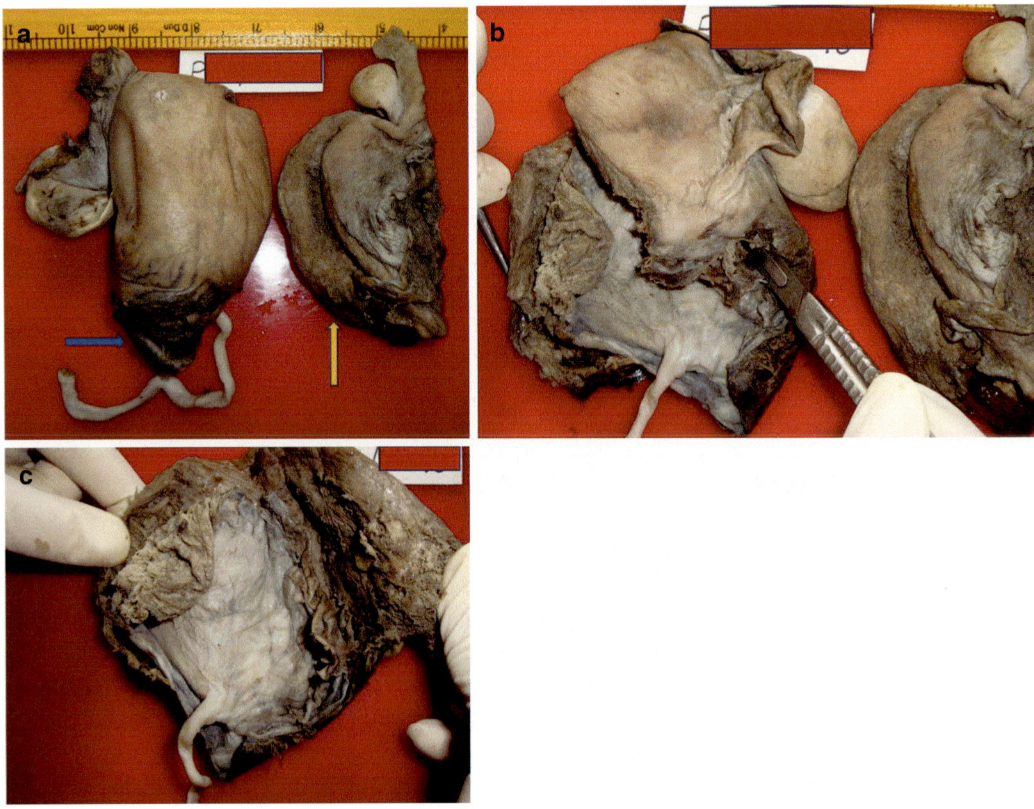

Fig. 12.1 Gross specimens of ruptured rudimentary horn with one-sided fallopian tube and the ovary. Umbilical cord jutting out of the rupture site below (blue arrow pointing to hemorrhagic rupture site) and the main uterus with cervix (orange arrow) with other side adnexa (**a**). (**b**) Internal surface of rudimentary horn showing attached placenta with umbilical cord. (**c**) Close up of the internal surface of the rudimentary horn

12.3 Final Cause of Death

Hemorrhagic shock due to ruptured uterine rudimentary horn pregnancy and hemoperitoneum

12.4 Clinicopathologic Discussion

Uterine rupture means a full-thickness disruption of the uterine wall that involves the overlying visceral peritoneum (uterine serosa) also. By definition, it is associated with the following:

- Clinically significant uterine bleeding
- Fetal distress
- Protrusion or expulsion of the fetus and/or placenta into the abdominal cavity

Uterine scar dehiscence, on the other hand, involves the disruption and separation of a preexisting uterine scar. Uterine scar dehiscence is more common than uterine rupture and does not usually result in major maternal or fetal complications. The vast majority of uterine ruptures occur in women who have uterine scars, usually from previous cesarean deliveries or a previous myomectomy or a single-layer hysterotomy closure. Congenital uterine anomaly, a macrosomic fetus, prostaglandin exposure, uterine instrumentation, and a failed previous trial of a vaginal delivery are other factors. Previous successful vaginal delivery and a prolonged interpregnancy interval after a previous cesarean delivery may act as deterrents. Onset of a prolonged and profound fetal bradycardia is the most consistent early indicator of uterine rupture as opposed to

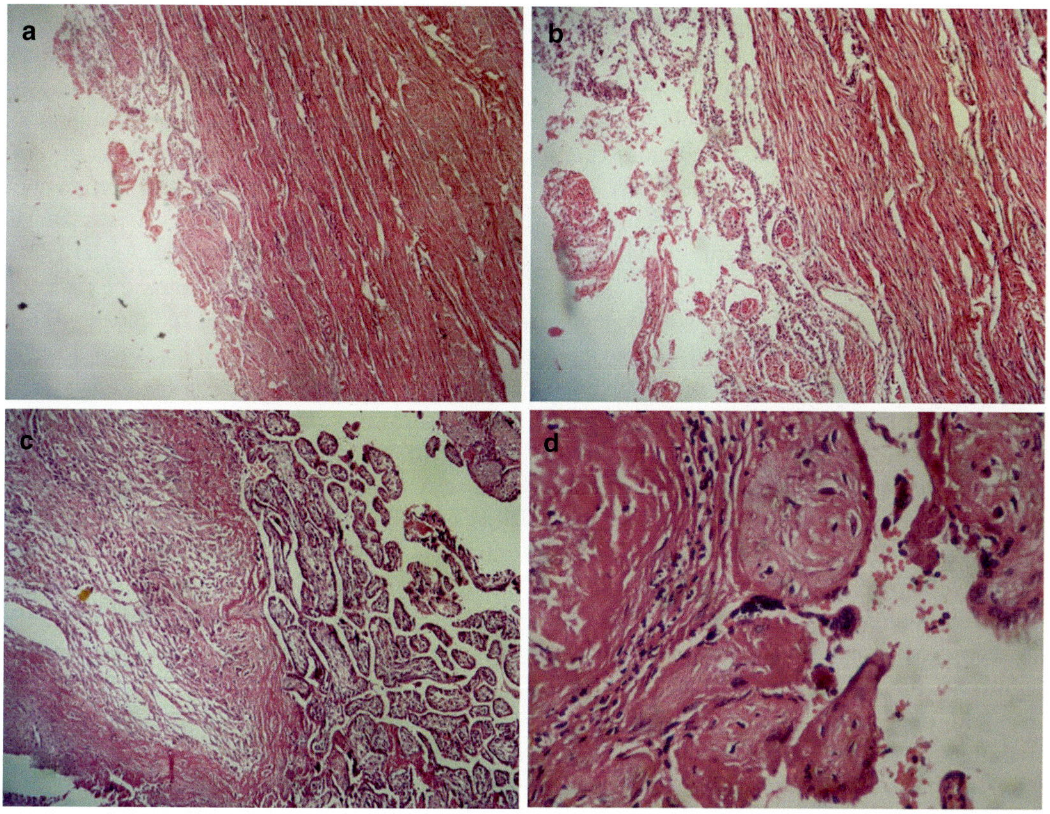

Fig. 12.2 Thin congested endometrium with underlying normal myometrium in the main uterus (**a**, **b**) H&E, 100× and 200×. Decidualized endometrium with overlying placental chorionic villi in rudimentary horn (**c**, **d**) H&E, 200× and 400×

abdominal pain, abnormal progress in labor, and vaginal bleeding. Definitive therapy for the fetus is delivery to avoid major fetal morbidity and mortality [1]. Fetal or placental extrusion through the uterine wall usually leads to irreversible fetal damage.

Conservative surgical management in the form of uterine repair should be reserved for women who are desirous for fertility, with no extension of the tear to the broad ligament, cervix, or paracolpos, easily controllable uterine hemorrhage, no evidence of an evolving DIC. Hysterectomy is the treatment of choice for intractable uterine bleeding or when the uterine rupture sites are multiple, longitudinal, or low lying. Severe maternal blood loss or anemia, hypovolemic shock, and maternal death are the consequences of uterine rupture. Maternal death as a consequence of uterine rupture occurs at a rate of 0–1% in developed nations, but the mortality rates in developing countries are 5–10%. Proper supportive and resuscitation measures may aid in preventing maternal death.

The Mullerian ducts are present in both sexes but regress under the influence of anti-Mullerian hormone (AMH) produced by the testes, which prevents the development of female internal organs in the male embryo. Without the influence of AMH, the ducts develop into the uterus, uterine tubes, cervix, and the upper one-third of the vagina in a female embryo. The development of the Mullerian ducts is regulated by many signaling molecules and gene expression. Disruption of any of these can result in anomalies like agenesis of the uterus, unicornuate uterus, bicornuate uterus, didelphys uterus, septate uterus, and arcuate uterus. The unicornuate uterus is due to the arrest of the development of one of the Mullerian ducts. There are four subtypes of the unicornuate uterus: absent rudimentary horn, non-cavitary rudimentary horn, cavitary communicating horn, and cavitary noncommunicating rudimentary horn. Mullerian abnormalities are present in 0.17% of fertile women and 3.5% of infertile women, and a unicornuate uterus is observed in 0.4% of women. Approximately 84% of unicornuate uteruses have a contralateral rudimentary horn. An embryo can implant in a uterus with a rudimentary horn or in a unicornuate uterus. Although these conditions are similar, their reproductive outcomes are completely different. Diagnosis of a rudimentary horn requires hysterosalpingography, hysteroscopy, and laparoscopy. MRI and 3-D ultrasound are the mainstays of diagnosis of Mullerian anomalies, with poor sensitivity (26%), compared to traditional ultrasound. The experience, skill, and awareness of uterine malformations of the radiologist are other important factors in this diagnosis.

Rudimentary horn pregnancy (RHP), being rare, with an incidence of one in 76,000 to one in 160,000, [2] results in the rupture of the horn by the second trimester in 80–90% of all cases, leading to emergency surgery, blood transfusions, and increased morbidity. Early diagnosis before rupture can lead to successful management and prevention of maternal morbidity and mortality. Clinical symptoms like pain in the abdomen with signs of rupture, peritonitis, and free fluid during their second trimester should be seriously considered, particularly in patients with a known diagnosis of a unicornuate uterus [3]. Laparoscopic removal of an accessory uterine horn (in the non-pregnant state) was first reported by Nezhat et al. in 1994, followed by several case reports subsequently. Three valid reasons justify this surgical excision: removal of the cause of dysmenorrhea, the prevention of possible endometriosis caused by transtubal menstrual reflux, and avoiding an intracornual pregnancy implantation. As the risk of rupture of a pregnant rudimentary uterine horn in the second trimester is very high, its excision is recommended as soon as possible. An RHP can cause heavy bleeding and threaten the patient's life. Excision of the ruptured rudimentary horn and ipsilateral salpingectomy has been done in some of these cases with an uneventful postoperative recovery of the patients [4].

The present case was a young primigravida whose ANC details were not available and who was brought to our institute in an unconscious gasping state and died within 55 min of admission. Timely USG revealed an intraabdominal fetus, confirming uterine rupture. However, RHP with rupture was the diagnosis on autopsy. This condition of uterine anomaly may not be detected till a young woman has difficulty getting pregnant or suffers from complications during pregnancy. Hence a high index of clinical suspicion is the key to preventing maternal mortality.

References

1. Togioka BM, Tonismae T. Uterine rupture. [Updated 2021 Jul 1]. In: StatPearls [Internet]. Treasure Island, FL: StatPearls Publishing; 2021.
2. Ghotra MK, Joshi B, Bhutani S. Ruptured rudimentary horn pregnancy: delayed diagnosis. Case Rep Cureus. 2021;13(6):e15873. https://doi.org/10.7759/cureus.15873.
3. Li X, Peng P, Liu X, Chen W, et al. The pregnancy outcomes of patients with rudimentary uterine horn: a 30-year experience. PLoS One. 2019;14(1):e0210788. https://doi.org/10.1371/journal.pone.0210788.
4. Rajbhandary S, Das A, Rai M, Sah AK. Rupture of non-communicating rudimentary horn pregnancy at 15 weeks with previous normal pregnancies: a case report. Case Rep JNMA J Nepal Med Assoc. 2020;58(228):614–7. https://doi.org/10.31729/jnma.5104.

13 Retained Products of Conception and Dilatation and Curettage: A Cause for Disseminated Intravascular Coagulation

Kusum D. Jashnani, Sushama A. Chandekar, and Rakesh R. Bhadade

13.1 Clinical History

A 19-year-old female, primigravida with 5 months of gestation, had been admitted to a private hospital with bleeding per vagina and pain in the abdomen for 10 to 12 days, where she was found to have retained products of conception and hence D & C was done. The histopathology report for this was not available to us. She had been given antibiotics and antimalarials and was transfused with one unit each of whole blood and platelets. History provided by her relatives was her having taken treatment first from some local doctor for bleeding per vagina 12 days back. After taking those tablets, she had passed three big clots per vagina. She was referred to our tertiary care hospital as a case of retained products of conception with disseminated intravascular coagulation with bleeding per vagina and hematuria. On admission, clinical examination revealed poor general condition. She was drowsy, afebrile, and very pale with blood pressure and pulse of 100/60 mm Hg and 100/min, respectively. Respiratory examination showed bilateral basal crepitations. Per abdomen was soft. Per vaginal examination showed a closed cervix with no active bleeding. Local examination revealed lower limb petechiae, subconjunctival hemorrhages, and ecchymotic patches over the trunk, upper limb, and lower limb. Later she developed one episode of generalized tonic convulsion; she became unconscious, not responding to deep painful stimuli. The patient was put on mechanical ventilation. She was transfused with four units each of platelets and fresh frozen plasma and two units of packed red cells.

Investigations: Ultrasonography revealed a bulky uterus with 3.4 × 1.4 cm echogenic material in the endometrial cavity. Hematological investigations showed a WBC of 15,400/cumm, falling hemoglobin of 6.6 gm/dl, and a platelet count of 26,000/cumm. Coagulation studies showed an activated partial thromboplastin time of 36 s (control was 25 s), while prothrombin time, bleeding time, and clotting time were within normal limits. FDP and D dimer reports were not available. Biochemical investigations showed blood urea nitrogen of 12 mg/dl, serum creatinine of 0.6 mg/dl, random blood sugar of 132 mg/dl, total protein 5.6 g%, total bilirubin of 1 mg%, and alkaline phosphatase 43 U/L. Peripheral blood smear was negative for the malarial parasite.

K. D. Jashnani (✉) · S. A. Chandekar
Department of Pathology, Topiwala National Medical College and BYL Nair Charitable Hospital, Mumbai, Maharashtra, India

R. R. Bhadade
Department of Medicine (Critical Care Unit), Topiwala National Medical College and BYL Nair Charitable Hospital, Mumbai, Maharashtra, India

K. D. Jashnani (ed.), *Maternal Mortality - Lessons Learnt from Autopsy*, https://doi.org/10.1007/978-981-19-3420-9_13

The clinical condition of the patient kept deteriorating, and the patient was declared dead within 24 h of admission. A complete autopsy was performed after due consent.

13.2 Autopsy Findings

She was averagely built and nourished, pale, with petechial hemorrhages present all over her body. Ecchymotic patches were also present over trunk, upper limb, and lower limb. Eyes showed periorbital oedema and subconjunctival hemorrhages. Frothy hemorrhagic fluid was seen oozing out of the mouth and nostrils. A tongue bite was seen. On opening of the abdomen, blood clots weighing 20 g were seen in the uterovesical and Douglas pouch. The meninges were congested with subarachnoid hemorrhages seen in the peri-pontine and superior cerebellar surface. The occipital lobe of the cerebrum showed few foci of intracerebral hemorrhages. Both the lungs were firm and hemorrhagic with oozing of blood-tinged frothy fluid and showed intra-alveolar hemorrhages (Fig. 13.1a, b) along with hyaline membrane formation on histology. The trachea, epicardium and myocardium of the heart, entire gastrointestinal tract, and pelvicalyceal system of both kidneys showed petechial hemorrhages (Figs. 13.1c, d and 13.2a, b). Kidneys also showed fibrin thrombi within glomerular capillaries, which were confirmed by special stain phosphotungstic acid hematoxylin (Fig. 13.2c, d). The stomach and small intestine also showed mucosal and serosal hemorrhages (Fig. 13.3a–d). The uterus was 10 × 6 × 4.5 cm in size; the endometrial cavity showed three small blood clots, confirmed on microscopy with no evidence of RPOCs. The cervix showed serosal hemorrhages.

13.3 Final Cause of Death

Multiorgan failure due to disseminated intravascular coagulation and acute respiratory distress syndrome in a postabortal case.

13.4 Clinicopathologic Correlation

Retained products of conception (RPOC-placental or fetal tissue) can happen after abortion (terminated pregnancy), cesarean birth, miscarriage, and vaginal delivery. RPOC are reported in 17% of first trimester miscarriages and 40% of second trimester miscarriages, compared to less than 3% of full-term deliveries. It is responsible for postpartum hemorrhage and infection and is a stimulating factor for DIC. Uterine bleeding, foul-smelling discharge, pelvic pain, fever, and/or uterine tenderness are some of the clinical manifestations of RPOC. These clinical findings are nonspecific, as some degree of postabortal bleeding and discomfort are common [1]. Dilation and curettage, the treatment of choice for RPOC, can have complications of uterine perforation, infection, adhesions, infertility, so also DIC.

DIC is not a specific illness; rather, it is a complication of other illnesses which include conditions like sepsis and severe infection (including COVID-19), trauma, malignancy (solid and lymphoproliferative/myeloproliferative malignancies), severe transfusion reactions, and varied obstetric complications. Bleeding from at least three unrelated sites is particularly suggestive of DIC. Acute and chronic are the two forms of DIC. Acute DIC results from sudden exposure of blood to procoagulants (e.g., tissue factor (TF) or tissue thromboplastin), leading to intravascular coagulation with generation and deposition of fibrin in the microvasculature of various organs. This is followed by severe consumptive coagulopathy, leading to bleeding from different sites. Chronic DIC is a compensated state that develops when blood is continuously or intermittently exposed to small amounts of TF. There is less obvious clinical or laboratory indication of the presence of DIC, frequently seen in patients with solid tumors.

(1) Thrombocytopenia, (2) prolongation of prothrombin time and activated partial thromboplastin time, (3) low fibrinogen concentration, and (4) increased levels of fibrin degradation

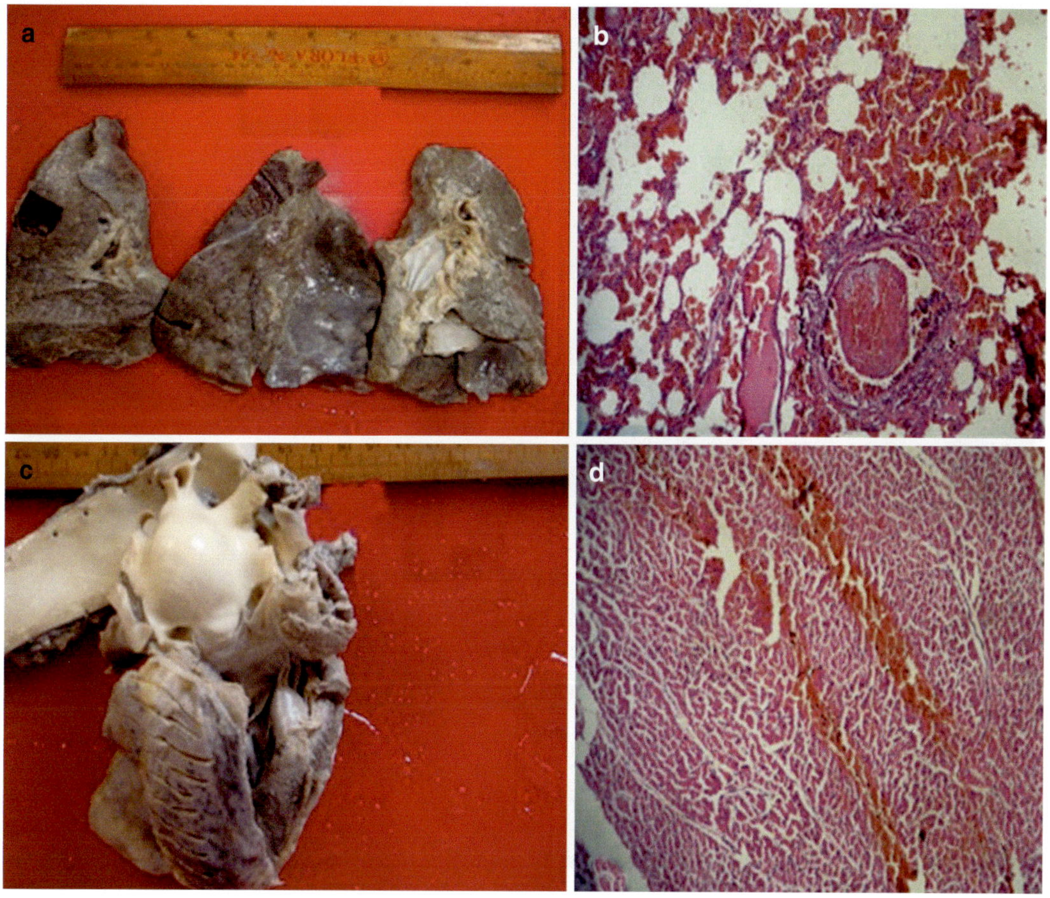

Fig. 13.1 (**a**) Gross photograph of lung showing firm areas of hemorrhage. (**b**) Microphotograph of lung showing intra-alveolar hemorrhages (H&E, 100×). (**c**) Gross photograph of heart with petechial hemorrhages over epicardium and on cut surface. (**d**) Microphotograph of heart showing areas of hemorrhages within the myocardial fibers (H&E, 100×)

products and D-dimer are some of the diagnostic investigations of DIC.

The massive fibrin deposition in DIC suggests that fibrinogen levels should be decreased as seen above in point (3). Fibrinogen, as a positive acute-phase reactant, is increased in inflammation, and one study has demonstrated that in up to 57% of DIC patients, the levels of fibrinogen may be within normal limits. Fibrinolysis being an important component of DIC, elevated levels of D-dimer and FDPs are an evidence of fibrin breakdown. Testing for D-dimer (the better test for DIC) or FDPs is helpful in differentiating DIC from other conditions associated with a low platelet count and prolonged clotting times, such as chronic liver disease [2].

DIC usually results from one of these two pathways:

1. A systemic inflammatory response, causing the activation of the cytokine network with subsequent coagulation activation (e.g., in sepsis or major trauma)
2. Exposure to procoagulant material (e.g., in cancer, crush brain injury, or obstetric cases)

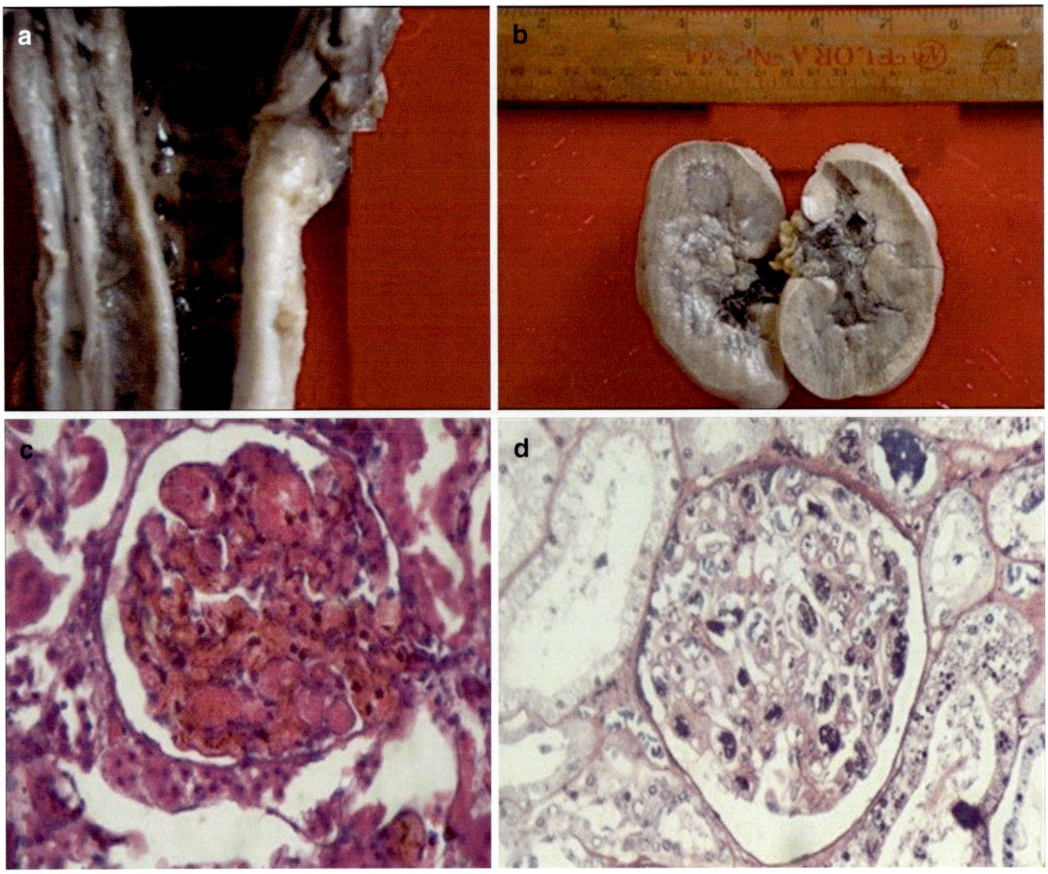

Fig. 13.2 (**a**) Gross photograph of trachea with mucosal surface showing petechial hemorrhages. (**b**) Gross photograph of kidney with hemorrhages in the pelvicalyceal system. (**c**) Microphotograph of kidney showing fibrin thrombi within glomerular capillaries (H&E, 400×). (**d**) Microphotograph of kidney with PTAH staining showing blue staining for fibrin thrombi (PTAH, 400×)

> Amniotic fluid embolism, abruptio placentae, acute peripartum hemorrhage, preeclampsia/eclampsia/HELLP syndrome, retained products of conception (also a cause for chronic DIC), septic abortion, and acute fatty liver of pregnancy are obstetric causes of acute (hemorrhagic) DIC [3].

Acute DIC often manifests as petechiae and ecchymosis, along with blood loss from intravenous lines. In postoperative DIC, bleeding can occur in the vicinity of surgical sites, drains, and tracheostomies, as well as within serous cavities. Histologic studies in patients with DIC show the presence of ischemia due to fibrin deposition in small vessels of various organs. Multiple organ dysfunction syndrome (MODS), shock, and death are the varied complications of DIC.

Thrombotic thrombocytopenic purpura (TTP)—hemolytic uremic syndrome (HUS) is a thrombotic microangiopathy like DIC, but distinctly different; results of blood coagulation assays in TTP-HUS are normal. Thrombocytopenia is a common feature of DIC and immune thrombocytopenic purpura (ITP); however, coagulation activation or microangiopathic hemolytic anemia is not seen in ITP [4].

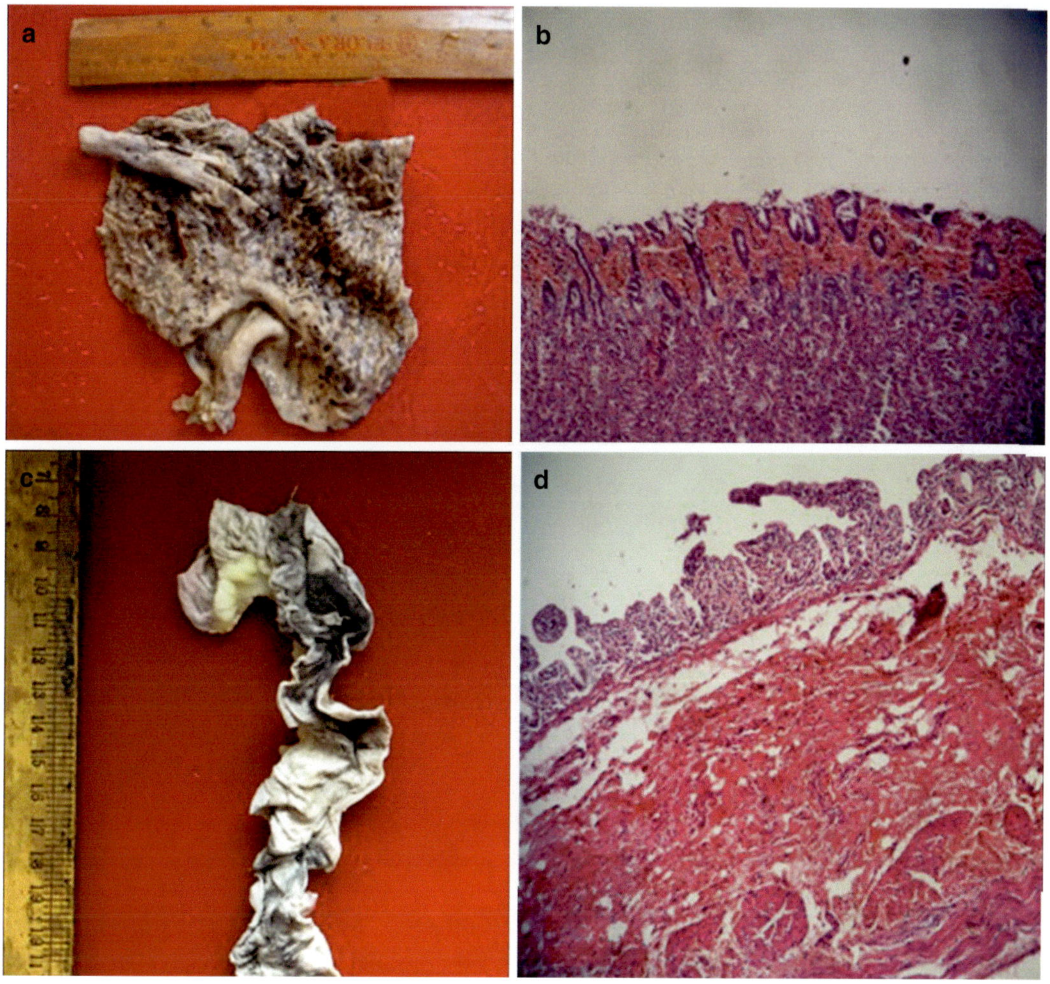

Fig. 13.3 (**a**) Gross photograph of stomach with mucosa showing multiple petechial hemorrhages. (**b**) Microphotograph of stomach showing mucosal hemorrhages (H&E, 100×). (**c**) Gross photograph of small intestine with mucosal hemorrhages. (**d**) Microphotograph of small intestine showing submucosal hemorrhages (H&E, 100×)

Patients with DIC should be treated at hospitals with appropriate critical care and available facilities of hematology, blood bank, or surgery [5]. Patients who present to hospitals without these resources should be transferred to a tertiary care hospital immediately if possible. Treatment primarily focusses on treating the underlying disorder. If infection is the causative etiology, the appropriate antibiotics are given with efforts taken for source control. In the case of an obstetric catastrophe, the primary approach is to provide appropriate obstetric care, in which case the DIC usually subsides. If the underlying cause of DIC is not known, a diagnostic workup can be initiated. Heparin is very occasionally used to treat the thrombosis that occurs with DIC. Platelet transfusion is to be considered in patients with DIC and severe thrombocytopenia, in particular, in patients with bleeding or in patients at risk for bleeding. Fresh frozen plasma (FFP) may be administered in an attempt to replenish coagulation factors and antithrombotic factors in patients with abnormal coagulation studies [5]. It should be remembered that DIC is a common complication of many obstetric events, so one should be alert to its occurrence.

References

1. Erez O, Mastrolia SA, Thachil J. Disseminated intravascular coagulation in pregnancy: insights in pathophysiology, diagnosis and management. Am J Obstet Gynecol. 2015;213(4):452–63. https://doi.org/10.1016/j.ajog.2015.03.054.
2. Sahin S, Eroglu M, Tetik S, Guzin K. Disseminated intravascular coagulation in obstetrics: etiopathogenesis and up to date management strategies. J Turk Soc Obstet Gynecol. 2014;11(1):42–51.
3. Adkins K, Minardi J, Setzer E, Williams D. Retained products of conception: an atypical presentation diagnosed immediately with bedside emergency ultrasound. Case Rep Emerg Med. 2016;2016:9124967. https://doi.org/10.1155/2016/9124967.
4. Kerns JL, Ti A, Aksel S, Lederle L, Sokoloff A, Steinauer J. Disseminated intravascular coagulation and hemorrhage after dilation and evacuation abortion for fetal death. Obstet Gynecol. 2019;134(4):708–13. https://doi.org/10.1097/AOG.0000000000003460.
5. Guha P. Disseminated intravascular coagulopathy following induced second trimester curettage abortion. ISRN Obstet Gynecol. 2011;2011:591760. https://doi.org/10.5402/2011/591760.

Part II

Indirect Maternal Deaths

14 Pulmonary Bone Marrow Embolism: The Uncommon but Fatal Complication of Sickle Cell Disease

Niyati N. Sangoi, Kusum D. Jashnani,
Lalita Yoganand Patil,
and Vandana Rajesh Saravade

14.1 Clinical History

A 28-year-old female, G3P1A1, was admitted from ANC OPD in view of raised blood pressure. On examination, there was no pain in abdomen/decreased or absent fetal movements/headache/nausea/vomiting or blurring of vision. Emergency LSCS was done in view of severe oligohydramnios (AFI-2.4) with premature rupture of membrane on the seventh day of admission, at 36.5 weeks. The baby delivered was alive and healthy.

Past history revealed that the patient was diagnosed with sickle cell anemia 3 years back, during her first pregnancy. She was hospitalized in view of fever at 5 months of gestation and subsequently suffered a pregnancy loss. During her second pregnancy, the patient had a history of nine units of packed cell transfusions in view of severe anemia. The patient had history of repeated episodes of hemoptysis every year for which she did not take any treatment. There was a history of blood transfusion when the patient was 10 years old, details of which were not available. The patient was transfused three units of packed cells during the current pregnancy and treated symptomatically. She was also diagnosed with hypothyroidism during the current pregnancy.

N. N. Sangoi · K. D. Jashnani (✉) · L. Y. Patil
Department of Pathology, Topiwala National Medical College and BYL Nair Charitable Hospital, Mumbai, Maharashtra, India

V. R. Saravade
Department of Obstetrics and Gynecology, Topiwala National Medical College and BYL Nair Charitable Hospital, Mumbai, Maharashtra, India

14.2 Investigations

Hemogram: Hb 9.2 g%, TLC 14,700/μL with polymorphonuclear leucocytosis, platelet count 269,000/μL. On peripheral smear examination, RBCs were predominantly microcytic, hypochromic with a number of target cells and occasional polychromatophils and sickle cells. There were 14 nucleated RBCs/100 WBCs. No parasite was seen. Retic count was 5.2%. Iron profile: serum ferritin 609.30 ng/ml, TIBC 502 μg/dl, serum iron 131 μg/dl, transferrin saturation 26.1%. Prothrombin time 12.5 s and prothrombin index 0.88. Her arterial blood gas analysis was suggestive of respiratory alkalosis. Her direct Coomb's test was negative, but her indirect Coomb's test was positive. Serum electrophoresis was not carried out during her entire hospital stay.

Biochemical profile: BUN 09 mg%, serum creatinine 0.5 mg%, random blood glucose 125 mg%, Na+ 140 mEq/L, K+ 5.4 mEq/L, total protein 6.4 g/dl, serum albumin 3.1 g/dl, SGOT 81 units/L, SGPT 24 units/L, total bilirubin 2.3 mg/dl, and direct bilirubin 0.4mg/dl.

On postoperative day 4 of LSCS, the patient developed breathlessness and severe joint pain at

K. D. Jashnani (ed.), *Maternal Mortality - Lessons Learnt from Autopsy*,
https://doi.org/10.1007/978-981-19-3420-9_14

multiple locations. The breathlessness progressed to NYHA grade III. It was not associated with trauma. In view of her deteriorating condition, she was transferred to the medical intensive care unit. On examination, the patient was afebrile. Her pulse rate was 101/min, blood pressure was 140/90 mmHg, and respiratory rate was 32/min. Within 24 h, her general condition deteriorated even further. The patient was put on ventilator support, but despite all resuscitative measures, she could not be revived and was declared dead. The total hospital stay was 12 days. A complete autopsy was performed on this patient, after due permission.

14.3 Autopsy Findings

The right lung weighed 250 g, and the left lung weighed 239 g. The pleura was thickened. On cut surface, the lungs were subcrepitant to rubbery in consistency. Multiple thrombi were seen occluding the pulmonary vessels (Fig. 14.1a). On micros-

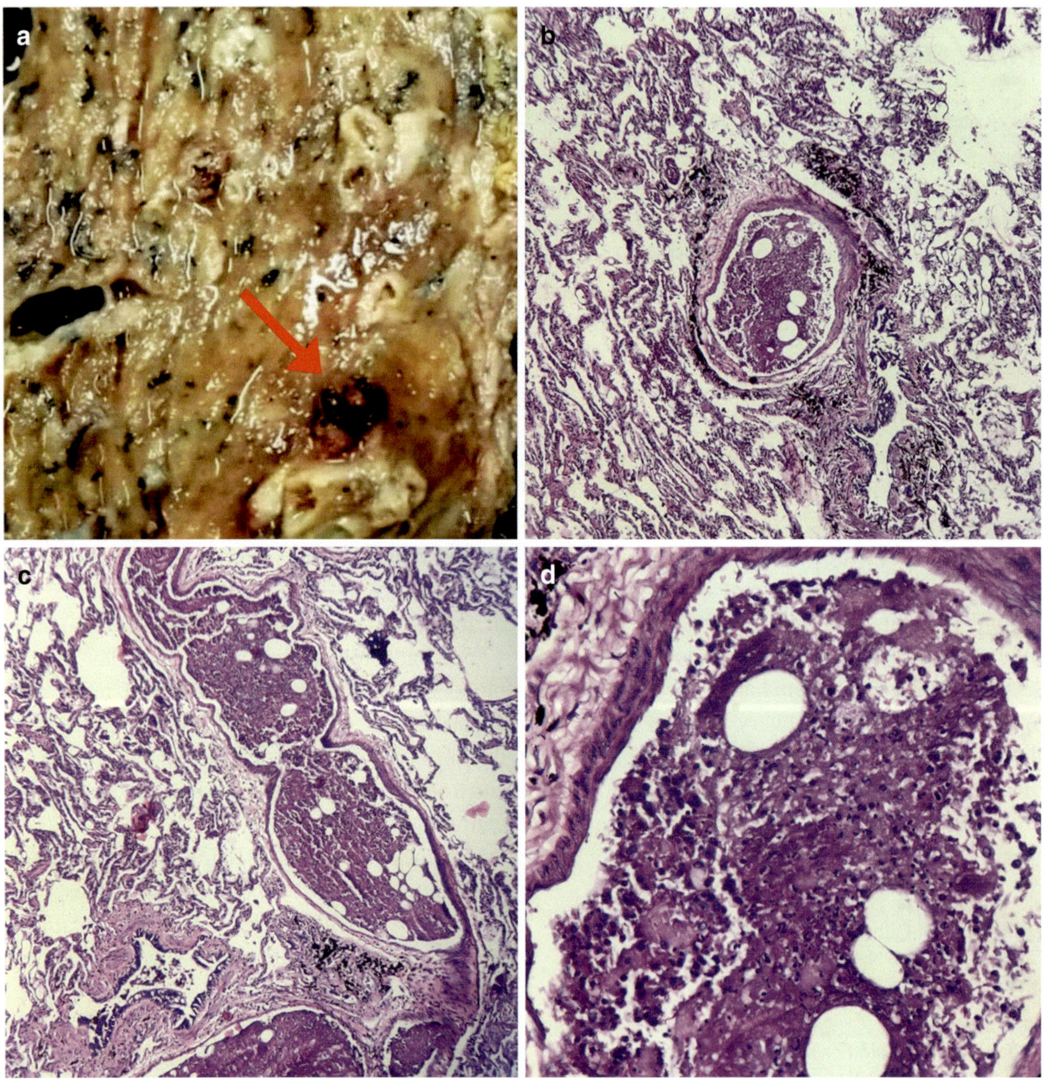

Fig. 14.1 (**a**) Gross picture of the lung with pulmonary vessel showing the presence of embolus (red arrow). (**b**, **c**) Microscopy (100×, H&E stain) of the lung showing the presence of bone marrow emboli in the pulmonary vasculature. (**d**) Microscopy (400×, H&E stain) of the bone marrow embolus showing fat spaces, few hematopoietic cells, and large areas of necrotic bone marrow

copy, the lung parenchyma showed multiple areas of fibrosis. The interstitium was widened and showed the presence of lymphocytes, macrophages, few plasma cells, and few neutrophils. There were few patchy areas of intra-alveolar macrophages with the rest of the alveolar spaces being empty. Small and medium-sized arteries showed the presence of bone marrow emboli, suggestive of pulmonary bone marrow embolism (Fig. 14.1b–d). These emboli showed focal areas of necrosis. Bronchioles were unremarkable. The spleen weighed 200 g with a thick capsule. The cut surface of the spleen was firm with multiple fibrotic bands, giving it a lobular appearance (Fig. 14.2a). On microscopy, the spleen showed thick fibrous bands forming multiple small and large lobular areas (Fig. 14.2b). The sinuses in these lobules showed the presence of sickled

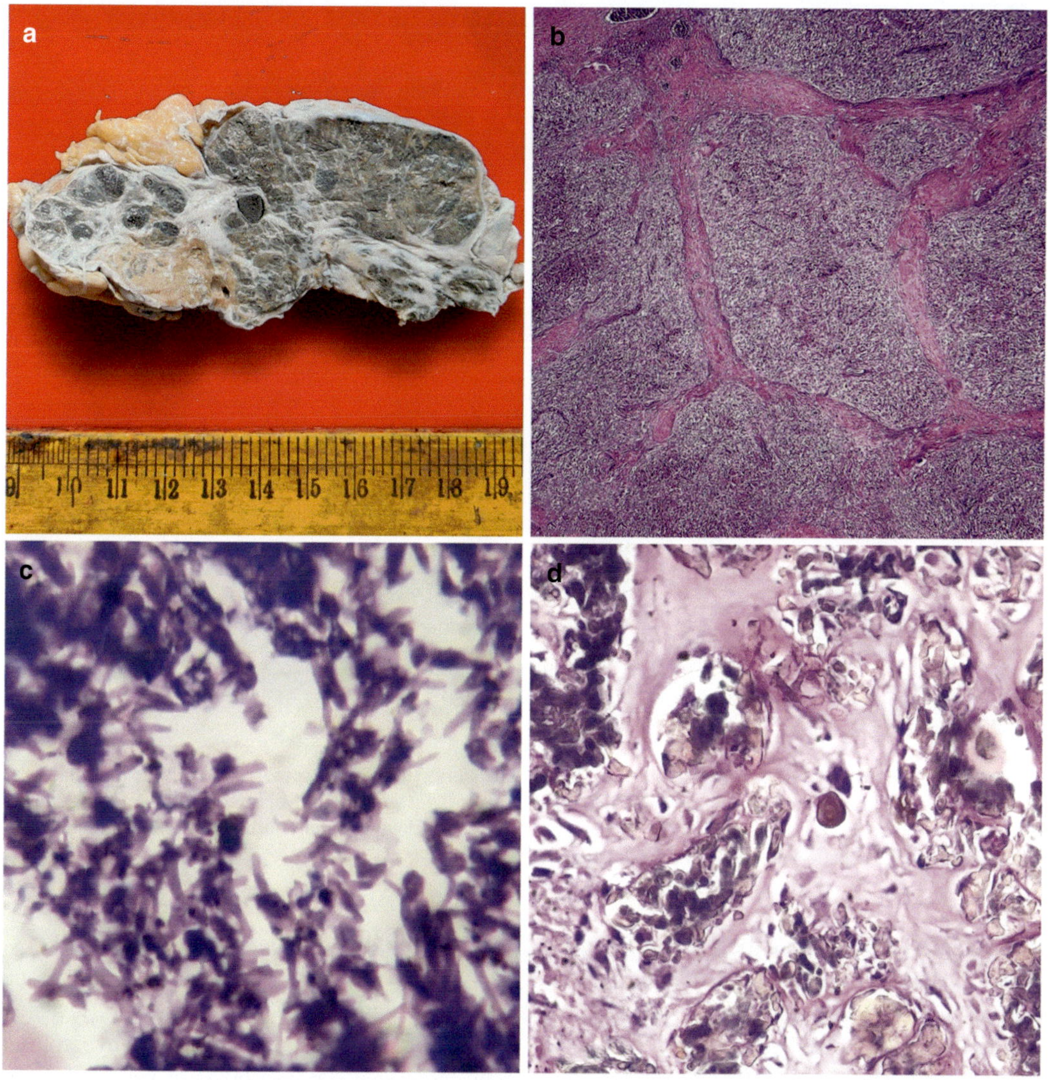

Fig. 14.2 (**a**) Coronal slice of the spleen showing the presence of multiple fibrotic bands dividing the spleen into multiple lobules. (**b**) Microscopy (100×, H&E stain) showing the lobular appearance of the spleen due to multiple fibrotic bands. The sinusoids are packed with sickled RBCs. (**c**) Microscopy (1000×, H&E stain) showing the presence of sickled RBCs in the sinusoids of the spleen. (**d**) Microscopy (400×, H&E stain) of the spleen showing the presence of Gamna-Gandy bodies

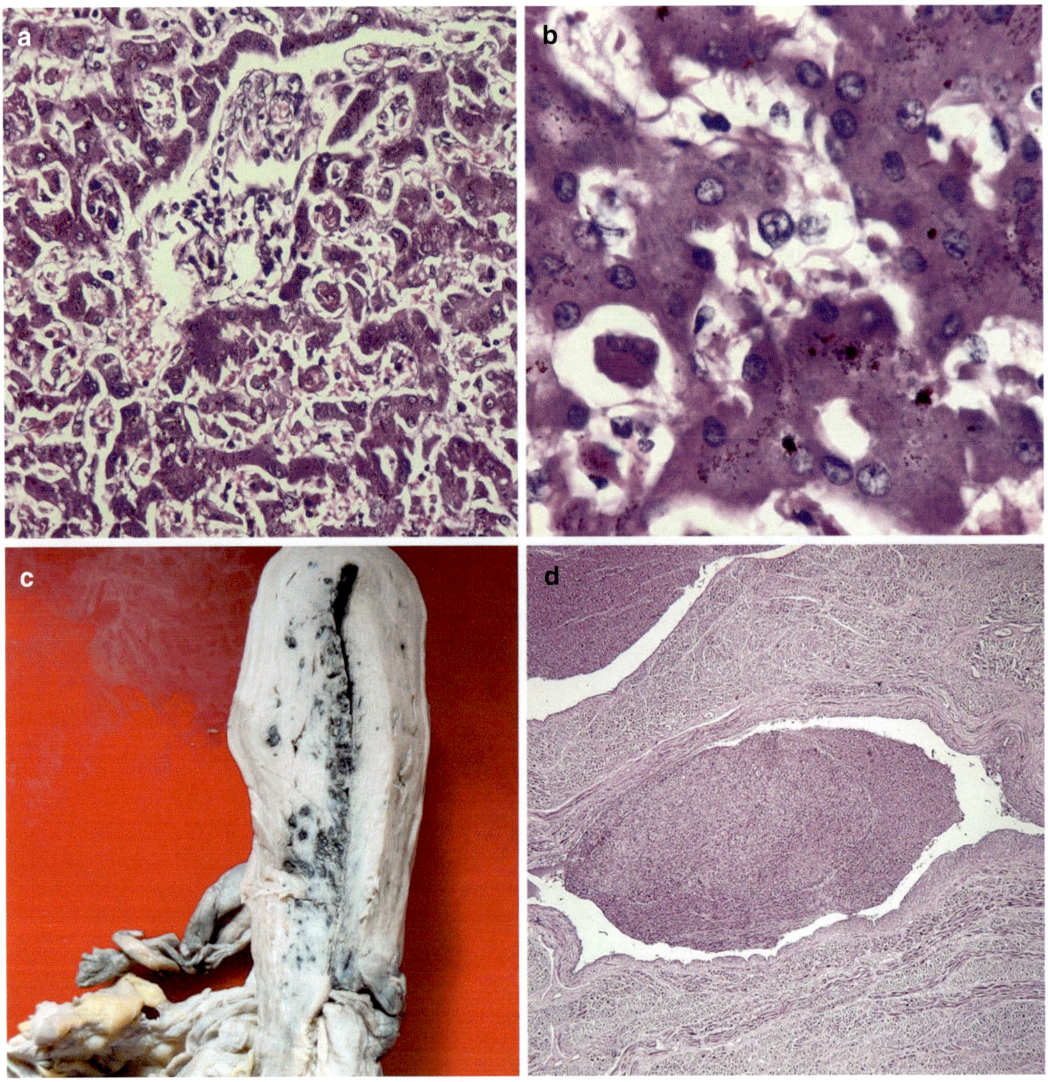

Fig. 14.3 (**a**) Microscopy (100×, H&E stain) of the liver showing hepatic sinusoids packed with sickled RBCs. (**b**) Microscopy (1000×, H&E stain) showing the presence of sickled RBCs in the hepatic sinusoids. (**c**) Gross picture of the uterus showing the presence of multiple thrombi in the myometrial vessels. (**d**) Microscopy (400×, H&E stain) of the uterus demonstrating fibrin thrombi in the myometrial vessels

RBCs (Fig. 14.2c). Multiple focal areas of Gamna-Gandy bodies with calcification and hemosiderin deposits were also seen (Fig. 14.2d). There was no evidence of infarct. The liver weighed 2.6 kg and was enlarged. The capsule and cut surface were unremarkable on gross examination. On microscopy, the normal hepatic lobular architecture was maintained. The sinusoids showed the presence of sickled RBCs (Fig. 14.3a, b). The kidney, adrenals, and thyroid appeared unremarkable on gross examination, but on microscopy, their blood vessels showed the presence of sickled RBCs. Bone marrow examination on microscopy revealed hypercellular marrow due to erythroid hyperplasia with large areas (almost 60%) of necrosis of the marrow cells. However, there was no evidence of any abnormal cells or epithelioid cells in the marrow. The myometrial vessels showed thrombi both grossly (Fig. 14.3c) as well as microscopically. These were fibrin thrombi and not bone marrow emboli (Fig. 14.3d). Examination of the heart showed mild dilatation of all four chambers with mild hypertrophy of the left ventricle. Microscopy was unremarkable. Examination of the rest of the organs was unremarkable on gross and microscopy.

14.4 Final Cause of Death

Pulmonary bone marrow embolism with respiratory failure in a postpartum female with sickle cell disease.

14.5 Clinicopathologic Discussion

Sickle cell disease is a hereditary hemoglobinopathy which occurs due to a missense mutation in the beta-globin gene. This leads to the replacement of glutamic acid by hydrophobic valine residue. It causes hemolytic anemia, which is associated with hyperbilirubinemia, increased reticulocytes, and the presence of sickled cells. The patient in discussion had increased bilirubin and reticulocyte count with the peripheral blood showing occasional sickled RBCs. The clinical manifestations of sickle cell disease are variable in terms of severity. Some individuals have mild symptoms, some have repeated vaso-occlusive crises, but in some individuals, symptoms are triggered in hypoxic states. The HbS molecules undergo polymerization when deoxygenated, leading to clinical manifestations and complications of sickle cell disease [1].

One of the commonest causes of patient morbidity and mortality in sickle cell disease is "vaso-occlusive crisis." They are also known as "pain crisis," are nearly the pathognomonic symptoms of the SCDs, and are precipitated by infection, operation, stress, or injuries. They occur due to hypoxic injury and subsequent infarction causing severe pain. A particularly dangerous type of vaso-occlusive crisis is the "acute chest syndrome." It involves the lungs and presents with chest pain, fever, cough, and pulmonary infiltrates. Pulmonary bone marrow embolism has been recognized as a significant cause of death in patients with acute chest syndrome and sickle cell disease [2]. The pathogenesis of pulmonary bone marrow embolism is not very clear. Bone marrow infarction is commonly seen in patients with sickle cell disease, and the emboli are thought to arise from the necrosis of bone marrow. This infarcted/necrotic marrow enters the venous vessels within the bone and further enters the venous circulation. The anatomical structure of the cancellous bone containing the red marrow makes this movement possible. These bone marrow emboli have usually been observed in medium and small-sized pulmonary vessels. They are constituted by marrow fat cells, megakaryocytes, and erythroid and myeloid precursors [3]. Fat embolism syndrome (FES) is another fatal complication of sickle cell anemia characterized by the release of fat globules into the circulation, leading to respiratory and neurologic damage. FES is also most often associated with long bone fractures. It is important to be able to distinguish bone marrow embolism from fat embolism. The former, as already stated, is seen mainly in the small and medium-sized branches of the pulmonary circulation, while the latter is seen within the pulmonary microvasculature [4].

In the case being discussed, the patient presented with severe breathlessness and multiple joint pains which worsened within 24 h. Autopsy findings revealed the presence of pulmonary bone marrow embolism with the presence of sickle cells in multiple organs including the spleen, kidneys, liver, thyroid, and adrenals. Initially during childhood, the spleen is enlarged due to congestion of red pulp by sickled red cells trapped in the sinuses. This phenomenon of painful enlargement is known as splenic sequestration crisis. However, with time, the spleen undergoes fibrosis, infarction, and progressive shrinkage due to chronic erythrostasis [1], aided by low pH and low oxygen tension in the sinusoids and splenic cords. This can be seen in the gross as well as microscopic examination of our case. This is autosplenectomy wherein a nonfunctional spleen is a major contributor to the immune deficiency that exists in these individuals. Failure of opsonization and an inability to deal with infective encapsulated microorganisms, particularly

Streptococcus pneumoniae, ensue, leading to an increased risk of sepsis in the future, which may be fatal.

In conclusion, women with sickle cell anemia are at a greater risk for complications including mortality, during pregnancy [5]. A more aggressive monitoring and follow-up of such patients is of utmost importance. A careful monitoring and good, supportive care can lead to successful pregnancy outcomes. These women should be counseled on the use of contraception in case pregnancy is not desired as well as the risks and potential outcomes for themselves as well as their children, in case they get pregnant. There is no specific treatment suggested yet, but just careful and aggressive monitoring and follow-up for pregnant women with sickle cell disease.

References

1. Kumar V, Abbas K, Aster J. Robbins and cotran pathologic basis of disease. 10th ed. London: Elsevier; 2020. p. 641–4.
2. Dang NC, et al. Bone marrow embolism in sickle cell disease: a review. Am J Hematol. 2005;79:61–7.
3. Selvi S, et al. A fatal case of bone marrow embolism of unknown cause masquerading clinically as dengue shock syndrome. Indian J Pathol Microbiol. 2012;55:572–3.
4. Targueta EP, Hirano ACG, Campos FPF, Martines JAS, Lovisolo SM, Felipe-Silva A. Bone marrow necrosis and fat embolism syndrome: a dreadful complication of hemoglobin sickle cell disease. Autops Case Rep. 2017;7(4):42–50. https://doi.org/10.4322/acr.2017.043.
5. Rizk S, et al. Perinatal maternal mortality in sickle cell anemia: two case reports and review of the literature. Hemoglobin. 2017;41:225–9.

15 Neurocysticercosis, Pregnancy, and Albendazole: The Unholy Trio

Sweety Shinde, Kusum D. Jashnani, and Rosemarie de Souza

15.1 Clinical History

A 27-year-old female with 8 months of amenorrhea complained of holocranial throbbing headache, generalized seizures, and projectile vomiting for 3 days. She had history of generalized tonic-clonic convulsions two years ago which was treated with Ayurveda medicines. Her previous two pregnancies resulted in full-term normal deliveries. On examination, she was irritable and drowsy and had neck rigidity and generalized hypertonia. She was able to move both her arms and legs. Her pupils were bilaterally reactive to light. There was no pedal edema or jaundice. Examination of the cardiovascular system and respiratory system was normal. There was no hepatosplenomegaly. Per abdomen showed a soft, non-tender gravid uterus. Her blood pressure was 112/84 mmHg. The clinical differential diagnoses included eclampsia, epilepsy, cranial hemorrhage, cranial tumor, superior sagittal sinus thrombosis, and meningitis.

S. Shinde · K. D. Jashnani (✉)
Department of Pathology, Topiwala National Medical College and BYL Nair Charitable Hospital, Mumbai, Maharashtra, India

R. de Souza
Department of Medicine, Topiwala National Medical College and BYL Nair Charitable Hospital, Mumbai, Maharashtra, India

On investigation, her renal and hepatic function tests were unremarkable. A complete hemogram showed all values within the normal range. Examination of cerebrospinal fluid (CSF) was unremarkable. Magnetic resonance imaging (MRI) revealed multiple, 8- to 12-mm-sized cerebral and cerebellar ring enhancing lesions. On radioimaging, the differential diagnoses for ring-enhancing lesions include tumors (glioblastoma, primary CNS lymphoma, metastases, etc.), infective lesions (tuberculoma, pyogenic abscess, neurocysticercosis, toxoplasmosis), demyelinating lesions (multiple sclerosis), and vascular lesions (subacute infarct, organizing hematoma). Being multiple with a targetoid appearance in the current case, the lesions were consistent with neurocysticercosis.

The patient was put on albendazole treatment. She developed status epilepticus and respiratory distress. On day three, she delivered a stillborn male child. Her condition deteriorated, and she expired on the fifth day after admission.

15.2 Autopsy Findings

The patient was averagely built and nourished. The brain weighed 1200 g. There was no evidence of meningeal exudate. Gyri were flattened, and sulci were obliterated, suggestive of cerebral

K. D. Jashnani (ed.), *Maternal Mortality - Lessons Learnt from Autopsy*,
https://doi.org/10.1007/978-981-19-3420-9_15

edema. Multiple cysts measuring 0.5–1.5 cm were seen on the cortical surfaces of the cerebral and cerebellar hemispheres (Fig. 15.1a, b), while ventricles were unremarkable. The right pleural surface showed a similar single 1 cm cyst (Fig. 15.1c). Both the lungs showed gray-white consolidation of the lower lobes, suggestive of lobar pneumonia. All other organs were in their normal anatomical position and showed a normal gross appearance. Histopathology of the cystic lesions showed encysted scolex within the bladder wall. The bladder wall consisted of an outer cuticle, a middle cellular, and an inner parenchymatous layer. Invagination of the thick segment in the stroma appeared as stacks (Fig. 15.2a). This microscopic appearance was consistent with cysticercosis. There was a pericystic tissue reaction in the form of multinucleate giant cells and a dense lymphocytic infiltrate (Fig. 15.2b). Lungs showed dense bronchial and alveolar neutrophilic exudate suggestive of bronchopneumonia. All other organs were essentially normal on microscopy.

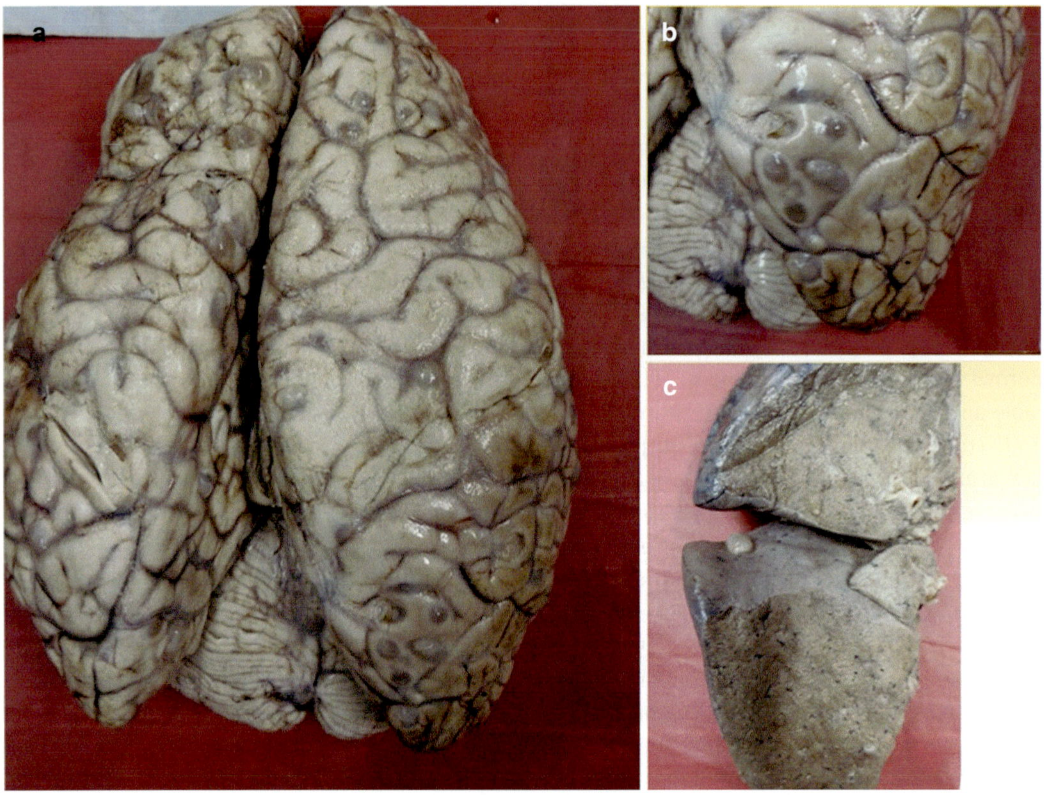

Fig. 15.1 (**a**) Multiple cysts involving cerebral and cerebellar hemispheres. The cysts are unilocular with single white specks within consistent with invaginated scolex of cysticercosis. Inset (**b**) shows closer view of cysts. (**c**) Gross image of the lung shows solitary cyst on pleural surface. Lungs show lower lobe consolidation

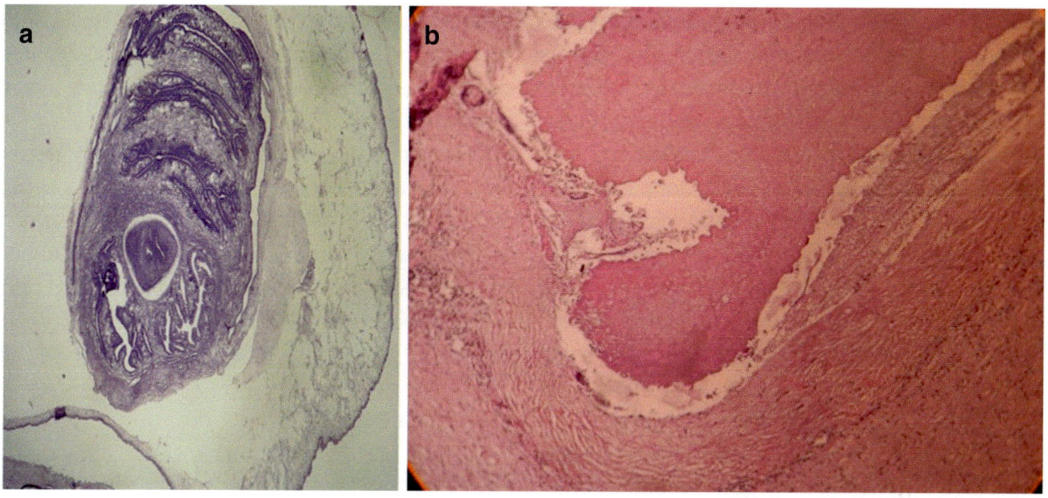

Fig. 15.2 (**a**) Photomicrograph, H&E, 400× shows cysticercal wall and invaginated scolex. (**b**) Photomicrograph, H&E, 100× shows pericystic fibrosis, mononuclear infiltration, and foreign body giant cell reaction

15.3 Final Cause of Death

Bilateral confluent bronchopneumonia and neurocysticercosis in a postpartum female.

15.4 Clinicopathologic Discussion

Neurocysticercosis (NCC) refers to involvement of the brain or spinal cord by the larval form of *Taenia solium* [1]. Indian studies show a prevalence of 1.3–4.5 per 1000 epilepsy patients [2]. In endemic countries like India, it can be the cause of one-third of the cases of acquired epilepsy [3]. Human beings and pigs can act as both definitive hosts and intermediate hosts. Human feces can contain proglottids and egg forms. On ingestion by pigs, these develop into larval forms which get encysted in pig muscles. Upon ingestion of cysticerci-infested pork by human beings, the larval forms develop into adult worms in the intestine. Taeniasis refers to the harboring of adult worms in the intestine [1, 3].

In endemic areas, >50% of cases are detected incidentally at autopsy since live larvae remain asymptomatic [1]. Symptoms develop when disintegrating larval forms incite a fibro-inflammatory response. Based on location, NCC is classified as subarachnoid-cisternal, parenchymal, intraventricular, and spinal. NCC can present with arachnoiditis, obstructive hydrocephalus, paraparesis, and Brun's syndrome, i.e. episodic ataxia and vertigo, due to intermittent obstruction of the foramina [1, 3, 4]. Multiple cysts can result in status epilepticus. Seizures in pregnancy can occur due to meningitis, dural sinus thrombosis, eclampsia, epilepsy, and intracranial tumor [1, 5]. Our case showed signs of meningeal irritation which are seen in <2% of cases. However, there was no meningeal thickening or exudate [1].

Developmental stages of cysticerci include vesicular, colloidal, granular, nodular, and calcified nodular [1, 3, 4]. Colloidal and granular forms appear hyperintense on T2-weighted MRI. Pericystic inflammatory response is seen as ring enhancement on T1-weighted contrast images [1, 3, 4].

Morphological forms of NCC include cellulose (often <2 cm size, remain clinically silent) and racemose (large sized with bunch-of-grapes appearance, often situated in ventricles, incite an intense inflammatory response and present with obstructive hydrocephalus) [1, 6, 7]. Del Brutto's criteria [7] for the diagnosis of NCC include radioimaging, histopathology, epidemiology, and serology. Enzyme immunotransfer blot detects antibodies, while the enzyme-linked immunosorbent assay detects cysticercal antigen. Other diagnostic modalities include fundoscopy and stool examination for proglottids. Our patient satisfied the absolute criteria for definitive diagnosis as she had characteristic MRI and histopathology. Treatment of NCC include anti-epileptics under due steroidal cover, cysticidal drugs (albendazole, praziquantel), and ventriculo-peritoneal shunt for intraventricular cysts [1].

Pregnancy and vegetarianism are two highlights of the present case. On enquiry, the patient was on a vegetarian diet. Ingestion of eggs by humans from feces-contaminated raw vegetables, feces-contaminated water, or autoinfection via ano-oral route leads to the development of larval forms. These can subsequently encyst in a subcutaneous tissue, muscle, eyes, or brain which is referred to as cysticercosis. Vegetarians are thus equally susceptible to NCC as non-vegetarians [1, 3, 5].

Studies indicate increased risk of seizures due to NCC during pregnancy. This is attributed to enhanced T-cell immune response and phagocytic activity, lowered B-cell response, and increased blood-brain barrier permeability, all of which may promote parasite survival during pregnancy [8–10]. Colloidal forms represent degenerating larvae that incite inflammation, while granular forms result in tissue fibrosis. Our patient already had NCC in colloidal and granular stages as evidenced by pericystic fibro-inflammatory response and ring enhancement on MRI. Albendazole, being cysticidal, can accelerate larval disintegration and worsen the fibro-inflammatory response, as in our case [3, 4]. Multiple degenerating cysts can catalyze status epilepticus. Hence, albendazole should be avoided in pregnancy [3, 4]. In this patient, albendazole could have been postponed till delivery or substituted by safer drugs like lamotrigine and levetiracetam.

Fetus can be affected in multiple ways during maternal NCC. It can develop hypoxia due to maternal seizures [3]. In addition, albendazole can cause congenital malformations and spontaneous abortion [11]. Praziquantel has lower teratogenic potential [8]. An infant can also develop cysticercosis during delivery via feco-oral transmission from a carrier mother. This can be prevented by administering non-absorbable drugs like niclosamide [3, 12].

Thus, neurocysticercosis in pregnancy needs vigilant and holistic therapeutic decisions. Cysticidal drugs can act as a double-edged sword in a pregnancy with NCC. Albendazole treatment has adverse effects on the mother-child unit and needs to be chosen with discretion.

References

1. Kimura-Hayama ET, Higuera JA, Corona-Cedillo R, Chávez-Macías L, Perochena A, Quiroz-Rojas LY, et al. Neurocysticercosis: radiologic-pathologic correlation. Radiographics. 2010;30:1705–19.
2. Amudhan S, Gururaj G, Satishchandra P. Epilepsy in India I: epidemiology and public health. Ann Indian Acad Neurol. 2015;18:263–77.
3. Webb C, La Rosa M, Olson G, Cabada M. Neurocysticercosis in pregnancy. Am J Perinatol Rep. 2018;8:e51–6.
4. D'Cruz CR, Ng SM, Dassan P. Neurocysticercosis in pregnancy: maternal and fetal outcomes. Oxf Med Case Reports. 2016;7:138–40.
5. Abdelwahab IF, Klein MJ, Hermann G, Abdul-Quader M. Solitary cysticercosis of the biceps brachii in a vegetarian: a rare and unusual pseudotumor. Skelet Radiol. 2003;32:424–8.
6. Singhal SR, Nanda S, Singhal SK. Neurocysticercosis as an important differential of seizures in pregnancy: two case reports. J Med Case Rep. 2011;5:206.
7. Del Brutto OH, Rajshekhar V, White AC Jr, Tsang VC, Nash TE, Takayanagui OM, et al. Proposed diagnostic criteria for neurocysticercosis. Neurology. 2001;57:177–83.
8. Pandian JD, Venkateswaralu K, Thomas SV, Sarma PS. Maternal and fetal outcome in women with epilepsy associated with neurocysticercosis. Epileptic Disord. 2007;9:285–91.
9. Bonney EA. Immune regulation in pregnancy: a matter of perspective? Obstet Gynecol Clin N Am. 2016;43:679–98.
10. Arce SA, Luquín ADD, Cárdenas G. Interleukin 10 and dendritic cells are the main suppression mediators of regulatory T cells in human neurocysticercosis. Clin Exp Immunol. 2016;183:271–9.
11. Gyapong JO, Chinbuah MA, Gyapong M. Inadvertent exposure of pregnant women to ivermectin and albendazole during mass drug administration for lymphatic filariasis. Tropical Med Int Health. 2003;8:1093–101.
12. Asnis D, Kazakov J, Toronjadze T, Bern C, Garcia HH, McAuliffe I, et al. Neurocysticercosis in the infant of a pregnant mother with a tapeworm. Am J Trop Med Hyg. 2009;81:449–51.

16 Lupus Nephritis and Pregnancy: Concern for Both Mother and Fetus

Kusum D. Jashnani, Mamta Vasudev Kripalani, Lalita Yoganand Patil, and Rakesh R. Bhadade

16.1 Clinical History

A 22-year-old multigravida with 5 months of amenorrhea came with complaints of facial rash (predominately on cheeks) and oral ulcers for 4 months and weight loss of about 17 kg in 3 months. She also had fever for a month and dry cough along with dyspnea on exertion—grade 3—and orthopnea for 3–4 days.

She took treatment for the same from a private hospital, but facial rash persisted and she eventually developed high-grade fever, bilateral pedal edema, and facial swelling. Following this, she was again admitted to a private hospital with diagnosis of dengue and typhoid fever. The edema didn't resolve, and the patient developed chest pain, orthopnea, PND, and DOE. The patient was then referred to our tertiary care hospital in view of anemia, thrombocytopenia, and pericardial effusion. After admission, various laboratory and radiological investigations were performed, and the patient was diagnosed with SLE. She was started on Inj. Lasix, Inj. Methylprednisolone, and Inj. Albumin. Antibiotics were given, and a blood transfusion was done. However, on the 17th day of admission, the patient became drowsy and disoriented, underwent spontaneous labor, and delivered stillborn baby—a male child, 390 g. The condition worsened, and she was declared dead on day 1 postpartum—after 6 h.

Investigations CBC revealed pancytopenia with hemoglobin of 7 g/dL, WBC count of 1300/mm^3, and a platelet count of 33,000/mm^3 on the day of admission, which eventually improved during the stay in the hospital, and on the day of death, CBC was suggestive of bicytopenia with hemoglobin of 6.4 g/dL, a platelet count of 30,000/mm^3, and a normal WBC count of 4500/mm^3 with raised ESR and BUN. The patient had hypoproteinemia, hypoalbuminemia, and hypocomplementemia. Urine routine microscopy revealed +++ proteinuria and hematuria.

Serological investigations revealed ANA + (speckled pattern) and anti-ds DNA (−). ANA blot test showed positivity for anti-RNP/Sm, anti-SSA, anti-nucleosome, and anti-histone. Direct Coomb's test was positive.

Radiology was suggestive of moderate/gross pericardial effusion, impending ARDS on 2D ECHO and HRCT, and USG revealed IUFD.

Clinical impression was CCF with LRTI with pericardial effusion with pancytopenia in a case of SLE with ARDS versus pulmonary hemorrhage in a 6-month pregnant female.

K. D. Jashnani (✉) · L. Y. Patil
Department of Pathology, Topiwala National Medical College and BYL Nair Charitable Hospital, Mumbai, Maharashtra, India

M. V. Kripalani
Shri Siddhivinayak Ganapati Cancer Hospital, Miraj, Maharashtra, India

R. R. Bhadade
Department of Medicine (Critical Care Unit), Topiwala National Medical College and BYL Nair Charitable Hospital, Mumbai, Maharashtra, India

K. D. Jashnani (ed.), *Maternal Mortality - Lessons Learnt from Autopsy*,
https://doi.org/10.1007/978-981-19-3420-9_16

16.2 Autopsy Findings

Butterfly rash on face and pallor were present; bilateral pitting edema over the foot was present on external examination. Internal examination revealed pale organs and 50 cc of pericardial fluid (yellow, clear). The lungs weighed 650 g each and appeared boggy, voluminous, and angry red looking. The cut surface was rubbery to firm in consistency (Fig. 16.4a). On microscopy, the pleura showed fibrous thickening and the presence of lymphoplasmacytic infiltrate. Multiple patchy areas of intra-alveolar edema fluid, hemorrhage, and mixed inflammatory infiltrates along with hemosiderin-laden macrophages were present. Presence of eosinophilic hyaline membrane lining the alveolar septae was noted (Fig. 16.4b). Few small-sized vessels showed fibrin thrombi. The impression was acute respiratory distress syndrome.

The heart weighed 450 g and was globular in shape. The epicardial surface was roughened

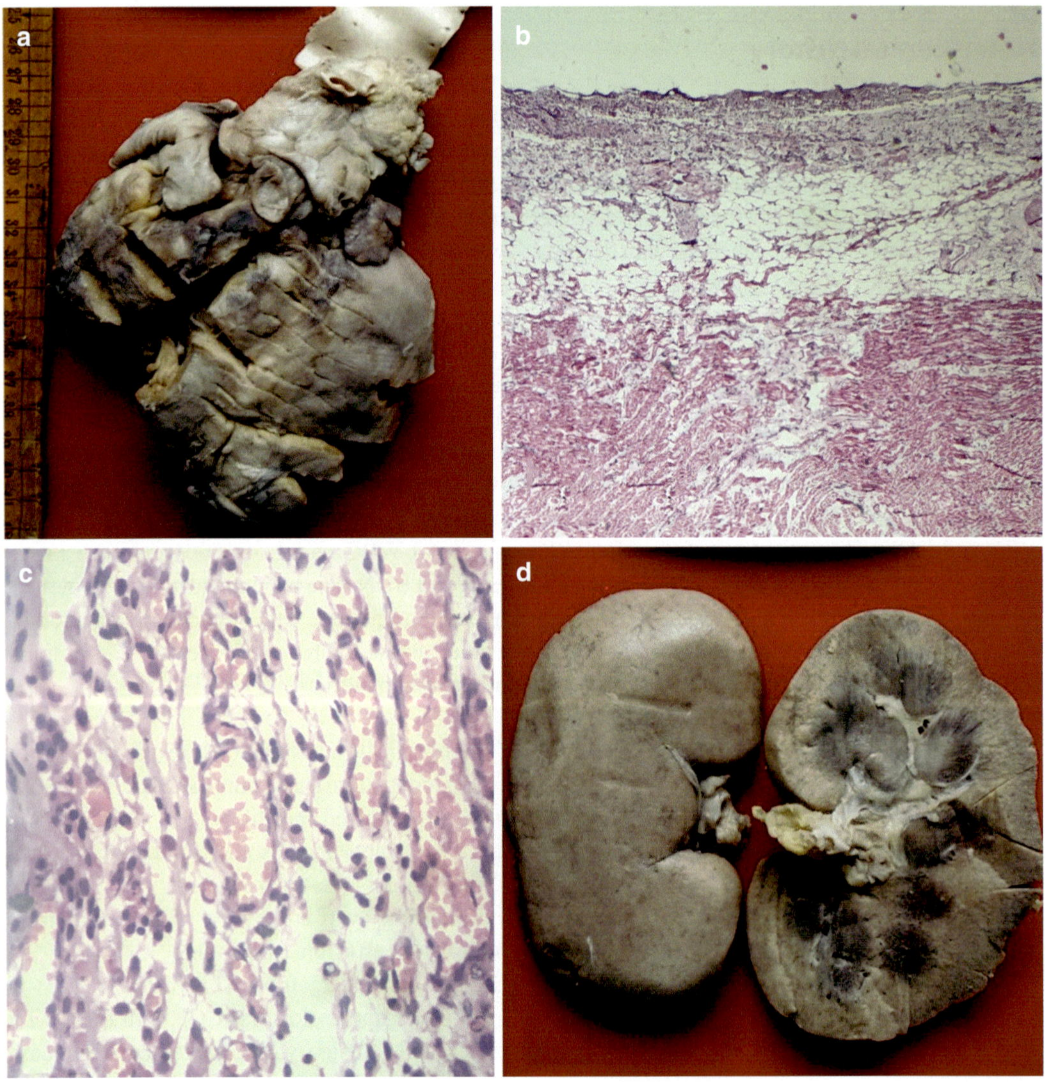

Fig. 16.1 (**a**) Gross specimen of heart with roughened and shaggy epicardial surface suggestive of pericarditis. (**b**, **c**) Epicardium showing fibrous thickening with presence of moderate degree of mixed inflammatory infiltrate, proliferating blood vessels suggestive of pericarditis (nonspecific). (H&E, 200x, 400×). (**d**) Gross specimen of kidney, appears enlarged and swollen. Cut surface shows normal cortex and congested medulla

and shaggy suggestive of pericarditis (Fig. 16.1a). The chambers were slightly dilated. Microscopic examination revealed the epicardium showing fibrous thickening with the presence of a moderate degree of mixed inflammatory infiltrate, proliferating blood vessels, and focal areas of fibrin deposition (Fig. 16.1b, c). The endocardium was unremarkable with mild hypertrophy of myocardial fibers. The impression was pericarditis (nonspecific).

The kidneys weighed 220 g each; they were enlarged and swollen. The medulla was congested on the cut surface (Fig. 16.1d). On microscopy, 40–45% of glomeruli were enlarged and hypercellular, showing the proliferation of endothelial and mesangial cells along with infiltration of leukocytes; occasional glomeruli showed cellular crescents (Fig. 16.3a, c). Many glomeruli showed fibrinoid necrosis, and few showed the presence of intracapillary thrombi (Fig. 16.2a–d). Few glomeruli showed mild GBM thickening, and few

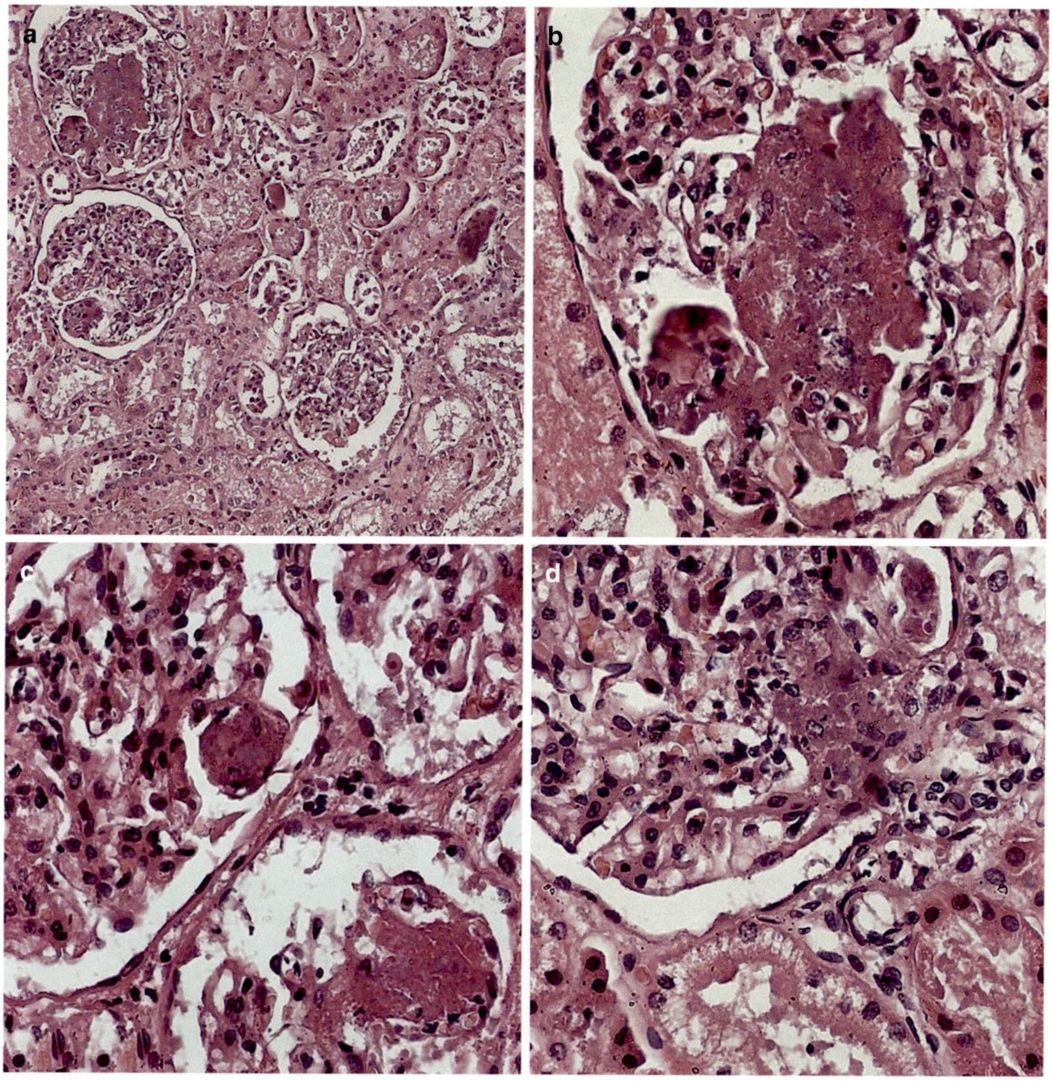

Fig. 16.2 (**a**) Glomeruli are enlarged, hypercellular showing proliferation of endothelial and mesangial cells along with infiltration of leukocytes. Glomerulus showing fibrinoid necrosis and intracapillary thrombus. Impression: Lupus nephritis (Class III) (H&E, 200×). (**b**) Glomerulus showing fibrinoid necrosis. (H&E, 400×). (**c**) Enlarged, hypercellular glomeruli showing proliferation of endothelial and mesangial cells along with fibrinoid necrosis and intracapillary thrombus (H&E, 400×). (**d**) Enlarged, hypercellular glomerulus showing infiltration of leukocytes (H&E, 400×)

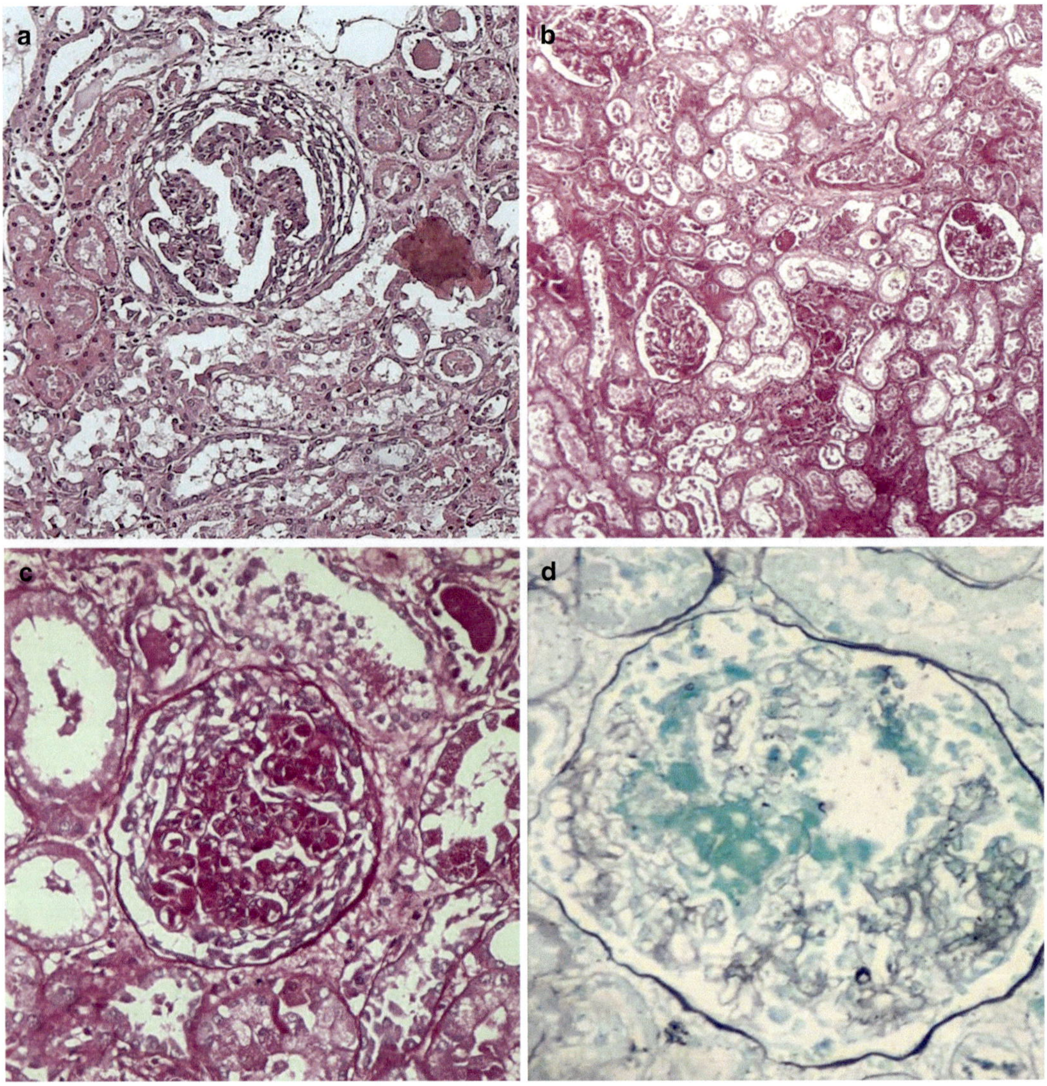

Fig. 16.3 (**a**) Glomerulus showing cellular crescent. Tubules showing cloudy change (H&E, 200×). (**b**) Enlarged, hypercellular glomeruli with mild GBM thickening (PAS, 100×). (**c**) Glomerulus showing crescent formation and mild GBM thickening (PAS, 400×). (**d**) Glomerulus showing segmental necrosis, breakdown of GBM (GMS, 400×)

showed segmental necrosis and breakdown of GBM (Fig. 16.3b, d). The tubules showed cloudy change, and the blood vessels were unremarkable. Impression was lupus nephritis (class III – focal proliferative glomerulonephritis).

Uterus under microscopy showed decidual change of endometrium with the presence of isolated intermediate trophoblastic cells. Myometrium showed physiological hypertrophy and pre-ischemic changes.

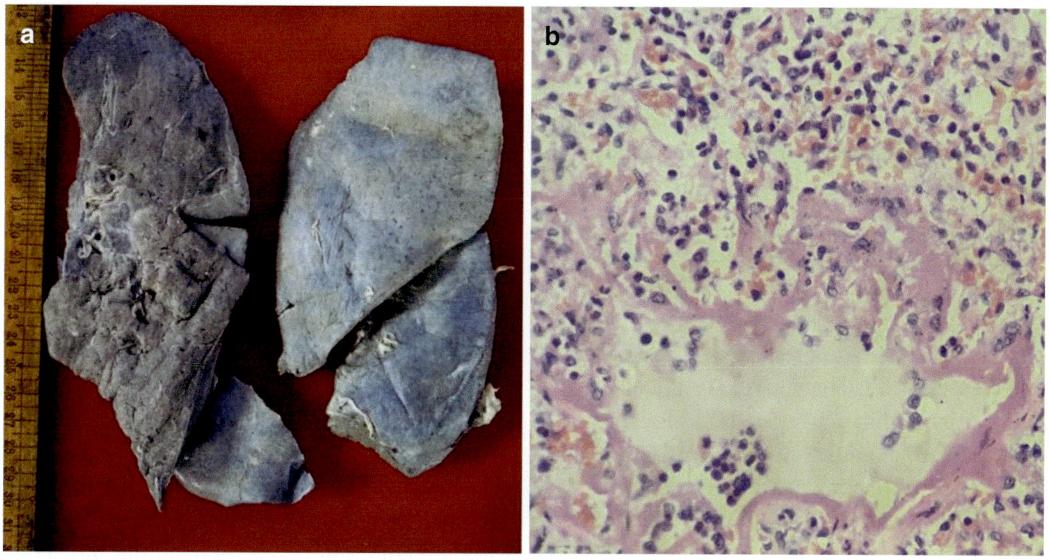

Fig. 16.4 (**a**) Gross specimen of lung- externally appeared boggy, voluminous, cut surface was rubbery to firm in consistency suggestive of ARDS. (**b**) Patchy area of intra-alveolar mixed inflammatory infiltrate noted. Presence of eosinophilic hyaline membrane lining the alveolar septa suggestive of acute respiratory distress syndrome (H&E, 400×)

16.3 Final Cause of Death

Acute respiratory distress syndrome and renal failure in a postpartum female with class III lupus nephritis.

16.4 Clinicopathologic Discussion

Amongst the autoimmune disorders, SLE is the one that most commonly affects women during their reproductive age. It is a multisystem disorder characterized by the production of autoantibodies and immune complex formation. The antibodies can be directed against many nuclear antigens (ANAs) of different organs. The immune complexes can be deposited or formed in diverse tissues, activating the complement and releasing proinflammatory cytokines that cause tissue damage. The diagnosis of SLE requires correlation of clinical (skin lesions, oral ulcers, renal disease, neurological affectation, hematologic disorders) and immunological alterations detected by the laboratory: anti-Sm antibodies, anti-DNA, and others [1].

SLE in pregnancy is considered to be a high-risk situation with higher maternal and fetal adverse outcomes. Opportunistic infections, sepsis, flares of lupus nephritis, and renal impairment are the common causes of maternal deaths in patients with SLE [2]. The most frequent adverse fetal events that can occur in lupus pregnancy are miscarriages, stillbirths, neonatal death, premature delivery, and intrauterine growth retardation [2]. The patient in discussion suffered from ARDS, nonspecific pericarditis, and lupus nephritis (LN); radiology revealed IUFD, and she delivered a stillborn baby.

Most patients (almost 50%) with SLE will have clinical evidence of kidney disease, usually an abnormal urinalysis, with or without an elevated plasma creatinine concentration, at some point in the course of their disease, as was seen in our case. Large, intact immune complexes of anti-double-stranded DNA antibodies are deposited in the mesangium and subendothelial space. There is the activation of complement with a resultant influx of neutrophils and mononuclear cells. The presence of subendothelial deposits in glomerular capillaries is crucial in the induction of severe damage, which correlates with endocapillary proliferation, necrosis, karyorrhexis, and crescents. It is characterized clinically by an active urine sediment (red cells, white cells, and cellular and granular casts), proteinuria, and, often, an acute decline in kidney function.

All patients with known SLE should undergo laboratory testing to assess for kidney involvement at regular intervals. The diagnosis of LN is ideally confirmed by a kidney biopsy. Treatment is guided by the histologic subtype (International Society of Nephrology/Renal Pathology Society [ISN/RPS] class, the degree of activity and chronicity) and by complicating lesions such as interstitial nephritis and thrombotic microangiopathy [3].

The revised ISN/RPS (2018) classification system divides glomerular disorders associated with SLE into six different patterns (or classes) based upon kidney biopsy histopathology [3].

Minimal mesangial LN (class I): Normal glomeruli by LM, but mesangial immune deposits by IF.

Mesangial proliferative LN (class II): Purely mesangial hypercellularity of any degree or mesangial expansion by LM, with mesangial immune deposits.

Focal LN (class III): Less than 50% of glomeruli are affected by light microscopy showing hypercellularity, karyorrhexis, fibrinoid necrosis, crescents.

Diffuse LN (class IV): Active disease shows hypercellular, necrotizing lesions and crescent formation, affecting more than 50% of glomeruli on light microscopy.

Lupus membranous nephropathy (class V): Lupus membranous nephropathy is present in 10 to 20% of patients with LN with usually normal or only slightly elevated creatinine. It is characterized by diffuse thickening of the glomerular capillary wall on light microscopy and by subepithelial immune deposits on immunofluorescence or electron microscopy.

Advanced sclerosing LN (class VI): It is characterized by global sclerosis of more than 90% of glomeruli. It represents healing of prior inflammatory injury, as well as the advanced stage of chronic class III, IV, or V lupus nephritis (LN). Active glomerulonephritis should not be observed, and immunosuppressive therapy is usually not beneficial.

The increased frequency of ARDS in lupus is because of increased immunological compromise from the SLE itself and also due to the immunosuppressant used for its treatment as well as the lung compromise caused by SLE [4]. The most common cause of ARDS is sepsis; others include lupus pneumonitis and diffuse alveolar hemorrhage [5].

The patient in discussion suffered from systemic lupus erythematosus and (1) was being treated with immunosuppressive agents like steroids, which may have led to secondary infections and ARDS, or (2) SLE could have led to IUFD and thus sepsis and hence ARDS, or (3) ARDS could be due to acute lupus pneumonitis with clinical features of shortness of breath and chest pain. (4) Another possibility is of ARDS being the causative agent and leading to hypoxia and IUFD. Thus, ARDS being the cause or the effect is an unsolved mystery in this case.

To conclude, pregnancy is not a contraindication in SLE; however conception can be delayed until the disease is in remission to ensure the best outcomes of pregnancy. Lupus activity, kidney function, and the presence of antiphospholipid antibodies are the factors on which the maternal and fetal outcomes depend [2]. Lupus flare in pregnancy leading to ARDS is a critical condition, and its treatment might be a challenge even in experienced hands [5].

References

1. Hochberg MC. Arthritis Rheum. 1997;40:1725.
2. Moroni G, Ponticelli C. Pregnancy in women with systemic lupus erythematosus (SLE). Eur J Intern Med. 2016;32:7–12.
3. Chen D, Hu W. Lupus podocytopathy: a distinct entity of lupus nephritis. J Nephrol. 2018;31(5):629–34.
4. Chen YA, Tseng JJ, Yang MJ, Tsao YP, Lin HY. Acute respiratory distress syndrome in a pregnant woman with systemic lupus erythematosus: a case report. Lupus. 2014;23(14):1528–32.
5. Banjar A, Rasheed J, Alkhatib K, Omran N. Systemic lupus erythematosus with pregnancy and acute respiratory distress. Saudi Crit Care J. 2017;1(2):70.

17 Disseminated Microthrombi in Pregnancy: Not Always DIC, Think of TTP

Sheetal Anil Ghugare, Kusum D. Jashnani, Lalita Yoganand Patil, and Vandana Rajesh Saravade

17.1 Clinical History

A 35-year-old multigravida (G4 P3 L2 D1) with 16 weeks of gestation had history of sudden onset of headache and one episode of seizure for 1 day. She was taken to a nearby hospital and given injectable drugs, her headache resolved, and she went home. But next day, she started shouting and was not able to speak properly, for which she was taken to two different hospitals. She was found to have IUFD with DIC; she was transferred to our hospital for further management. She had no history of fever, breathlessness, vomiting, chest pain, loss of consciousness, bowel bladder incontinence, or any major medical and surgical illness. Her general condition was poor, she was pale and icteric, and her blood pressure was 130/90 mmHg. Per abdomen was soft and tender, and a vertical scar was present. On central nervous system examination, she was conscious, not fully oriented, and not following verbal commands, pupils bilateral reacting to light; neck rigidity was absent. On the second day, extraocular movements were normal, deep tendon reflexes ++, movement of all four limbs ++, pupils slowly reacting to light and the absence of facial weakness. On the fourth day, she was not oriented and not responding to commands, with hemiparesis + and aphasia+. On the sixth day, she was drowsy and disoriented, suffered two episodes of generalized tonic clonic seizures (GTCS), and was seen in a gasping state. So, she was intubated, and CPR started. Despite all attempts, her condition deteriorated, and she expired on day 6 of hospital admission.

Obstetrics history: The first child was dead after 3 months of birth, the second child was 3 years old, and the third child was 20 months old. Each were full-term and delivered by LSCS. Now she was 16 weeks registered ANC.

17.2 Investigations

On the first day, hemoglobin was 4.7 g/dL, total WBC count was 6300/mm^3, and platelet count was 75,000/mm^3. On the sixth day, hemoglobin and TLC were raised and reached up to 9.1 g/dl and 18,600/mm^3, respectively. But platelets had gone down to 31,000/mm and again rose to 174,000/mm^3 on the sixth day. Coagulation screening test showed raised prothrombin time (16.7 s, control was 12 s), prothrombin index (1.26) and APTT (42.8 s, control was 25 s), but fibrinogen was within normal limits (112.2 mg/dl). Total and direct bilirubin levels were 4.9 and 1 mg/dl, respectively; SGOT and SGPT were

S. A. Ghugare · K. D. Jashnani (✉) · L. Y. Patil
Department of Pathology, Topiwala National Medical College and BYL Nair Charitable Hospital, Mumbai, Maharashtra, India

V. R. Saravade
Department of Obstetrics and Gynecology, Topiwala National Medical College and BYL Nair Charitable Hospital, Mumbai, Maharashtra, India

K. D. Jashnani (ed.), *Maternal Mortality - Lessons Learnt from Autopsy*,
https://doi.org/10.1007/978-981-19-3420-9_17

raised (2288 U/L and 1962 U/L, respectively), and alkaline phosphate was within normal limits. Serum albumin was slightly low (3.1 g/dl), and BUN, creatinine, and total protein were within normal limits. Electrolytes (Na and K) and glucose were normal. Serum LDH and uric acid were raised (11,396 IU/L and 8.7 mg/dl, respectively). Peripheral smear showed a picture of hemolytic anemia consisting of target cells, tear drop cells, pencil cells, schistocytes, nucleated RBC 111/100 WBC, corrected WBC count of 616/μl, macrovalocytes, toxic granules, polychromasia, Howell-Jolly bodies, and occasional giant platelets. Reticulocyte count was raised to 32%. Urine routine microscopy showed 18–20 RBC/hpf, and occult blood test was positive. On ultrasonography, a single intrauterine fetus was seen, but fetal heart sounds and fetal movements were absent, suggesting abruptio placentae and IUFD. Clinical impression was DIC, HELLP and posterior reversible encephalopathy syndrome. She received a total of six units of packed red cells, nine units of platelets and four units of FFP during her total hospital stay.

17.3 Autopsy Findings

On gross examination, the brain weighed 1.2 kg, meninges congested with mild cerebral edema and cerebellar tonsillar herniation. Microscopic examination showed cerebral edema, thrombi in small blood vessels, and mild lymphocytic infiltrate in the subarachnoid space (Fig. 17.1a, b). The heart weighed 460 g and was enlarged, globular and apex formed by both ventricles. Petechial

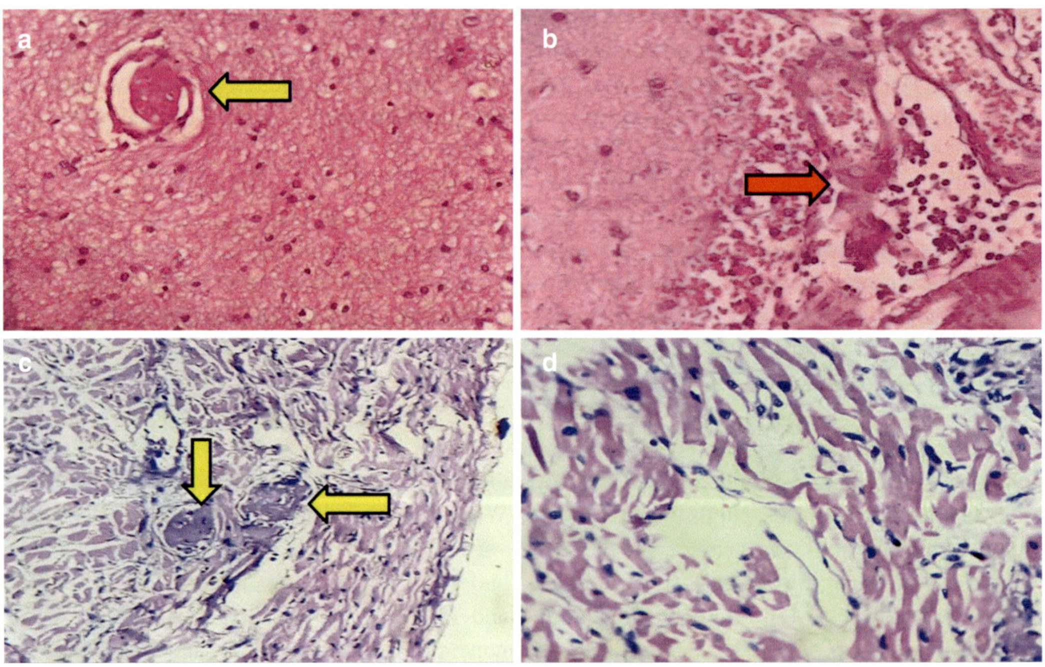

Fig. 17.1 (**a**, **b**, **H&E**, **200×**) Microscopic examination of the brain showing cerebral edema, thrombi in blood vessels (yellow arrow), mild lymphocytic infiltrate in the subarachnoid space and congested meningeal vessels (red arrow). (**c**, **H&E**, **100×**, **d**, **H&E**, **200×**) Microscopy of the heart showing thrombi in interstitial blood vessels (yellow arrow), myofibre disarray and mild lymphocytic infiltrate in focal areas

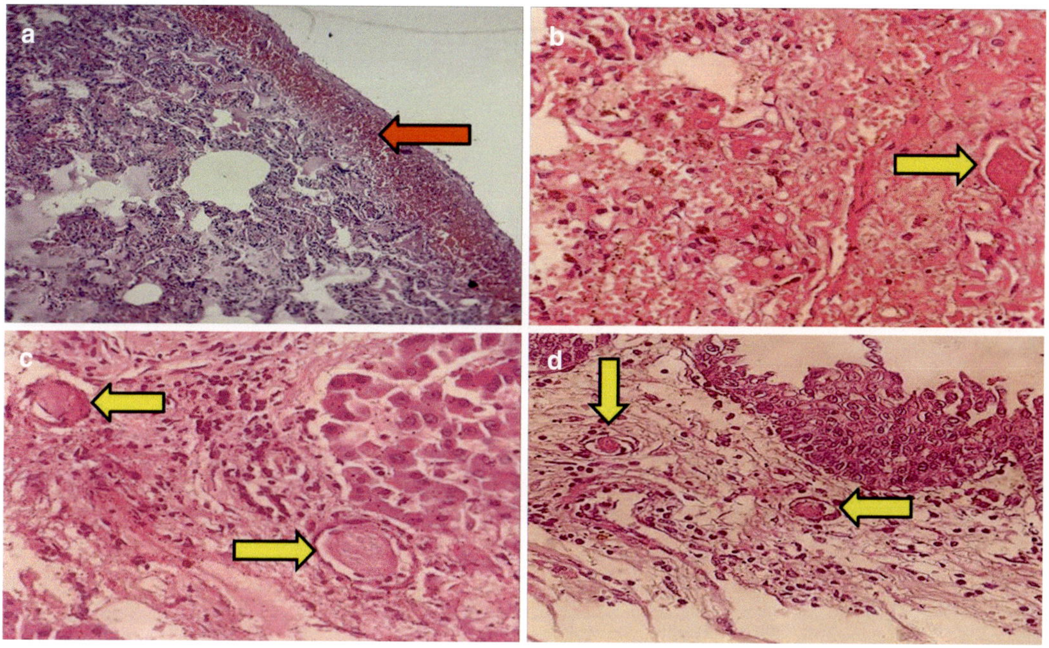

Fig. 17.2 (**a**, **b**) Microscopic examination of the lungs showing subpleural hemorrhage (red arrow), patchy areas of intra-alveolar edema fluid and thrombi in few small blood vessels (yellow arrow) H&E, 200×. (**c**) Microscopic examination of the liver showing thrombi in small blood vessels in portal tract (yellow arrow) H&E, 100×. (**d**) Microscopic examination of the esophagus showing thrombi in small blood vessels (yellow arrow) and mild mixed inflammatory infiltrate in the underlying wall of the esophagus H&E, 200×

hemorrhages were seen on the anterior and posterior surfaces of the heart, and a hemorrhagic area measuring 1 × 0.5 cm was seen on posterior surface, near the apex. Microscopy showed epicardial hemorrhages, hyaline thrombi in interstitial blood vessels, myofibre disarray and mild lymphocytic infiltrate in focal areas (Fig. 17.1c, d). The lungs weighed 430 g each; petechial hemorrhages were seen over the pleural surface. Microscopy showed subpleural hemorrhages, patchy areas of intra-alveolar edema fluid and thrombi in small blood vessels (Fig. 17.2a, b). The liver weighed 1.9 kg and was enlarged; multiple petechial hemorrhages were seen on the capsular and cut surface of the liver parenchyma. On microscopy, central hemorrhagic necrosis and thrombi in small blood vessels in portal tracts were seen (Fig. 17.2c). Similar thrombi in small blood vessels were also seen in the stomach, esophagus, pancreas, kidneys, and adrenals (Figs. 17.2d and 17.3a–d). Bone marrow, on microscopy, showed hypercellular marrow, micronormoblastic erythropoiesis and normal numbers of megakaryocytes. The uterus with a fetus weighed 578 g, and the microscopic examination of the uterus, cervix, and bilateral ovaries was unremarkable. The rest of the organs were remarkable.

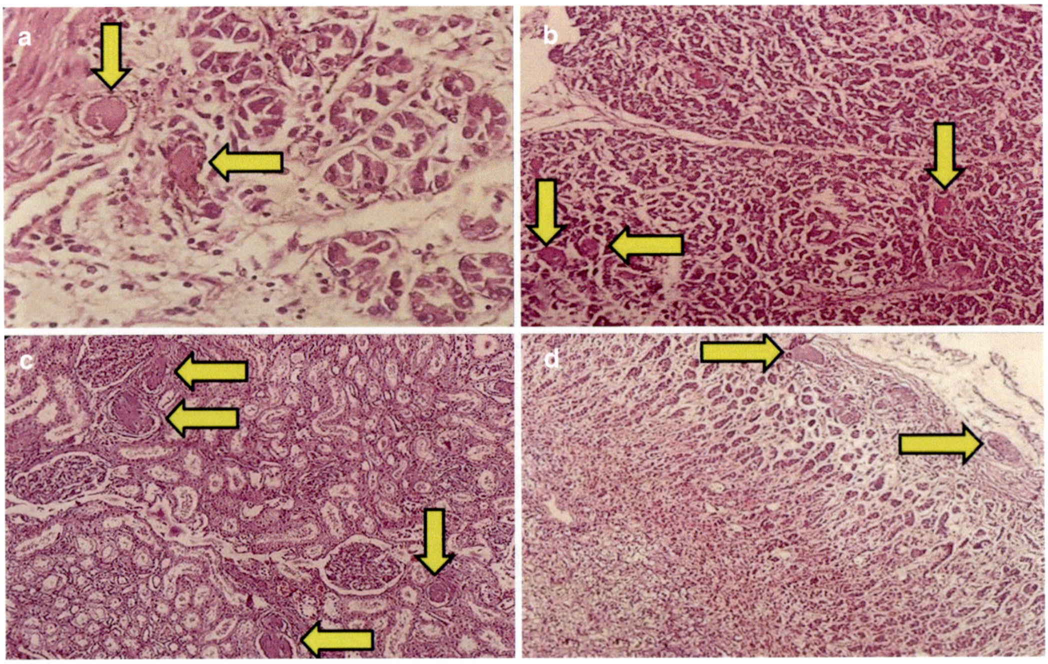

Fig. 17.3 (**a**) Microscopic examination of the stomach showing thrombi in small blood vessels (yellow arrow) and mild mixed inflammatory infiltrate in the mucosa of the stomach. (**b**) Microscopic examination of the pancreas showing normal lobular architecture, thrombi in tiny vessels in the parenchyma (yellow arrow). (**c**) Microscopic examination of the kidney showing thrombi in interstitial small blood vessels (yellow arrow), cloudy change seen in renal tubules. (**d**) Microscopic examination of adrenal gland showing thrombi in small vessels in adrenal cortex (yellow arrow). All H&E, 200×

17.4 Final Cause of Death

Multiple organ failure due to TTP in a 4-month pregnant female with intrauterine fetal death.

17.5 Clinicopathologic Discussion

As per clinical history and autopsy findings on gross and microscopy, we had differential diagnosis of DIC, HUS, HELLP syndrome and TTP. HELLP syndrome is characterised by hemolysis, elevated liver enzymes and low platelet count, without neurological symptoms or thrombi in vessels on microscopy. So, HELLP syndrome was ruled out. HUS shows microangiopathy of the kidney involving glomerular capillaries and arterioles, microangiopathic hemolytic anemia and thrombocytopenia. However, neurological symptoms are uncommon, thrombi are localised to the kidney only, with no thrombi in other organs, so HUS was also ruled out. DIC usually shows abnormal coagulation parameters, i.e. low platelet, low fibrinogen, raised PT/APTT, high D-dimer and petechial hemorrhages on the serosal surface of organs. Following DIC, fibrinolysis gets activated, and FDP formed have an inhibitory effect on clot formation, thereby ruling out DIC. In TTP, classic pentad, i.e. microangiopathic hemolytic anemia, thrombocytopenia, renal insufficiency, neurologic abnormalities, and fever are seen. Disseminated microthrombi are characteristic of TTP, and these microthrombi are found in arterioles and capillaries in a variety of organs including the brain, heart, gastrointestinal tract, pancreas, skin, adrenal gland, and kidney. All of these findings were present clinically as well as on microscopy in our case, whereby a diagnosis of TTP was offered on autopsy.

Thrombotic thrombocytopenic purpura is a rare disorder that results in the formation of platelet-rich thrombi in small blood vessels (arterioles and capillaries most frequently affected) throughout the body. This results in a low platelet count, low red blood cell count due to their breakdown and kidney, heart and brain dysfunction due to organ ischemia. Cause of TTP is unknown, but the two best understood causes of TTP are due to autoimmunity (autoantibody-mediated inhibition or clearance of ADAMTS13 activity) and inherited deficiency or reduced activity of ADAMTS13, a metalloprotease responsible for cleaving large multimers of VWF into smaller units [1]. Acquired TTP accounts for more than 90% of cases of TTP in adults. Predisposing factors include cancer, pregnancy, bone marrow transplantation, medication use (antiviral drugs, chemotherapy, medications, platelet aggregation inhibitors, immunosuppressants, etc.), HIV-1 infection and bacterial infection. The mechanism of TTP is spontaneous aggregation of platelets and activation of coagulation in the small blood vessels. The increase in circulating multimers of VWF increases platelet adhesion to areas of endothelial injury, particularly where arterioles and capillaries meet, which in turn results in the formation of small platelet clots called thrombi, in the absence of ADAMTS13. Normally, this tendency of VWF and platelets to form microthrombi is alleviated by ADAMTS13, which cleaves VWF before it is activated by shear stress to cause platelet aggregation in the circulation [2, 3]. As platelets are used up in the formation of thrombi, this then leads to a decrease in the number of overall circulating platelets, which may then cause life-threatening bleeds. RBCs passing through the microscopic clots are subjected to shear stress, which damages their membranes, leading to rupture of RBCs within blood vessels, which in turn leads to anemia and schistocyte formation. The presence of these blood clots in the small blood vessels reduces blood flow to the organs, resulting in cellular injury and end organ damage. Due to the high mortality of untreated TTP, a presumptive diagnosis of TTP is made even when only microangiopathic hemolytic anaemia and thrombocytopenia are seen, and therapy is started. Plasmapheresis is the treatment of choice for TTP. If apheresis is not available, fresh frozen plasma can be infused, but the volume that can be given safely is limited due to the danger of fluid overload. Corticosteroids (prednisolone) are usually given. Immunosuppressive therapy (e.g. vincristine, cyclophosphamide, cyclosporine A), or splenectomy is tried for the people with refractory or relapsing TTP. The mortality rate is around 95% for untreated cases, but the prognosis is reasonably favourable (80–90% survival) for people with idiopathic TTP diagnosed and treated early with plasmapheresis. Common causes of death in patients with TTP are cardiovascular disease [4] (like sudden cardiac death, heart failure, arrhythmias, myocardial infarction), cancer, infections and some other unknown causes [5].

References

1. Rosai J. Genitourinary pathology. Kidney: non-neoplastic diseases. In: Rosai and Ackerman's surgical pathology. 11th ed. Mosby: Elsevier; 2018. p. 935–1013.
2. Veyradier A, Stepanian A, Coppo P. ADAMTS13, thrombotic thrombocytopenic purpura and pregnancy. Hered Genet. 2012;1:002. https://doi.org/10.4172/2161-1041.S1-002.
3. Elayoubi J, Donthireddy K, Nemakayala DR. BMJ Case Rep. https://doi.org/10.1136/bcr-2017-221648.
4. Nichols L, Berg A, Rollins-Raval MA, Raval JS. Cardiac injury is a common postmortem finding in thrombotic thrombocytopenic purpura patients: is empiric c cardiac monitoring and protection needed? Ther Apher Dial. 2015;19(1):87–92.
5. Hosler GA, Cusumano AM, Hutchins GM. Thrombotic thrombocytopenic purpura and hemolytic uremic syndrome are distinct pathologic entities. A review of 56 autopsy cases. Arch Pathol Lab Med. 2003;127:834–9.

18 HEV-Associated Hepatic Necrosis and Hepatic Encephalopathy in Pregnancy: Should Hepatitis E Virus Surveillance Be Made Mandatory in Pregnancy?

Sushama A. Chandekar,
Padmaja Vishwadeep Patil, Kusum D. Jashnani,
and Rosemarie de Souza

18.1 Clinical History

A 25-year-old female, in her second pregnancy (G2P0L0A1) with 20 weeks of gestation, presented to the hospital as a referral from a peripheral hospital. She had been unwell with altered sensorium and uprolling of eyeballs for 1 day. She had history of fever with chills, vomiting and yellowish discolouration of urine in the last 5 days. She had past history of hepatitis 2–3 years back, details of which were not known. She was not registered for any antenatal care (ANC).

The patient had induced abortion in the peripheral hospital, the reason for which was not known. From there, she was referred to our hospital in view of hepatic encephalopathy grade IV. There was no history of oliguria, loose motions or trauma. Clinical examination revealed a deeply jaundiced patient with poor general condition. Central nervous system examination showed a deeply unconscious patient who was not responding to deep painful stimuli. She was afebrile, with pallor and icterus ++, bilateral pedal edema, with blood pressure and pulse of 120/70 mm Hg and 107/min, respectively. Respiratory examination showed bilateral harsh breath sounds. Per abdomen- uterus corresponded to 14 weeks of size, per vaginal examination showed blood clots, and blood-tinged urine was seen approximately of volume 500cc on catheterization.

Hematological investigations showed a WBC of 4300/cumm, falling haemoglobin of 8.5 gm/dl, and a platelet count of 1.79 lakhs/cumm. Coagulation studies showed prothrombin time of >60 s (control was 14 s). Biochemical investigations showed blood urea nitrogen of 10 mg/dl, serum creatinine of 8 mg/dl, fasting blood sugar of 711 mg/dl, sodium 142 mEq/L, and potassium 4.3 mEq/L. Liver function test results were not available. HIV, HCV and HBsAg were non-reactive. Clinical impression was acute fulminant hepatitis with hepatic encephalopathy grade IV with sepsis and coagulopathy in a case of induced complete abortion. The clinical condition of the patient deteriorated, and the patient was declared

S. A. Chandekar · K. D. Jashnani (✉)
Department of Pathology, Topiwala National Medical College and BYL Nair Charitable Hospital, Mumbai, Maharashtra, India

P. V. Patil
Rajmata Jijau Hospital, Navi Mumbai, Maharashtra, India

R. de Souza
Department of Medicine, Topiwala National Medical College and BYL Nair Charitable Hospital, Mumbai, Maharashtra, India

K. D. Jashnani (ed.), *Maternal Mortality - Lessons Learnt from Autopsy*,
https://doi.org/10.1007/978-981-19-3420-9_18

dead within 18 h of admission. A complete autopsy was performed.

18.2 Autopsy Findings

She was averagely built and nourished, with icterus ++ and pedal edema +. Serosanguinous frothy fluid was seen oozing out from the mouth and nostrils. The liver was shrunken in size, weighing 800 g with a wrinkled capsule. It was soft, foldable and focally friable with small yellowish areas on the cut surface (Fig. 18.1). On histopathological examination, there was loss of normal lobular architecture with evidence of massive necrosis of hepatocytes. Apoptotic bodies were present (Figs. 18.2, 18.3, and 18.4). The portal tract and surrounding necrosed hepatocytes showed mild mononuclear cell infiltrate. Few preserved hepatocytes were swollen with pale staining, finely granular cytoplasm. Lungs weighed 600 g each, with frothy fluid oozing out on pressure on the cut surface. Histopathology showed eosinophilic edema fluid within the alveolar spaces with fibrin thrombi in few small-sized branches of the pulmonary artery. Bilateral kidneys weighed 150 g each and showed prominent cortical striations with a maintained corticomedullary ratio. The pelvicalyceal system was dilated with mucosal hemorrhages in bilateral kidneys. Histopathologic examination showed multiple patchy areas of acute tubular necrosis, with congested glomerular and interstitial

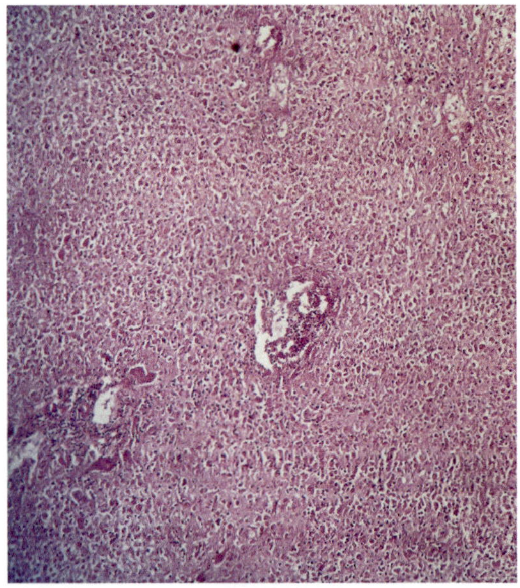

Fig. 18.2 Microphotograph of the liver showing massive hepatic necrosis (H & E, 100×)

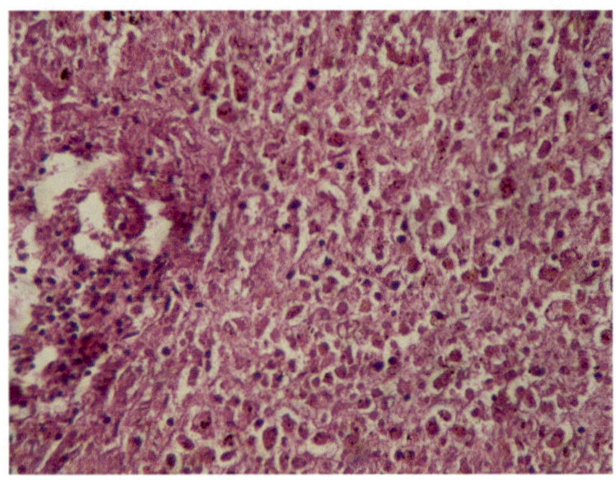

Fig. 18.3 Microphotograph of the liver showing several hypereosinophilic necrotic hepatocytes and cholestasis (H&E, 400×)

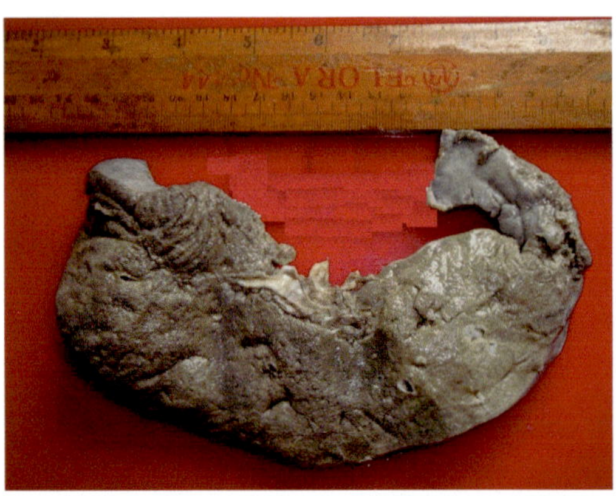

Fig. 18.1 Gross photograph of small shrunken and limp liver slice with wrinkled capsule

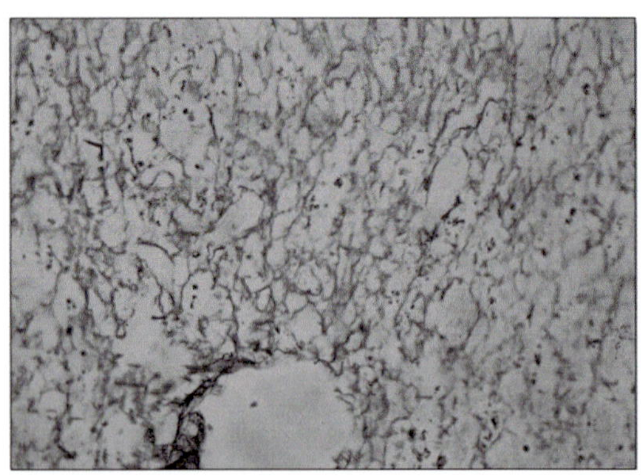

Fig. 18.4 Microphotograph of the liver showing collapse of reticulin network (Reticulin stain, 400×)

capillaries with unremarkable arteries. Uterine myometrium showed physiologic changes of hypertrophy and preischaemia on histopathology. The rest of the organs were unremarkable. On evaluating the hepatitis E status of the autopsy blood sample, it was found to be positive.

18.3 Final Cause of Death

Acute renal failure and hepatic encephalopathy due to massive hepatic necrosis in a case of induced abortion with HEV infection.

18.4 Clinicopathologic Discussion

In pregnancy, the spectrum of liver disease may range from mild asymptomatic cases to fatal and irreversible deterioration in liver functions, leading to significant morbidity and even mortality [1]. The fatality rate among pregnant women with acute liver failure (ALF) is reported to be high in India at 22.2% with the maximum severity occurring during the third trimester (41.4%). ALF, also referred to as FHF, is defined as the development of severe acute liver injury with encephalopathy and elevated prothrombin time/international normalized ratio (INR) in a patient without cirrhosis or pre-existing liver disease. In our case, the leading cause of death was cerebral edema, which occurs commonly as the acute presentation of fulminant liver failure. Spontaneous bleeding occurs in less than 10% of cases in ALF. It is secondary to liver failure, when the failing liver cannot make enough coagulation/clotting factors due to massive hepatic necrosis. Acute renal failure in the present case was because of hypovolemia. Hypotension occurs following massive hepatic necrosis as hypoalbuminemia causes a shift of fluid from the intravascular compartment to the extravascular space. In a study by Patra et al., it was found that death from fulminant hepatic failure (FHF) has been seen to be more common in HEV-infected pregnant women or have worse fetal outcomes than in pregnant women with jaundice and acute viral hepatitis caused by other hepatitis viruses [2, 3]. Hepatitis E virus (HEV) infection in pregnancy is also associated with high rates of spontaneous abortion, intrauterine fetal death and preterm labour. Clinical outcomes associated with HEV infection are quite diverse. It most commonly manifests as self-limiting, acute icteric hepatitis, which is indistinguishable from acute hepatitis caused by other hepatotropic viruses. The illness usually lasts for a few weeks, although some patients have a somewhat prolonged illness with prominent cholestatic manifestations. In a proportion of patients, the illness is particularly severe and presents as fulminant hepatitis [4, 5]. Pregnancy is associated with increased risk of severe disease with these patients rapidly progressing to encephalopathy, coagulopathies, progressive weakness and fulminant hepatitis needing close follow-up. The cause of ALF in pregnant women may be reduced immunity or altered hormonal status in pregnancy [6]. Pregnancy is associated with high levels of steroid hormones (estrogen and progesterone). These hormones may promote viral replication and also have a direct inhibition on hepatic cells which may predispose to hepatic dysfunction/failure when exposed to infectious pathogens. With regard to high mortality rate of jaundice in pregnancy, especially HEV infection, simple measures like healthy diet and maintaining good personal hygiene would definitely reduce the disease occurrence. In a study carried out in our department [7], fulminant hepatic failure due to submassive to massive hepatic necrosis was the predominant cause of death in 16 (27.59%) out of 58 cases, with positive serology for HEV infection in six cases. Fulminant hepatic failure due to hepatitis E infection as the leading cause of maternal mortality in our institute was explained by close proximity of a municipal corporation hospital for infectious diseases to our tertiary care centre. We wonder if testing for HEV should also be made a part of mandatory investigations in pregnant women.

References

1. Pandey CK, Karna ST, Pandey VK, Tandon M. Acute liver failure in pregnancy: challenges and management. Indian J Anaesth. 2015;59:144–9.
2. Patra S, Kumar A, Trivedi SS, Puri M, Sarin SK. Maternal and fetal outcomes in pregnant women with acute hepatitis E virus infection. Ann Intern Med. 2007;147:28–33.
3. Jashnani KD, Rupani AB, Wani RJ. Maternal mortality: an autopsy audit. J Postgrad Med. 2009;55(1):12–6.
4. Anitha P, Shruti C. Autopsy study of maternal death in a tertiary care centre. Indian J Obst Gynecol Res. 2018;5(4):504–10.
5. Butler DC, Lewin DN, Batalis NI. Differential diagnosis of hepatic necrosis encountered at autopsy. Acad Forensic Pathol. 2018;8(2):256–95.
6. Navaneethan U, Mohajer A, Shata MT. Hepatitis E and pregnancy: understanding the pathogenesis. Liver Int. 2008;28:1190–9.
7. Jashnani KD, Chandekar SA, Pawar A, Dalal AR, Wani RJ. Hepatitis E infection and pregnancy: a fatal combination. Int J Basic Appl Med Sci. 2015;5(2):264–9.

H1N1 Influenza in Pregnancy: Yet Another Dreaded Flu

19

Gayathri Prashant Amonkar
and Kusum D. Jashnani

19.1 Clinical History

A 28-year-old female patient $G2P_1L_1$ day 7 post LSCS on ventilatory support in a critical condition was referred from a private hospital to our tertiary care center where the patient succumbed on the way and was brought dead to our hospital. Indication for LSCS was non progression of labor and bleeding PV. She had delivered a healthy female child weighing 3.8 kg, and subsequently on day 3 post LSCS, she developed severe breathlessness. Clinical diagnosis of ARDS was made, and the patient was intubated and put on ventilatory support.

On investigating in the private hospital, the patient was detected to be H1N1 (swine flu) RT-PCR positive. The patient was negative for malaria, leptospirosis, and dengue. Her Hb was 7.3 g/dL, total WBC count was 9000/cumm, blood sugar was 108 mg/dl, BUN was 18 mg/dl, and serum creatinine was 1.2 mg/dl. Since the patient was brought dead to our hospital, a complete autopsy was performed.

19.2 Autopsy Findings

On gross examination during the autopsy, both the lungs were voluminous, boggy, each weighing 400 g, and markedly congested, angry red, and firm in consistency (Fig. 19.1). Examination of the uterus revealed the LSCS suture line which was intact. There was no gaping of the incision wound, sutures were intact, and there was an absence of any exudate. The endometrial cavity was dilated and congested with no evidence of retained products of conception. Histopathological examination of the lungs showed the presence of a bright pink eosinophilic hyaline membrane lining the alveolar septae in multiple areas, confirming the diagnosis of diffuse alveolar damage (DAD)—acute respiratory distress syndrome (Fig. 19.2). Occasional alveolar septae showed the presence of type II pneumocyte hyperplasia (Fig. 19.3). There was evidence of focal intra-alveolar edema, hemorrhages, and fresh fibrin thrombi in the small blood vessels. The uterine endometrium showed decidual change, and the myometrium showed physiological hypertrophy and preischemia. The rest of the organs showed congested blood vessels and no other significant pathology.

G. P. Amonkar · K. D. Jashnani (✉)
Department of Pathology, Topiwala National Medical College and BYL Nair Charitable Hospital, Mumbai, Maharashtra, India

K. D. Jashnani (ed.), *Maternal Mortality - Lessons Learnt from Autopsy*,
https://doi.org/10.1007/978-981-19-3420-9_19

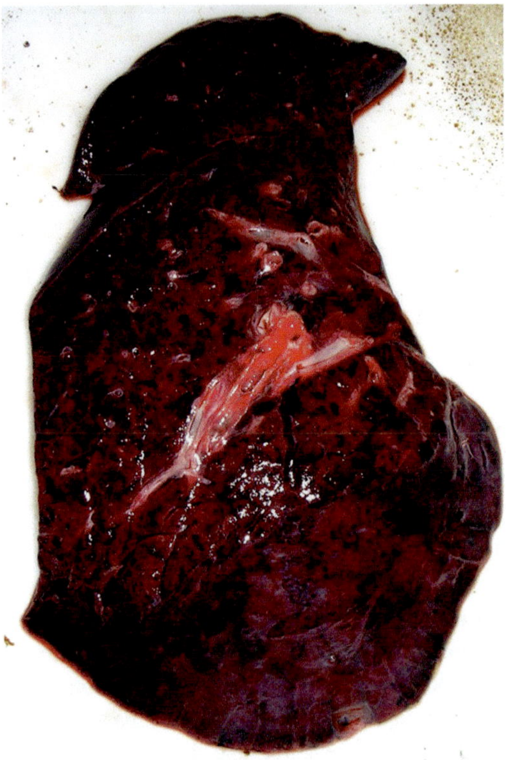

Fig. 19.1 Gross specimen of lung which is markedly congested, voluminous, and boggy (angry red)

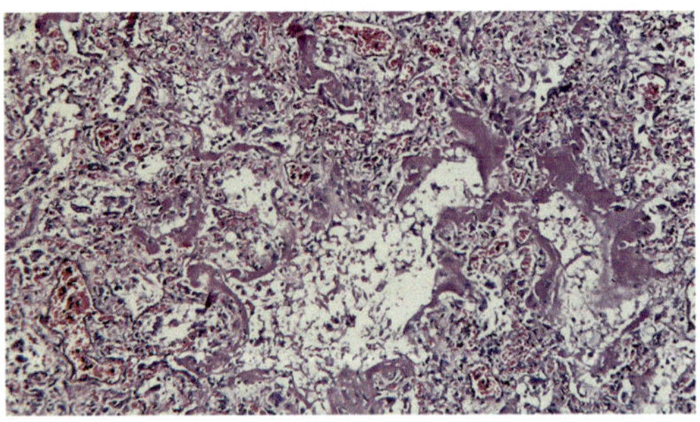

Fig. 19.2 Histopathology of the lung showing the presence of eosinophilic hyaline membranes along the alveolar septae (100×, H&E)

19.3 Final Cause of Death

Acute respiratory distress syndrome in a known case of a H1N1-infection positive female post lower segment cesarean section.

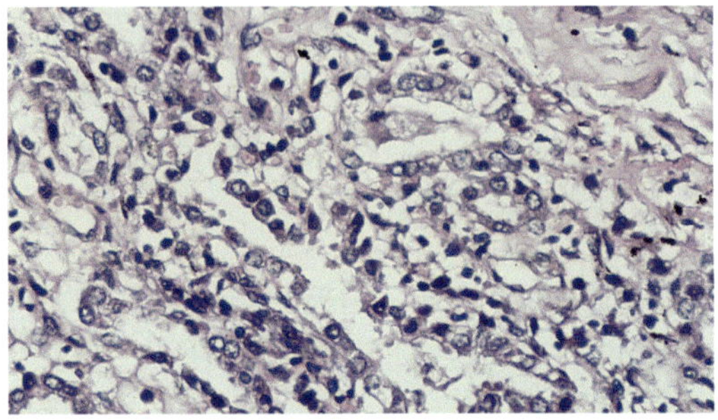

Fig. 19.3 Type 2 pneumocyte hyperplasia seen showing mild to moderate anisonucleosis (400×, H&E)

19.4 Clinicopathologic Discussion

H1N1 Influenza A virus infection can be a cause for maternal and perinatal mortality [1]. Pregnancy causes alterations in the maternal immunological and pathophysiological mechanisms which leads to increased susceptibility to bacterial, viral, and parasitic infections and autoimmune diseases [2]. The severity of the disease is usually higher with an advanced pregnancy. Human infection with the novel H1N1 influenza A virus, previously known as "swine flu," was first reported in April 2009 in Mexico. Influenza A viruses are classified based on the viral surface proteins, hemagglutinin (HA or H) and neuraminidase (NA or N) such as H1N1 and H5N1. The H1N1 influenza A virus causes increased morbidity and mortality in pregnant females. Pregnant women usually suffer a four- to fivefold increase in the incidence of major illness and hospitalization following influenza infection, compared to the general public. Mortality rates are highest if the infection occurs during the third trimester of pregnancy. Patients may present with cough, fever, and chills—the most common symptoms; shortness of breath, hemoptysis, hypoxia, wheezes, tachypnea, and decreased air entry are found in patients with severe symptoms who may require oxygen therapy and intubation with intensive management.

It may also be a cause of increased perinatal mortality and morbidity in the form of spontaneous miscarriages, stillbirths, premature rupture of membranes leading to preterm birth, small for gestational age, and increased NICU admissions with pneumonia.

These pregnant women, due to their increased risk, usually develop primary viral pneumonia and subsequently ARDS requiring mechanical ventilation. Pulmonary histopathology changes include acute lung injury, edema, hemorrhages, congestion, small vessel microthrombi, bronchopneumonia, and type 2 pneumocyte hyperplasia [3–7]. Acute lung injury in the form of hyaline membrane and organized diffuse alveolar damage with fibrosis may be encountered [5]. These histopathological changes may be focal or diffuse in nature. Diffuse alveolar damage (DAD) is the prototype of the acute lung injury pattern and is the histopathological manifestation of ARDS. ARDS includes three stages, with the first being an early acute exudative phase, the second is the subacute proliferative organizing stage, and the last is the late fibrotic stage. The earliest phase is seen in the first week of injury and histologically shows the presence of edema fluid, fibrin, and hemorrhage. Hyaline membranes are usually seen in the proliferative phase, 3–7 days after the initial lung injury. Mild interstitial mononuclear cell infiltration and fibrin thrombi may be seen in this phase. Hyaline membranes are slowly resorbed at the end of this phase. There may be complete resolution, or it may progress to the development of fibrosis; loose clusters of fibroblasts may be seen in the alveolar spaces. In extreme cases, extensive honeycombing of the lung may be seen residually. The organizing phase is marked by the reactive hyperplasia of the type II pneumocytes which may be focal or extensive, and the marked nuclear atypia may mimic malignancy histologically. Bronchioles may show squamous metaplasia. Our case was in the proliferative phase of ARDS going into the organizing phase as histopathology showed the presence of both classic hyaline membranes and type II pneumocyte hyperplasia.

Cytophagocytosis and hemophagocytosis have been reported in some cases. The trachea and bronchi histologically can show the presence of mixed inflammation, desquamation of the epithelium, hemorrhages, and in severe cases necrotizing tracheobronchitis [3, 5]. Other organ findings include myocarditis, brain edema, encephalopathy with hemorrhage, renal acute tubular necrosis, centrilobular necrosis of the liver, and hemorrhagic necrosis of the adrenal glands [8]. No specific inclusion bodies have been described in this infection. In our case, hyaline membranes, edema, hemorrhage and thrombi in small vessels were noted. Cytopathic effects in the form of occasional multinucleated giant cells with enlarged smudged nuclei were seen; however no specific inclusions were noted (Fig. 19.4). A healthy female child of 3.8 kg birth weight was delivered, thus confirming no fetal complications of H1N1 infection.

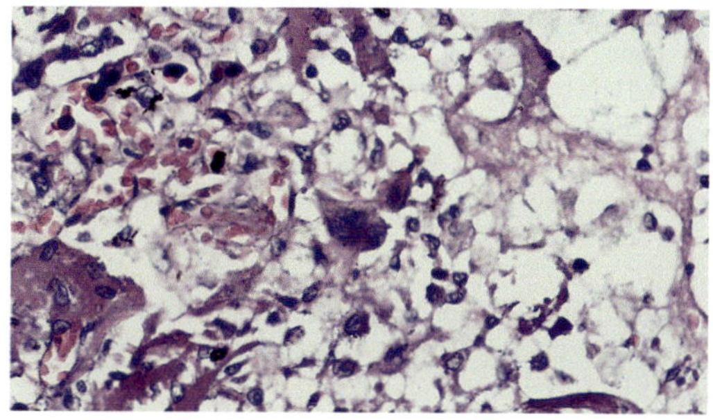

Fig. 19.4 Occasional multinucleated giant cells with enlarged smudged nuclei seen (400×, H&E)

The influenza viral antigen can be demonstrated by immunohistochemistry in the epithelial cells of the trachea, bronchi, bronchial glands, and alveolar epithelial cells [5]. The virus can be detected by electron microscopy and by tissue RT-PCR. Early treatment with Oseltamivir within 48 h of symptom onset, or as early as possible, is associated with fewer complications in hospitalized patients; this was the observation during the 2009 influenza A (H1N1).

References

1. Rasmussen SA, Jamieson DJ, Uyeki TM. Effects of influenza on pregnant women and infants. Am J Obstet Gynecol. 2012;207:S3–8.
2. Kourtis AP, Read JS, Jamieson DJ. Pregnancy and infection. N Engl J Med. 2014;370(23):2211–8.

3. Gill JR, Sheng ZM, Ely SF, et al. Pulmonary pathologic findings of fatal 2009 pandemic influenza A/H1N1 viral infections. Arch Pathol Lab Med. 2010;134:235–43.
4. Rosen DG, Lopez AE, Anzalone ML, et al. Postmortem findings in eight cases of influenza A/H1N1. Mod Pathol. 2010;148:1–9.
5. Nakajima N, Sato Y, Katano H, et al. Histopathological and immunohistochemical findings of 20 autopsy cases with 2009 H1N1 virus infection. Mod Pathol. 2012;25:1–13.
6. Mauad T, Hajjar LA, Callegari GD, et al. Lung pathology in fatal novel human influenza A (H1N1) infection. Am J Respir Crit Care Med. 2010;181(1):72–9.
7. Harms PW, Schmidt LA, Smith LB, et al. Autopsy findings in eight patients with fatal H1N1 influenza. Am J Clin Pathol. 2010;134(1):27–35.
8. Öcal Demir S, Atıcı S, Kepenekli Kadayifci E, et al. Influenza A (H1N1)-associated severe complications; hemolytic uremic syndrome, myocarditis, acute necrotizing encephalopathy. J Infect Dev Ctries. 2019;13(1):83–6.

“Über Diffuse” Myocarditis: Still a Giant Mystery!

20

Sneha Debbarma, Kusum D. Jashnani, Lalita Yoganand Patil, and Vrinda Kiran Kulkarni

20.1 Clinical History

A 26-year-old mother of a 3 1/2-year-old child, registered in the antenatal clinic as second gravida with a history of 6 1/2 weeks of amenorrhea, was admitted with complaints of sudden onset breathlessness, palpitation, vomiting, and bleeding per vagina for 1 day. She was scheduled for an voluntary termination of pregnancy and further treatment. She had received two rounds of DC shock and also amiodarone in view of ventricular tachycardia before she was referred to our tertiary hospital. Her general condition was poor during admission. Her physical examination revealed a pulse rate of 170 beats/min, blood pressure of 90/60 mmHg, respiratory rate of 35/min, and bilateral crepitation on chest auscultation with audible S1 and S2. She was shifted to the ICU, intubated, and initiated on mechanical ventilation.

Her laboratory investigations were as follows: hemoglobin 13.8 g/dL, hematocrit 42.7%, total leukocyte count 22.57 × 10^3/ml, platelets 354 × 10^3/ml, serum potassium 4.58 meq/l, serum creatinine 1.58 mg/dl.

Her ECG showed normal sinus rhythm with a right bundle branch block.

On 2D echocardiography, global left ventricular dysfunction with reduction in ejection fraction (35–40%) was seen, along with right ventricular aneurysmal dilatation with dyskinesia. An echogenic structure measuring 2.3 × 3.4 cm involving the right ventricle was viewed, which was suggestive of a thrombus. Mitral regurgitation was moderate, whereas tricuspid regurgitation was severe. An impression likely of arrhythmogenic right ventricular cardiomyopathy was drawn.

An early obstetric scan done on the day of onset of symptoms was suggestive of twin live intrauterine gestation of an average of 6 weeks and 2 days. Ultrasonography of the whole abdomen showed minimal ascites with gallbladder wall edema, right-sided mild pleural effusion, and mild hepatosplenomegaly.

Clinically, two differentials were considered: arrhythmogenic right ventricular dysplasia or right ventricular clot in situ. The patient's condition kept deteriorating, and in about 7 h of admis-

S. Debbarma
Shrimati Diwaliben Mohanlal Mehta Maa Sarvasadharan Rugnalay, Mumbai, Maharashtra, India

K. D. Jashnani (✉) · L. Y. Patil
Department of Pathology, Topiwala National Medical College and BYL Nair Charitable Hospital, Mumbai, Maharashtra, India

V. K. Kulkarni
Department of Medicine and Clinical Hematology, Topiwala National Medical College and BYL Nair Charitable Hospital, Mumbai, Maharashtra, India

K. D. Jashnani (ed.), *Maternal Mortality - Lessons Learnt from Autopsy*,
https://doi.org/10.1007/978-981-19-3420-9_20

sion, she expired. As per protocol, an autopsy with the necessary permission was performed.

20.2 Autopsy Findings

Grossly, the heart appeared enlarged and weighed 480 g, while the apex was formed by both the right and left ventricles. The right atrium and left ventricle were dilated with the latter appearing thinned out. A normal whitish aortomitral fibrous band was seen between the aortic and mitral valves (Fig. 20.1). No aneurysmal dilatation or organized thrombi were seen within the heart chambers. All coronaries were patent, and the aorta was unremarkable.

On histopathological examination, sections from the left ventricle showed marked destruction of myocardium by diffuse inflammatory cell infiltrate composed of lymphocytes, plasma cells, histiocytes, and many multinucleated giant cells (Figs. 20.2 and 20.3). This infiltration was also seen to extend to the epicardium. Evidence of myocytolysis was present, and fibrosis was also noted in places. The endocardium appeared unremarkable. There was no evidence of epithelioid cell granulomas, necrosis, bacterial colonies, or any other infective etiological agent. Sections from the right ventricle showed normal endocardium, myocardium, and epicardium. PAS and GMS stains were negative for fungi or any other infective organisms. Histopathological impression was that of giant cell myocarditis.

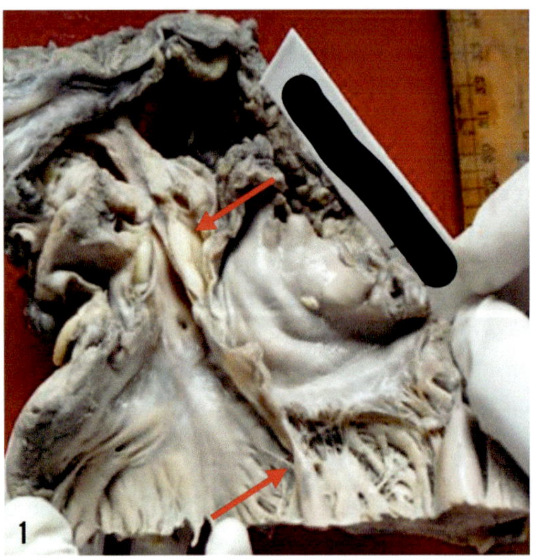

Fig. 20.1 Gross morphology of the heart showing the dilated left ventricle with a whitish aortomitral fibrous band seen between the aortic and mitral valves (arrows)

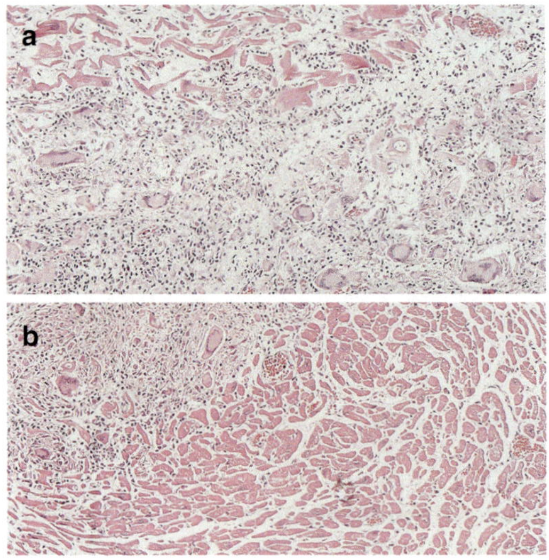

Fig. 20.2 (**a**, **b**) (H&E 100×): low power appearance of extensive damage to myocytes and infiltration by diffuse inflammatory cell infiltrate. Many multinucleated giant cells can be identified in (**a**)

Each lung weighed about 240 g. The pleura appeared smooth and shiny, and a focal area of collapse was seen. The lungs were rubbery in consistency with no evidence of pulmonary emboli. Microscopically, pleura showed mild fibrous thickening, interstitium was widened showing lymphocytes and congested capillaries, and alveolar spaces showed the presence of foamy macrophages and few multinucleated giant cells. Blood vessels and bronchioles were unremarkable. There was no evidence of epithelioid cell granulomas or necrosis. An impression of interstitial pneumonia was made. The rest of the organs were unremarkable on gross and microscopy.

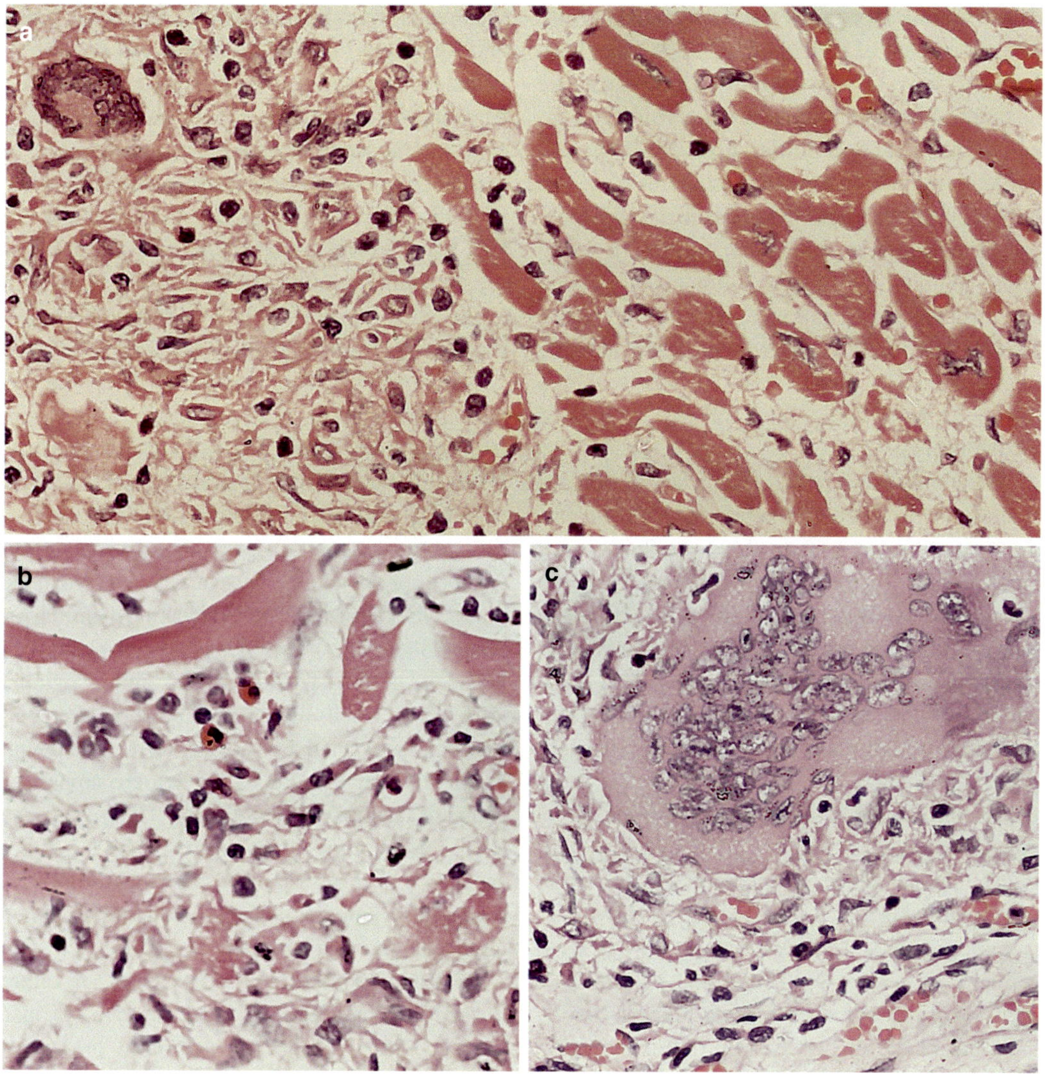

Fig. 20.3 (**a**, **b**) (H&E 400×): on higher power, the infiltration can be seen consisting of lymphocytes, plasma cells, histiocytes, few eosinophils (**b**), and multinucleated giant cells (**a**). (**c**) (H&E 400×): a giant cell can be seen consisting of more than 20 nuclei

20.3 Final Cause of Death

Cardiogenic shock in a case of giant cell myocarditis with interstitial pneumonitis.

20.4 Clinicopathologic Discussion

GCM is a rare entity, and symptomatic individuals can present with cardiac failure, dysrhythmias, heart block, dyspnea, acute coronary syndromes, cardiogenic shock, acute febrile illnesses, fatigue, or sudden death. The progression is rapid, and it frequently proves fatal. Noncardiac complaints like painless hematemesis have also been reported [1–4]. It is known to usually occur in the relatively young and otherwise healthy adults [5]. Ever since the early 1970s, GCM has been recognized as a separate entity from cardiac sarcoidosis, rheumatic heart disease, and Wegener's granulomatosis [6] with its etiology being predominantly unknown. GCM in the fulminant form should be considered separate from the isolated atrial GCM which is an indolent variant and is usually an incidental finding in surgical atrial specimens [7, 8]. Twenty percent of patients with GCM have been found to have an association with autoimmune disorders like ulcerative colitis, cryofibrinogenemia, rheumatoid arthritis, myasthenia gravis, hyperthyroidism, or hypothyroidism. It may also be associated with drug hypersensitivity, Wegener granulomatosis, thymoma, sarcoidosis, or infections. Without aggressive immunosuppression and cardiac transplantation, along with supportive therapy for congestive heart failure, tachyarrhythmias, and heart block, death occurs within a period of weeks or months since the onset of symptoms [2].

The clinical differential diagnoses to be considered for ARVD/C in the present case are cardiac sarcoidosis, idiopathic outflow tract tachycardias, some congenital heart disease with RV volume overload, and, if LV is involved, any type of idiopathic nonischemic dilated cardiomyopathy [9]. The differential diagnosis of an echogenic right heart mass on 2D echo, apart from thrombus, includes tumor and tricuspid valve vegetations [10, 11].

A final diagnosis in the living is possible by histopathological study of endomyocardial biopsy, apical-wedge samples, or sections from the explanted heart.

Serpiginous and grayish patches in the myocardium are seen, which represent confluent or multifocal areas of necrosis and allow a convenient naked eye diagnosis on gross examination [5, 6, 12]. The weight of the heart may be normal or increased slightly, with a uniform involvement of the four chambers of the heart in most cases. Mural thrombi may be present. The process essentially involves the myocardium, but endocardial and pericardial involvement can also occur [13, 14].

As proposed by Litovsky et al. [13], GCM can be classified into acute, healing, and healed phases. The acute phase is characterised by abundant inflammatory response, loose connective tissue stroma, and numerous giant cells. In the healing or resolving stage, the giant cells and inflammatory cells are reduced in number, while the myocardium is replaced by granulation tissue and immature fibrosis. Myocytes can be seen as islands of isolated cells or in small clusters, with surrounding scar tissue. There is an overlap to some extent seen between the different stages, in explanted or postmortem heart specimens, which is suggestive of temporal heterogeneity in GCM. A caution is warranted to be taken in this regard while scrutinizing an EMB specimen to grade the response to immunosuppressive therapy.

The differential diagnoses for GCM are the various granulomatous diseases which may present itself with clinical and morphological similarities, but the absence of granulomas along with the presence of giant cells on histopathological examination aid in diagnosing GCM. Immunohistochemical studies (not done in the present case) show that the giant cells stain with CD68, indicating their macrophage/monocyte origin. They do not stain with muscle markers like actin, desmin, and myoglobin [15]. CD3+ T cells are the predominant inflammatory cell type, whereas B cells are rare or absent. During the active phase, CD8 cytotoxic/suppressor cells are far more numerous than CD4 cells. The sequel of inflammatory injury to myocytes is represented by the occasionally found actin-positive myogenic-type giant cells at the edge of inflamed and viable myocytes in the healing stage.

In a country like India, most cases are either missed or diagnosed only on autopsy because biopsies from the endomyocardium or apical-wedge samples in such cases are rarely acquired [16]. Better understanding of the etiopathophysiology means enabling appropriate management of the condition.

References

1. Vaideeswar P, Cooper LT. Giant cell myocarditis: clinical and pathological features in an Indian population. Cardiovasc Pathol. 2013;22(1):70–4. https://doi.org/10.1016/j.carpath.2012.06.003.
2. Cooper LT Jr, Berry GJ, Shabetai R. Idiopathic giant-cell myocarditis–natural history and treatment. N Engl J Med. 1997;336(26):1860–6. https://doi.org/10.1056/NEJM199706263362603.

3. Cooper LT. Giant cell myocarditis in children. Prog Pediatr Cardiol. 2007;24(1):47–9. https://doi.org/10.1016/j.ppedcard.2007.08.002.
4. Anderson K, Carrier M, Romeo P, Pelletier GB, Liszkowski M, Racine N, White M, et al. An unusual case of giant cell myocarditis missed in a Heartmate-2 left ventricle apical-wedge section: a case report and review of the literature. J Cardiothorac Surg. 2013;8:12. https://doi.org/10.1186/1749-8090-8-12.
5. Permi HS. Idiopathic giant cell myocarditis presenting as sudden cardiac death- a rare case report. Nitte Univ J Health Sci. 2014;4(2):142–3.
6. Davies MJ, Pomerance A, Teare RD. Idiopathic giant cell myocarditis–a distinctive clinico-pathological entity. Br Heart J. 1975;37(2):192–5. https://doi.org/10.1136/hrt.37.2.192.
7. Ahmad I, Craig MD, Berry GJ, et al. Isolated giant cell myocarditis in the atrium: an incidental finding? Pacing Clin Electrophysiol. 2006;29:1179–80.
8. Larsen BT, Maleszewski JJ, Edwards WD, et al. Atrial giant cell myocarditis: a distinctive clinicopathologic entity. Circulation. 2013;127:39–47.
9. Corrado D, Link MS, Calkins H. Arrhythmogenic right ventricular cardiomyopathy. N Engl J Med. 2017;376:61–72.
10. Woodridge JD, Healey J. Echocardiographic diagnosis of right ventricular thromboembolism. Am Heart J. 1983;106:590–1.
11. Come PC, Kurland GS, Vine HS. Two-dimensional echocardiography in differentiating right atrial and tricuspid valve mass lesions. Am J Cardiol. 1978;44(1207-1):2.
12. Murty OP. Giant cell myocarditis with cardiac tamponade: a rare combination. Am J Forensic Med Pathol. 2008;29(3):245–8. https://doi.org/10.1097/PAF.0b013e318183d55f.
13. Litovsky SH, Burke AP, Virmani R. Giant cell myocarditis: an entity distinct from sarcoidosis characterized by multiphasic myocyte destruction by cytotoxic T cells and histiocytic giant cells. Mod Pathol. 1996;9:1126–34.
14. Berry GJ, Marboe CC. Idiopathic giant cell myocarditis. In: Mills SE, editor. Heart. Sternberg's diagnostic surgical pathology, vol. 1. Philadelphia: Wolters Kluwer Health; 2015. p. 2764–6.
15. Ariza A, Lopez MD, Mate JL, et al. Giant cell myocarditis: monocytic immunophenotype of giant cells in a case associated with ulcerative colitis. Hum Pathol. 1995;26:121–3.
16. Shanmugam J, Kumar PS, Panicker VK, Duvooru P. Sudden death due to giant cell myocarditis: a case report. Cardiol Res. 2015;6(6):372–5. https://doi.org/10.14740/cr446e.

21 Liver: A Fatal Target of Sepsis-Related Organ Dysfunction

Niyati N. Sangoi, Kusum D. Jashnani, Lalita Yoganand Patil, and Rosemarie de Souza

21.1 Clinical History

A 26-year-old female, primigravida, came with presenting complaints of high colored urine for 15 days, altered sensorium for 1 day, and abdominal pain for 4 days. The patient had history of one episode of generalized tonic-clonic seizure in the past 24 h. The patient had a full-term vaginal delivery of a stillborn male fetus weighing 2 kg at a local hospital, following which she was transferred to another hospital in view of clinical impression of hepatitis and, finally, to our hospital, where she had a hospital stay of 19 h. The patient had history of excessive blood loss post-delivery. The patient had no significant past medical history. She had no history of any bleeding from other sites, rash, melena, cold, or cough.

On examination, the patient was febrile and icteric. Her pulse rate was 90/min and regular and blood pressure was 150/90 mmHg. Her central nervous system examination revealed altered behavior and decerebrate posturing. Her abdomen was non-tender. The patient was transfused with four units of fresh frozen plasma during her hospital stay. Her condition deteriorated rapidly, and despite all resuscitative measures, the patient was declared dead after 19 h of hospital admission.

N. N. Sangoi · K. D. Jashnani (✉) · L. Y. Patil
Department of Pathology, Topiwala National Medical College and BYL Nair Charitable Hospital, Mumbai, Maharashtra, India

R. de Souza
Department of Medicine, Topiwala National Medical College and BYL Nair Charitable Hospital, Mumbai, Maharashtra, India

21.2 Investigations

Hemogram Hemoglobin 6.9 g/dL, total leucocyte count 41,000/μL with polymorphonuclear leukocytosis, platelet count 140,000/μL. Serology tests for hepatitis A, B, C, and E were negative. Biochemical profile: BUN 40 mg/dl, S. creatinine 1.94 mg/dl, random blood glucose 168 mg/dl, Na+ −120 mEq/L, K+ −5.2 mEq/L, total protein 5.7 g/dl, SGOT 115 U/L, SGPT 62 U/L, total bilirubin 16.7 mg/dl, direct bilirubin 8.7 mg/dl, prothrombin time 31.8 s (control was 14 s), and international normalized ratio (INR) 2.67. Her arterial blood gas analysis was suggestive of metabolic acidosis. Her fever profile was negative. Blood was sent for culture, and the report which was available after the autopsy revealed E coli organisms.

Cerebrospinal fluid examination showed no cells under microscopy. Ascitic fluid examination revealed 200 cells/mm^3 with 74% polymorphs and 26% lymphocytes. Pleural fluid examination revealed 150 cells/mm^3 with 55% polymorphs

K. D. Jashnani (ed.), *Maternal Mortality - Lessons Learnt from Autopsy*,
https://doi.org/10.1007/978-981-19-3420-9_21

and 45% lymphocytes. Her ECG was within normal limits.

Clinical impression was given as hepatitis with hepatic encephalopathy with coagulopathy and sepsis.

21.3 Autopsy Findings

A complete autopsy was performed on this patient, after due permission. On external examination, the skin and sclera showed the presence of icterus. Internal examination revealed the presence of approximately 1 l of blood mixed fluid in the thoracic cavity with the presence of a blood clot in the right mediastinum. The clot weighed 250 g and measured 11 × 10 × 2 cm. On microscopy, this clot showed large areas of hemorrhage with intervening foci of fibrin and a dense neutrophilic infiltrate. All the organs appeared pale on gross examination. The liver weighed 900 g. The capsule showed mild wrinkling with the liver appearing very pale on the cut surface (Fig. 21.1a). On histopathologic examination, the normal lobular hepatic architecture was maintained. Multiple tiny foci of hepatocytic necrosis were seen, along with the presence of lympho-

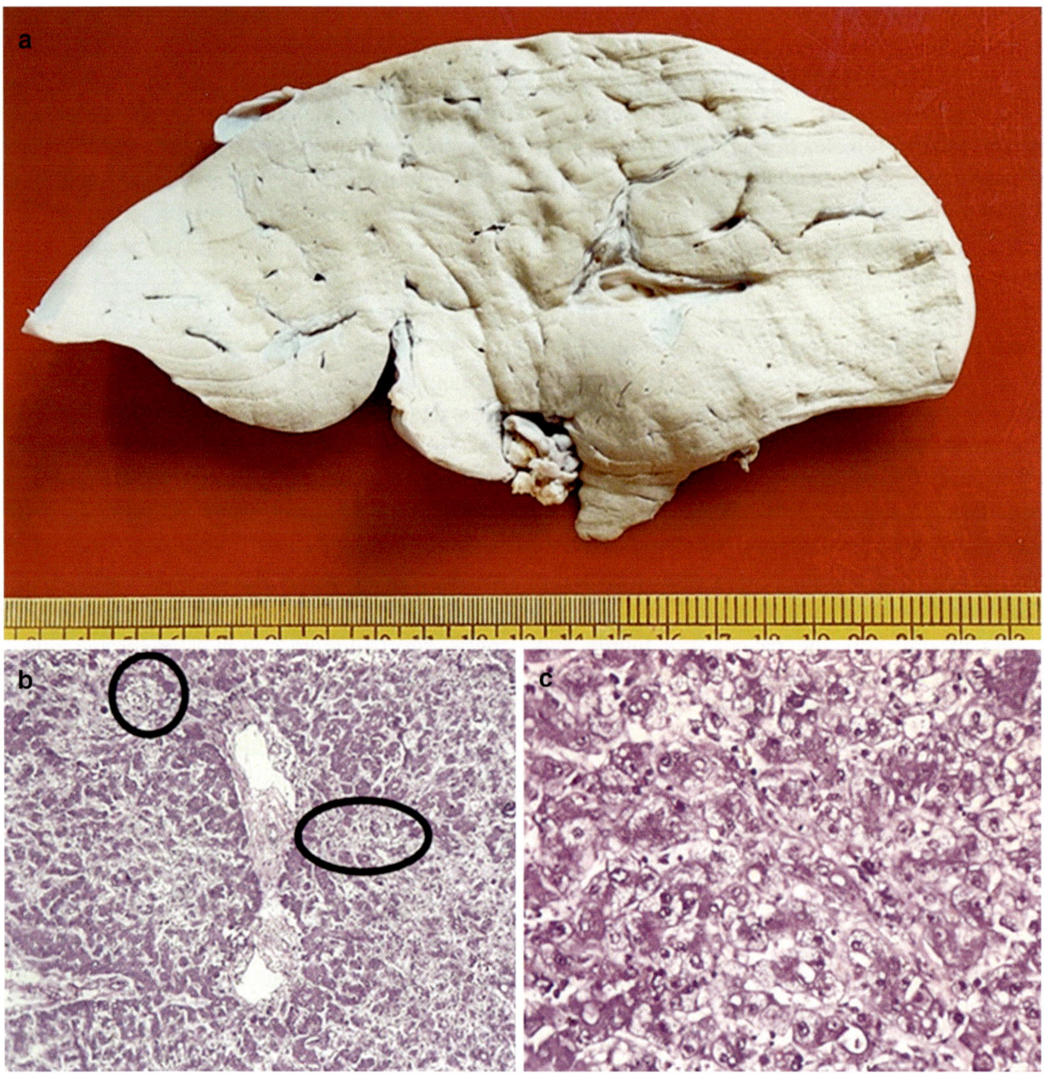

Fig. 21.1 (**a**) Coronal gross slice of the liver which is very pale. (**b**, **c**) Liver showing tiny foci of hepatocytic necrosis with the presence of lymphocytes (circled). Surrounding hepatocytes show balloon degeneration (**b**). The sinusoids are dilated and show the presence of lymphocytes; surrounding hepatocytes show balloon degeneration (**c**) (H&E, 100×, 400×)

cytes. Areas of bridging necrosis were also seen. Thirty percent of the hepatocytes showed balloon degeneration, and 20% of the hepatocytes showed microvesicular fatty change, rest were unremarkable. The sinusoids were dilated and congested and showed the presence of few lymphocytes (Fig. 21.1b, c). Focal areas of intrahepatocyte cholestasis were also seen. All these features suggested acute hepatitis. The pancreas weighed 70 g with the cut surface showing preserved normal lobular architecture with areas of chalky white necrosis in interstitial and peripancreatic fat. On microscopy, the normal architecture of the pancreas was maintained with multiple areas showing acinar destruction and the presence of a dense neutrophilic inflammatory infiltrate along with apoptotic bodies. The pancreatic ducts showed luminal obstruction by inspissated eosinophilic secretions with a dense neutrophilic infiltrate in some ducts. The intervening and surrounding fatty tissue showed multiple foci of fat necrosis with surrounding areas of inflammation (Fig. 21.2a, b). These features were suggestive of acute pancreatitis with fat necrosis. The kidneys were unremarkable on gross. Microscopy

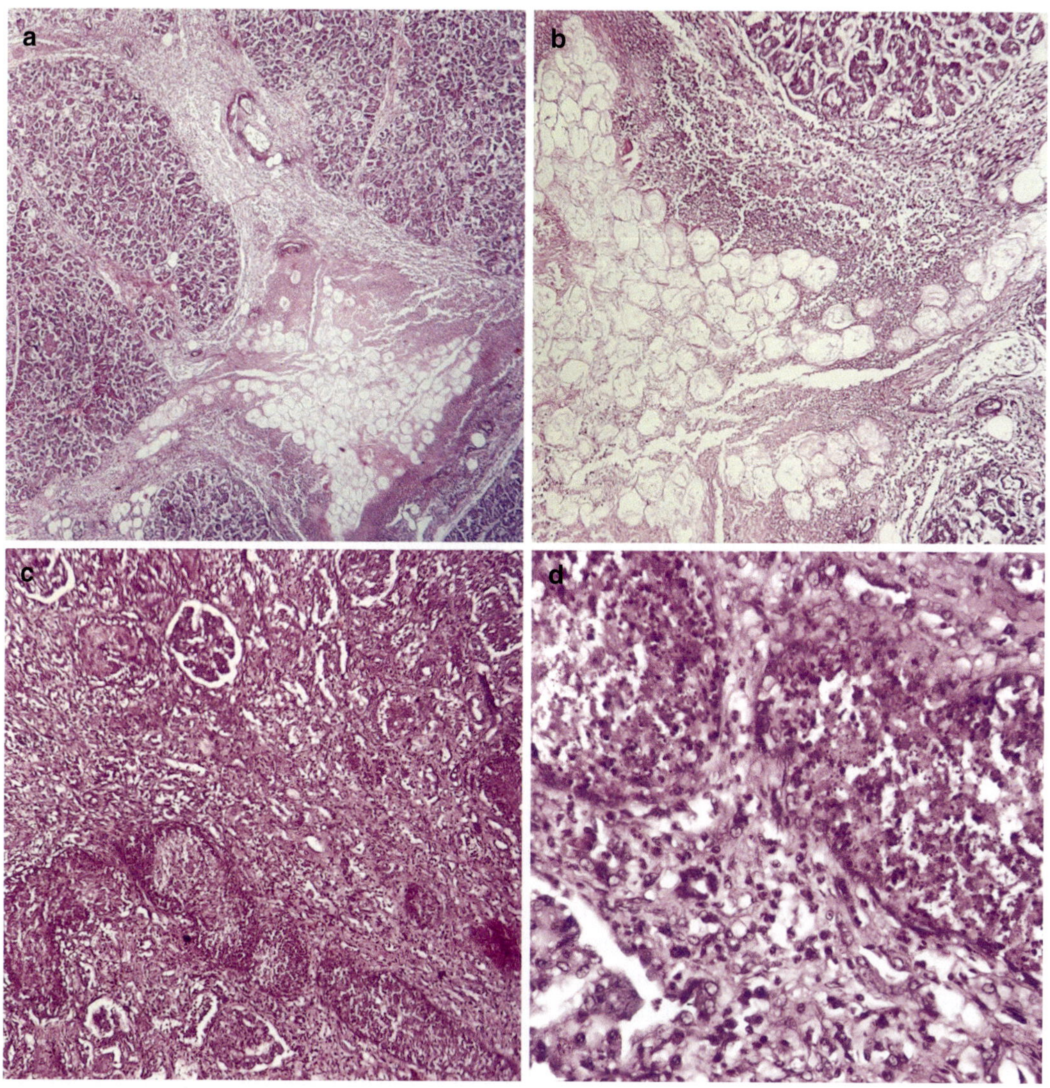

Fig. 21.2 (**a**, **b**) Pancreas showing foci of destruction of pancreatic acini with surrounding areas showing fat necrosis and inflammation (H&E, 100×, 200×). (**c**, **d**) Kidney showing the presence of a mixed inflammatory infiltrate in the interstitium with the tubules showing presence of pus casts (H&E, 100×, 400×)

showed congested glomerular and interstitial capillaries along with focal areas of interstitial mixed inflammatory infiltrate. The tubules showed the presence of pus casts and foci of acute tubular necrosis. Blood vessels were unremarkable (Fig. 21.2c, d). These features were suggestive of acute tubulointerstitial nephritis. The right lung weighed 150 g and appeared collapsed (confirmed on microscopy). The left lung weighed 220 g, with frothy fluid oozing out under pressure on the cut surface, suggestive of pulmonary edema (confirmed on microscopy). Gross examination of the uterus was unremarkable. On microscopy, the endometrium was decidualized with the attached fibrin clot showing neutrophilic infiltrate. The rest of the organs were unremarkable on gross and microscopy.

21.4 Final Cause of Death

Sepsis-associated encephalopathy with multiorgan failure in a postpartum female.

21.5 Clinicopathologic Discussion

Septic inflammatory response leads to brain dysfunction (septic encephalopathy), which is independent of other coexistent causes such as liver or renal dysfunction. Up to 60–70% of patients with sepsis have some degree of encephalopathy. Hepatitis in pregnancy can have various etiologies ranging from infections, autoimmunity, drugs, acute fatty liver of pregnancy, and portal thrombosis. Hepatitis A, B, C, and E, dengue, cytomegalovirus, HTLV, brucellosis, and rubella are the main infectious agents. Hepatitis can manifest as acute or chronic and can lead to liver damage, acute liver cell failure, or even liver carcinoma. The most common specific liver disease observed during pregnancy is intrahepatic cholestasis of pregnancy, whose commonest presenting symptom is pruritis. Acute fatty liver of pregnancy is a rare but fatal pathology. Preeclampsia can lead to HELLP [1].

Sepsis is a rare occurrence in pregnancy, and there has been an increase in sepsis related maternal mortality indicated by recent studies. Advanced age, comorbidities such as obesity, diabetes mellitus, and hypertension are the risk factors responsible for the increase in sepsis-related deaths. Complications of sepsis during pregnancy include premature delivery, infection in the fetus, higher fetal mortality, and increased necessity to perform a cesarean section delivery [2].

The liver plays a key role in maintaining homeostasis. The incidence of sepsis-associated liver dysfunction (SALD) is not well established. Metabolism of hepatocytes is modified towards the inflammatory response in the case of sepsis. Interleukin-6 is the main cytokine of the liver inflammatory response. It is responsible for synthesizing acute phase proteins whose increased concentration leads to protein C pathway inhibition, causing increased coagulation factor activity. Sepsis can show a wide range of coagulopathies ranging from mild abnormalities in the laboratory results of clotting time, prothrombin time, and platelet count to severe coagulopathy and disseminated intravascular coagulation. Histopathological examination of the liver in patients with jaundice occurring due to bacterial infections shows the presence of intrahepatic cholestasis. This occurs due to alterations in genes activating transcription and modifying posttranslational treatment of bile acids transporting proteins caused by lipopolysaccharide and proinflammatory cytokines [3]. When acute liver failure complicates pregnancy, mortality approaches 40% and the only viable alternative is liver transplantation [4]. Pancreatic injury is commonly seen in patients with sepsis and septic shock. The main cause for the same is tissue hypoperfusion. Other causes include oxidative stress, overwhelming inflammatory response, cellular apoptosis, and/or metabolic derangements [5].

In the present case, the patient presented with jaundice, fever, and altered sensorium. Her total leucocyte count was high with neutrophilic leukocytosis. Her serum creatinine, total bilirubin, direct bilirubin, prothrombin time, and international normalized ratio were elevated. Serum transaminases were mildly elevated. Her autopsy findings revealed multiple organ involvement – liver, pancreas, and kidney with the presence of serous effusions showing polymorphonuclear predominance. Her hemoglobin was low, which was reflected by all organs being pale during autopsy. The patient thus went into septic shock with multiorgan involvement.

Sepsis as a possible cause of liver dysfunction in pregnancy should be kept in mind when the patient presents with jaundice, deranged liver function tests, and all serology tests for hepatitis being negative. Early diagnosis of sepsis and its related complications can lead to immediate therapeutic action and possibly reduce the incidence of mortality.

References

1. Sarmento AMP, Oliveira ACT, Barbosa APXP, et al. Acute hepatitis in pregnancy: a case report. Asp Biomed Clin Case Rep. 2020;3(3):225–33.
2. Cordioli RL, Cordioli E, Negrini R, Silva E. Sepsis and pregnancy: do we know how to treat this situation? Rev Bras Ter Intensiva. 2013;25(4):334–44.
3. Woźnica EA, Inglot M, Woźnica RK, Łysenko L. Liver dysfunction in sepsis. Adv Clin Exp Med. 2018;27(4):547–51.
4. Pandey CK, Karna ST, Pandey VK, Tandon M. Acute liver failure in pregnancy: challenges and management. Indian J Anaesth. 2015;59:144–9.
5. Chaari A, Abdel Hakim K, Bousselmi K, et al. Pancreatic injury in patients with septic shock: a literature review. World J Gastrointest Oncol. 2016;8(7):526–31.

22 Complicated Malaria in Pregnancy

Daksha Piyush Prabhat,
Tejaswini Priyadarshan Waghmare,
and Pradeep Vaideeswar

22.1 Clinical History

A 26-year-old female with 5 months of amenorrhea was referred from a peripheral hospital (hospitalization for 2 days) with complaints of fever with chills and vomiting for 6 days and altered sensorium for 2 days. On examination, her pulse was 88 per minute and blood pressure 100/60 mm Hg. She was afebrile, pale, had mild icterus, and there was abdominal tenderness. She was disoriented but was responding to simple commands. Her pupils were sluggishly reacting to light. There was no neck stiffness.

Obstetric history: She had two earlier pregnancies. Her first child, a 5-year-old-male child, was a FTND. In her second pregnancy, she delivered twins, but both had expired on their day of birth. The third is the present pregnancy. She had not registered for antenatal care in any of her pregnancies.

Laboratory investigations: The salient abnormalities noted included hemoglobin of 5.4 g%, total count of 5400/mm^3, and a platelet count of 40,000/mm^3 with occasional trophozoites, and few gametocytes of *Plasmodium falciparum* identified on peripheral smear (Fig. 22.2a). In addition, the serum creatinine was 2.3 mg/dL and total bilirubin 3.5 mg/dL. Ultrasonography of the abdomen had been reported as hepatosplenomegaly with multiple splenic abscesses/infarcts and medical renal disease.

The clinical impression was *Plasmodium falciparum* malaria with thrombocytopenia with 5 months of amenorrhoea with splenic abscess and anemia. She was administered intravenous anti-malarials and antibiotics and was also transfused with 4 units of platelets and 1 unit of whole blood. However she developed breathlessness and hypotension and succumbed on the third day of hospitalization.

22.2 Autopsy Findings

A complete autopsy was performed on an averagely built and nourished woman. Mild pallor and icterus were noted on external examination. Linea nigra was noted on the abdomen that was distended (circumference 82 cm) with a uterine enlargement of approximately 20 weeks. The brain showed corticovenous congestion and mild edema. The heart weighed 220 g and showed mild left ventricular hypertrophy. The lungs were voluminous, rubbery and firm and showed patchy red congestion, suggestive of acute respiratory distress syndrome (ARDS). The vasculature was prominent; the bronchial tree was normal.

D. P. Prabhat (✉) · T. P. Waghmare
Department of Pathology (Clinical Pathology and Hematology Division), Seth G.S. Medical College and K.E.M Hospital, Mumbai, Maharashtra, India

P. Vaideeswar
Department of Pathology (Cardiovascular and Thoracic Division), Seth GS Medical College and KEM Hospital, Mumbai, Maharashtra, India

K. D. Jashnani (ed.), *Maternal Mortality - Lessons Learnt from Autopsy*,
https://doi.org/10.1007/978-981-19-3420-9_22

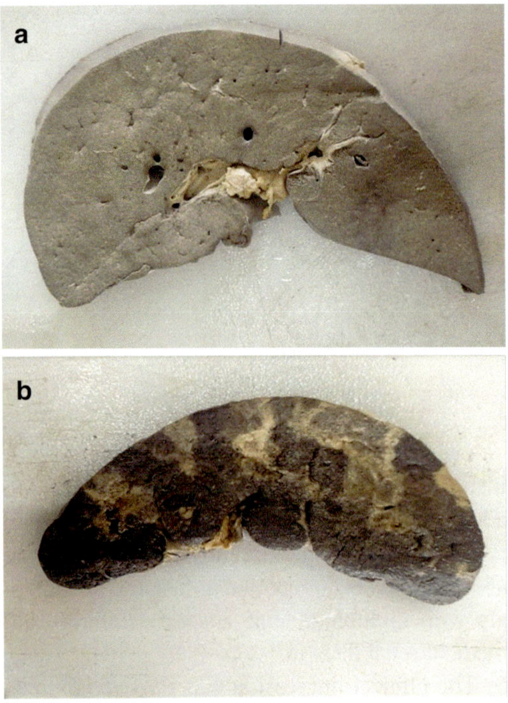

Fig. 22.1 (**a**) Gross: shows an enlarged liver with slate grey discolouration. (**b**) Gross: shows an enlarged spleen with multiple irregular pale infarcts

Pulmonary embolism was not noted. The liver was markedly enlarged (2.3 kg), congested, soft, foldable, and slate grey in colour (Fig. 22.1a). The spleen was enlarged (360 g) and showed the presence of multiple irregular pale firm areas of infarcts ranging from 1 × 1 cm to 4 × 5 cm and had hyperaemic borders (Fig. 22.1b). Some of these showed small areas of central necrosis. The kidneys were slightly enlarged, bilaterally weighed 130 g each and showed few irregular pale areas externally and prominent cortical striations on the cut surface. Petechiae were present on the pelvicalyceal mucosa. An enlarged uterus of size 26 × 20 × 5 cm contained a male fetus weighing 600 g in a breech position. The placenta appeared normal, and no abnormality was noted in the uterus. All other organs appeared normal.

On microscopic examination, the cerebrum revealed multiple Dürck's granulomas (Fig. 22.2c), petechial hemorrhages and congested vessels with occasional parasitized red blood cells (Fig. 22.2d). In the heart, the left ventricle showed mild hypertrophy of fibres. Sections of the lungs showed diffuse alveolar damage with focal bronchopneumonia. Edema fluid was noted in the alveolar spaces along with a few neutrophils in a fibrinous background and a few hyaline membranes (Fig. 22.3d). The liver showed marked Kupffer cell hyperplasia with blackish brown hemozoin pigment deposition (Fig. 22.3c), congested sinusoids with few parasitized red cells. Multiple areas of infarction along with marked sinusoidal congestion and reticuloendothelial cell hyperplasia with malarial pigment deposition were present in the spleen (Fig. 22.3a, b). Bone marrow exhibited erythroid hyperplasia and prominent macrophages with malarial pigment (Fig. 22.2b). Kidneys revealed patchy tubular necrosis. The placenta also showed the deposition of malarial pigment.

22.3 Final Cause of Death

Complicated malaria (cerebral malaria with ARDS) in a female with 5 months' amenorrhoea.

22.4 Clinicopathologic Discussion

Malaria, a parasitic infection transmitted by female anopheles mosquitoes, is one of the most devastating amongst infectious diseases. It is the second most common cause of infectious disease-related deaths in the world, after tuberculosis [1]. Malaria is caused by one or more of the four species of *Plasmodium* that infect humans: vivax, ovale, malariae and falciparum. Of these, *Plasmodium falciparum* is the most deadly [1].

The ability of *Plasmodium falciparum* to cause cytoadherence of erythrocytes to vascular walls causes sequestration of infected cells in small blood vessels. This further leads to end organ damage via hemorrhage or infarct [1]. Phagocytosis of infected blood cells in the spleen not only helps clear infection but also contributes to profound anemia and folic acid deficiency.

Pregnant women, children and immunocompromised individuals are seen to have the highest

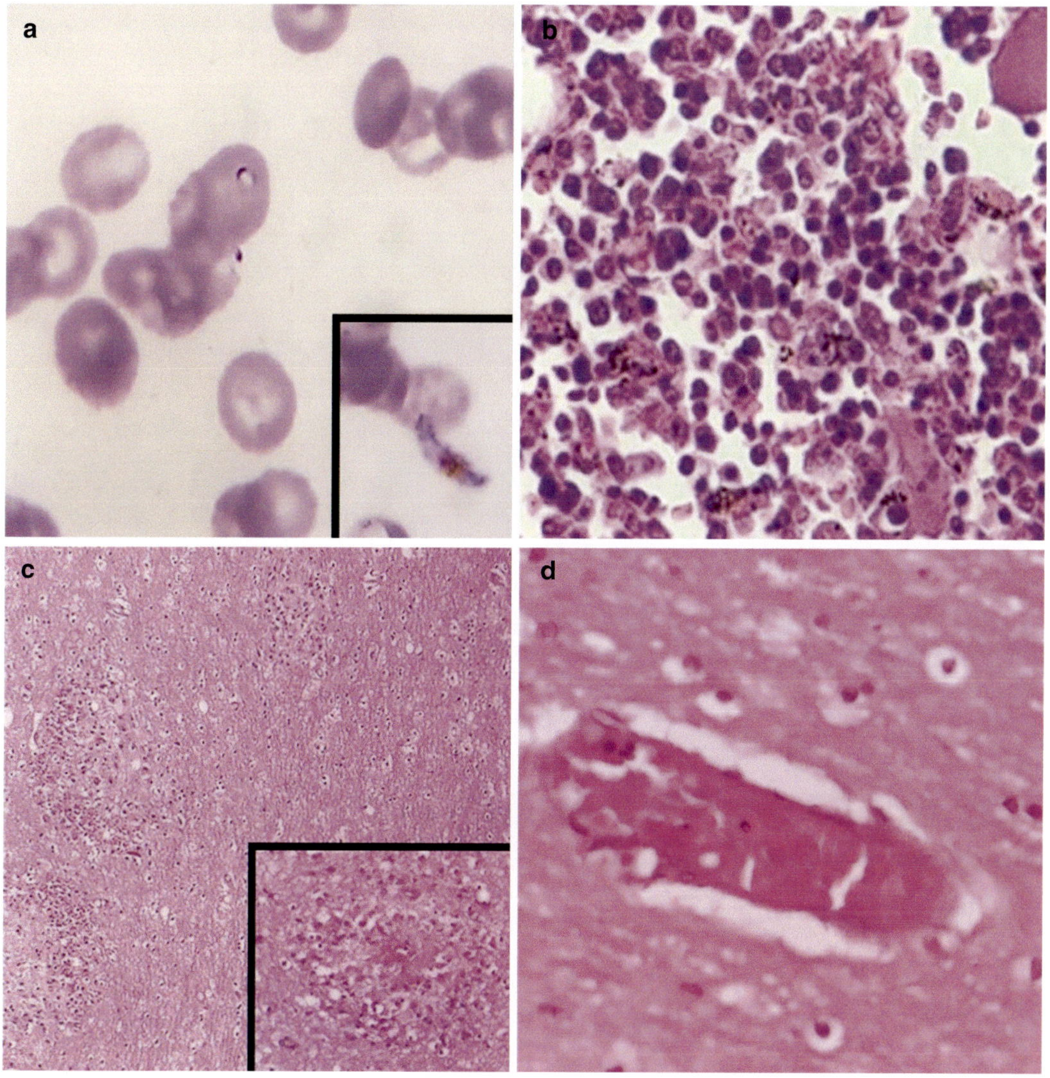

Fig. 22.2 (**a**) Peripheral smear (Leishmann, 100×) showing trophozoites of *P. falciparum*. Inset: gametocyte of *P. falciparum*. (**b**) Bone marrow (H&E 400×) showing the presence of granular brown hemazoin pigment. (**c**) Cerebrum (H&E 400×) showing multiple Dürck's granulomas inset: Dürck's granuloma. (**d**) Cerebrum (H&E 400×) showing congested vessels with an occasional parasitized RBC

morbidity and mortality. Pregnant women infected with malaria are three times more likely to suffer from severe disease as a result of malarial infection compared with their non-pregnant counterparts [1]. They have severe symptoms and outcomes, with higher rates of miscarriages, intrauterine fetal demise, premature delivery, low-birth-weight neonates and neonatal death [1]. They are also at a higher risk for severe anemia and maternal death, with mortality rates of approximately 50%. It is hypothesized that the majority of sequelae in pregnancy results from two main factors: the immunocompromised state of pregnancy and placental sequestration of infected erythrocytes. It is also thought that infected erythrocytes collected in the placenta stimulate pancreatic cell production of insulin, leading to hyperinsulinemia and hypoglycemia during infection [2]. This contributes to increasing the severity of disease during pregnancy. Other maternal effects of malarial infection result from the "stickiness" of the infected erythrocytes that become trapped in small vessels, resulting in cerebral malaria, renal failure and thrombocytopenia.

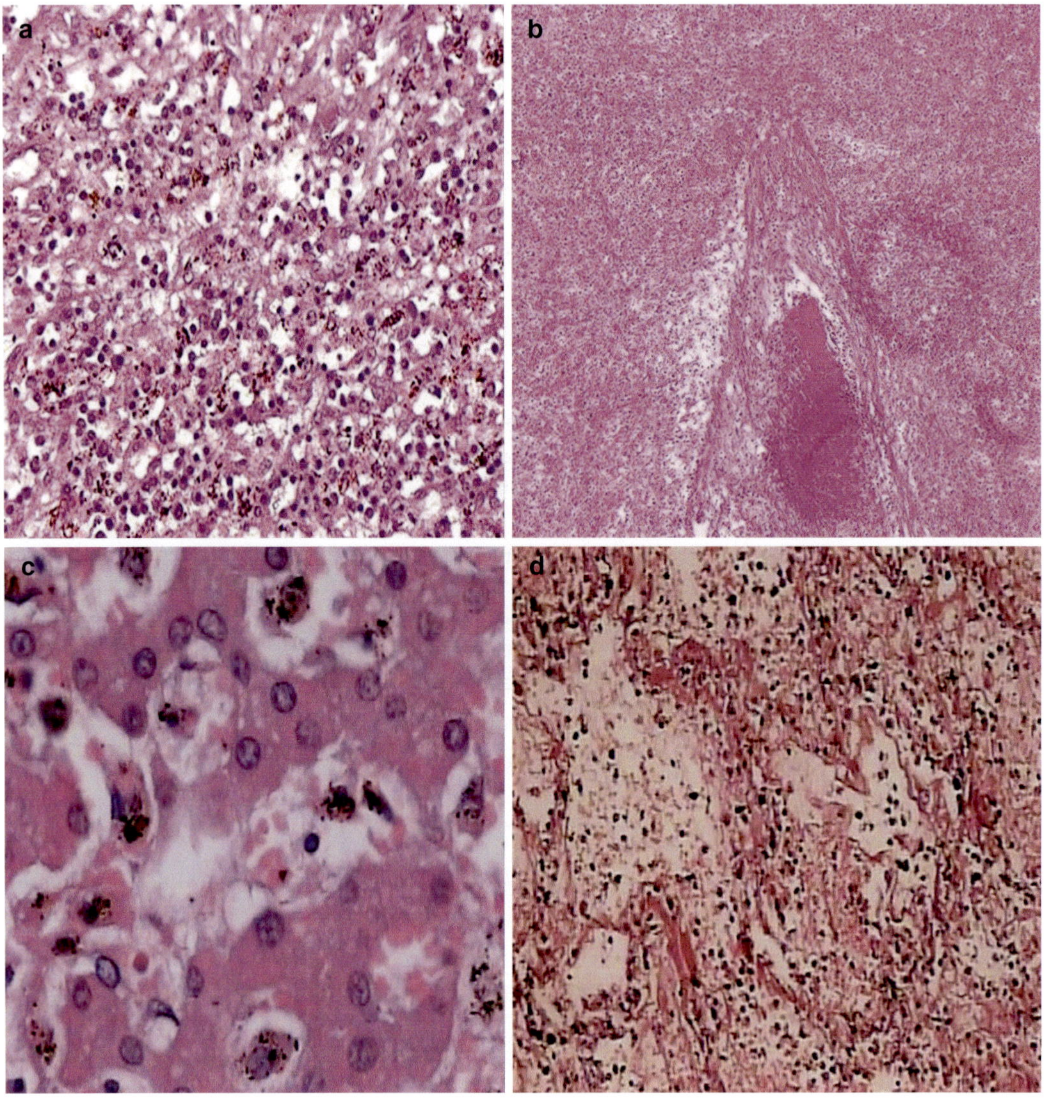

Fig. 22.3 (**a**) Spleen (H&E 400×) showing the presence of abundant hemazoin pigment. (**b**) Spleen (H&E 400×) shows an infarct with a vessel showing the presence of a thrombus. (**c**) Liver (H&E 400×) showing marked Kupffer cell hyperplasia with blackish brown hemozoin pigment deposition. (**d**) Lung (H&E 400×) shows diffuse alveolar damage with a few hyaline membranes suggestive of ARDS

Malaria is an intraerythrocytic parasite, so there is destruction of red cells containing parasites due to schizont rupture [3]. However, a more important contributor is the accelerated destruction of non-parasitized red cells that parallels disease severity. The hemolytic anaemia of malaria is aggravated by bone marrow dyserythropoiesis during and immediately after the acute illness.

Cerebral malaria is one of the most dreadful complications and leading cause of death in infections due to *Plasmodium falciparum*, accounting for around 13% of all malaria-related deaths [4]. The diagnosis requires the presence of neurologic symptoms in addition to the presence of asexual forms of the parasite on peripheral blood smears. All patients with *P. falciparum* malaria with neurologic manifestations of any degree should be treated as cases of cerebral malaria. The central neuropathological feature of cerebral malaria is the sequestration of parasitized red blood cells (PRBCs) in the microvasculature. Other neuropathological features include petechial hemorrhage in the brain parenchyma, ring hemorrhages and Dürck's granulomas; the latter are circumscribed cellular reactions, are comprised of collections of astrocytes and microglia containing iron pigment and are probably related to resorption of ring hemorrhages [5]. Our patient was disoriented at the time of presentation, and microscopy of the cerebrum revealed many Dürck's granulomas (Fig. 22.2c), petechial hemorrhages and congested vessels with occasional PRBC.

Splenic infarction, as was seen in our case, is a rare complication of malaria. Splenic complications other than infarction identified in cases of malaria are spontaneous splenic rupture, hyperreactive malarial syndrome, hypersplenism and splenic cysts [6]. Splenic infarction is not usually noted and is likely to be underdiagnosed in many cases of complicated malaria. Reports of malaria-associated splenic infarctions are rare; splenic infarction is a result of parenchymal ischemia from the occlusion of the arterial or venous circulation. Our case showed the presence of thrombi within the splenic vessels (Fig. 22.3b). However, the mechanism by which malaria results in splenic infarction is not clearly understood. Based on an investigation of the literature on malaria, one of the studies hypothesizes that the following factors would contribute to a hypoxic state attributable to splenic infarction: (1) hypercoagulable state; (2) intrasplenic structural change by adhesion of malaria-infected red blood cells to endothelial cells, with rosetting of PRBCs and non-PRBCs and splenic cellular hyperplasia; and (3) anemic hypoxia [6].

ARDS is an important complication in severe and complicated falciparum malaria infection. Pregnant women and non-immune individuals are observed to be more prone to developing this condition. Our case also had developed ARDS and was probably the cause of death. Literature studies reveal increased alveolar capillary permeability resulting in intravascular fluid loss into the lungs to be the key pathophysiologic mechanism. ARDS due to malaria is a disease with a very high mortality [7]. Malaria is endemic in our country and is one of the most challenging parasitic infections to eradicate. It is still one of the major contributors to maternal death. While the present case exhibited classical features of complicated falciparum malaria in the form of cerebral malaria, ARDS, severe anaemia and thrombocytopenia, it also showed a rare complication of multiple splenic infarcts.

References

1. Schantz-Dunn J, Nour NM. Malaria and pregnancy: a global health perspective. Rev Obstet Gynecol. 2009;2(3):186–92. https://doi.org/10.3909/riog0091.
2. Rogerson SJ, Hviid L, Duffy PE, Leke RF, Taylor DW. Malaria in pregnancy: pathogenesis and immunity. Lancet Infect Dis. 2007;7(2):105–17.
3. White NJ. Anaemia and malaria. Malar J. 2018;17:371. https://doi.org/10.1186/s12936-018-2509-9.
4. Mundhra S, Parmar U, Shukla D. A prospective study to identify the co-relation of a disease severity of complicated malaria & clinical outcome. Paripex-Ind J Res. 2016;4(7).
5. Chimelli L. A morphological approach to the diagnosis of protozoal infections of the central nervous system. Pathol Res Int. 2011;2011:290853. https://doi.org/10.4061/2011/290853.
6. Hwang JH, Lee CS. Malaria-induced splenic infarction. Am J Trop Med Hyg. 2014;91(6):1094–100.
7. Mohan A, Sharma SK, Bollineni S. Acute lung injury and acute respiratory distress syndrome in malaria. J Vector Borne Dis. 2008;45(3):179–93. PMID: 18807374.

Adrenal Hemorrhage: A Dark Horse in Maternal Mortality

23

Niyati N. Sangoi, Kusum D. Jashnani, and Lalita Yoganand Patil

23.1 Clinical History

A 26-year-old female, G2P1, was brought dead to our hospital. Two days back, she complained of abdominal pain and was admitted to a nearby hospital for the same, where her ultrasound examination showed evidence of intrauterine fetal death. She was in the 24th week of gestation, and the fetus was delivered at the same hospital. A few hours after delivery, her condition deteriorated, and she was found in a gasping state. In view of this, she was transferred to our hospital, where she was declared dead on arrival.

Investigations: Hemoglobin: 11.9 g/dL, total leucocyte count: 5380 cells/mm^3, platelet count: 175,000/mm^3, BUN: 0.6 mg/dl, serum creatinine: 0.9 mg/dl, SGOT: 55 U/L, SGPT: 36 U/L, total bilirubin: 0.5 mg/dL, direct bilirubin: 0.3 mg/dL, prothrombin time: 14 s (control of 12 s), INR (international normalized ratio): 1.1. A complete autopsy was performed on this patient, after due permission.

23.2 Autopsy Findings

The external examination was unremarkable. On internal examination, bilateral adrenals were enlarged with hemorrhagic external and cut surfaces (Fig. 23.1a). Microscopy of the adrenal glands showed extensive areas of hemorrhage in the cortex and medulla with the preservation of few tiny areas of normal cortical cells. Extra-adrenal fibrofatty tissue also showed the presence of hemorrhage (Fig. 23.1b–d). Gross examination of the heart showed the presence of subendocardial hemorrhages. Microscopy showed patchy areas of subendocardial hemorrhage and mild myofiber hypertrophy. The liver was foldable. The capsule of the liver showed plenty of pinpoint hemorrhages. On microscopy, the normal hepatic lobular architecture was preserved. Majority of the perivenular hepatocytes showed hemorrhagic necrosis (Fig. 23.2a). Some areas of periportal hepatocyte hemorrhagic necrosis were also seen (Fig. 23.2b, c). Blood vessels in the portal tract showed marked congestion. Hemorrhagic areas were seen in the serosa of the large intestine and lungs. The uterus showed the presence of placental tissue on the posterior wall. Microscopic examination of the endometrium showed decidual change with the presence of intermediate

N. N. Sangoi · K. D. Jashnani (✉) · L. Y. Patil
Department of Pathology, Topiwala National Medical College and BYL Nair Charitable Hospital, Mumbai, Maharashtra, India

K. D. Jashnani (ed.), *Maternal Mortality - Lessons Learnt from Autopsy*,
https://doi.org/10.1007/978-981-19-3420-9_23

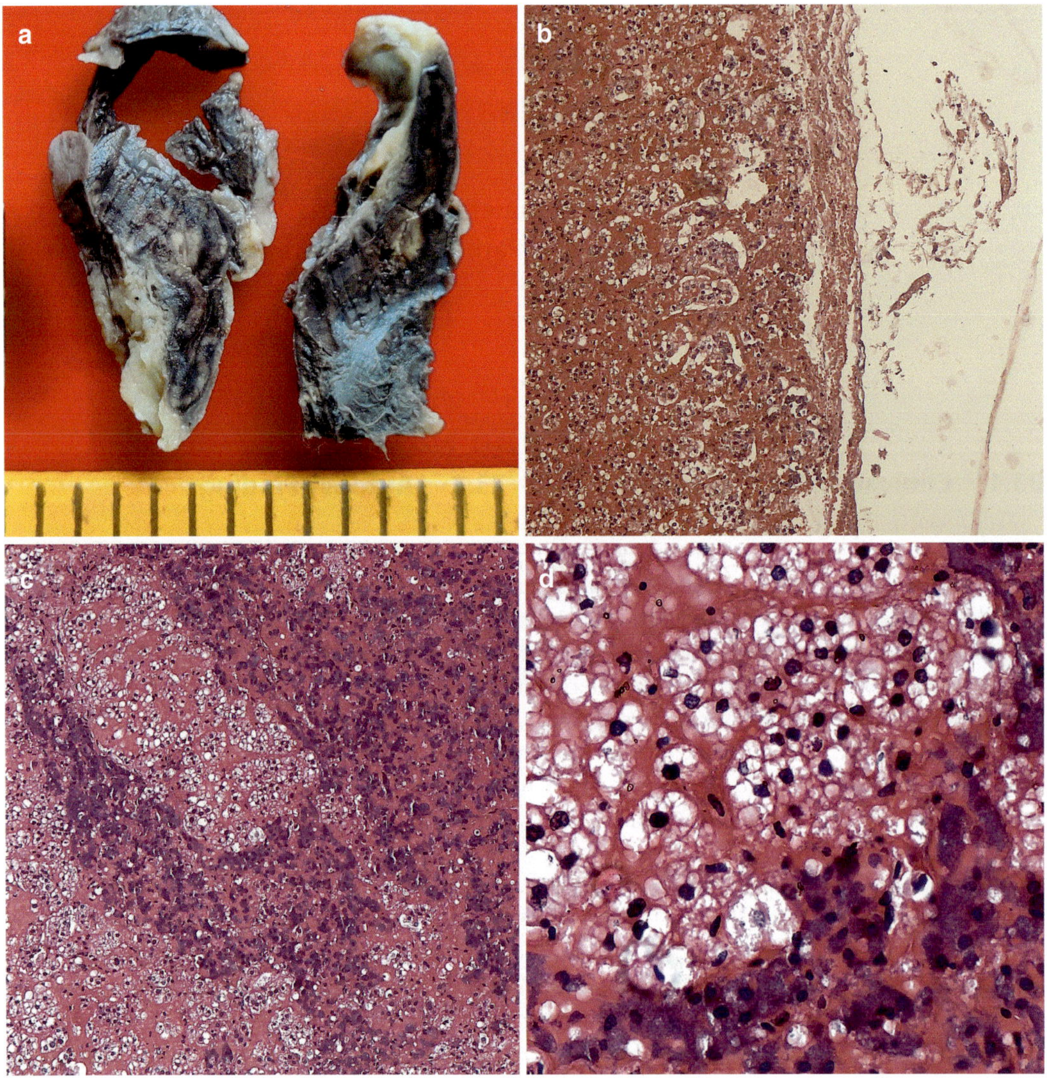

Fig. 23.1 (**a**) Gross picture of the adrenals showing an increased size with hemorrhagic cut surface. (**b**) Adrenal gland with capsule showing areas of hemorrhage (H&E, 100×). (**c**) Adrenal gland showing areas of hemorrhage (H&E, 200×). (**d**) Adrenal gland showing areas of hemorrhage (H&E, 400×)

trophoblastic cells and few chorionic villi near the endometrium with surrounding areas of hemorrhage. Myometrium showed a moderate degree of physiologic hypertrophy and pre-ischemic changes and presence of few intermediate trophoblast cells. Microscopy of the cervix showed few areas of hemorrhage and congested blood vessels. Bilateral ovaries and fallopian tubes were unremarkable. The rest of the organs were unremarkable.

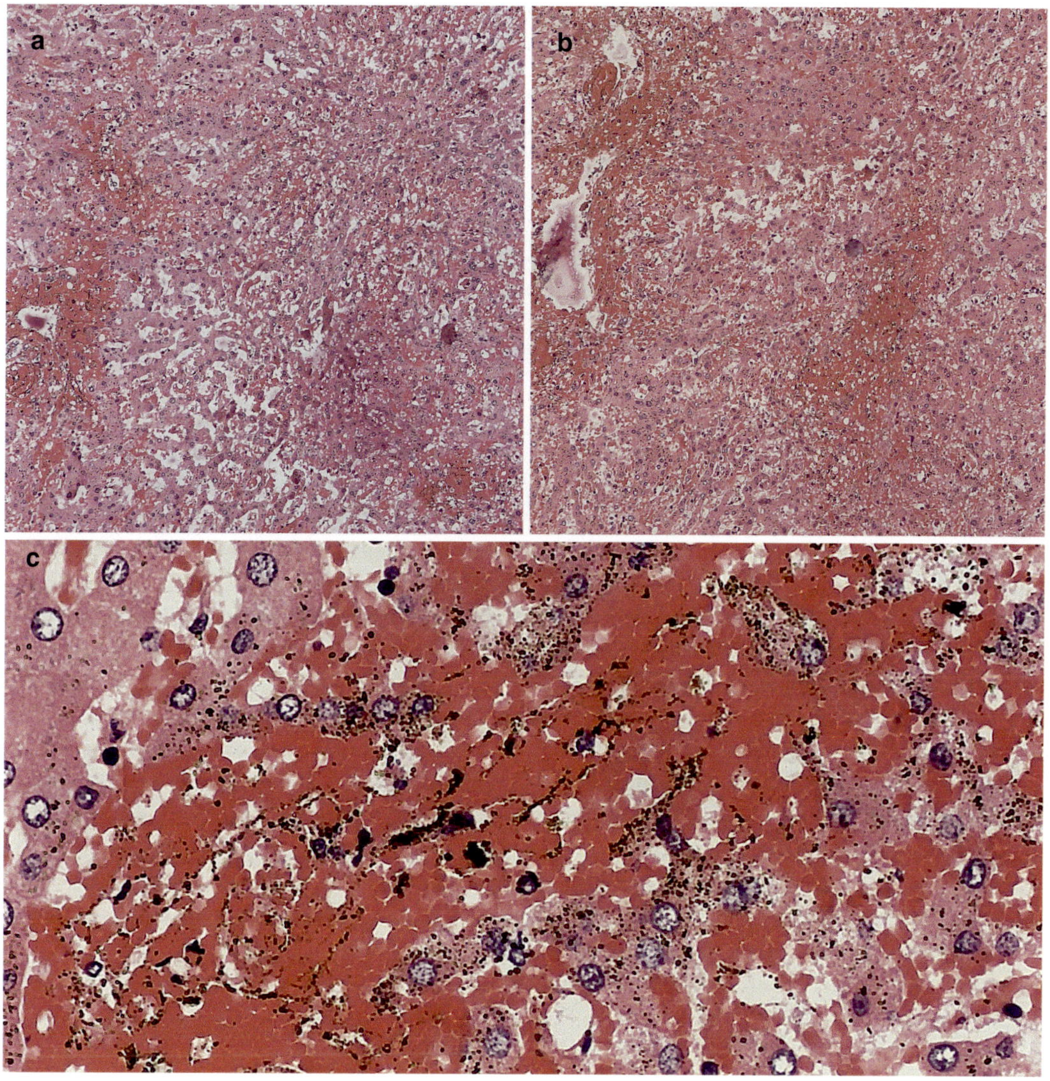

Fig. 23.2 (**a**) Perivenular hepatocytes showing hemorrhagic necrosis (H & E, 200×). (**b**) Periportal hepatocytes showing hemorrhagic necrosis (H & E, 200×). (**c**) Periportal hepatocytes showing hemorrhagic necrosis (H & E, 400×)

23.3 Final Cause of Death

Bilateral adrenal hemorrhage and shock with disseminated intravascular coagulation in a postpartum female with intrauterine fetal death.

23.4 Clinicopathologic Discussion

Adrenal hemorrhage is a rare but potentially fatal disorder which is characterized by bleeding into the adrenal glands. It may be unilateral or bilateral. The clinical symptoms can range from a nonspecific pain in the abdomen to catastrophic circulatory collapse. There are many causes of adrenal hemorrhage which include septicemia, blunt abdominal trauma, coagulopathies, pregnancy, stress, use of anticoagulants, essential thrombocytosis, and antiphospholipid syndrome [1].

The incidence of adrenal hemorrhage amongst pregnant women is unknown [2]. In the general population, its incidence is estimated to be 0.3–1.8% [3]. The adrenal glands have a rich arterial blood supply, and the arteries abruptly transition into a capillary bed with drainage through relatively limited venous branches at the corticomedullary junction. This predisposes the adrenal medulla, under stress conditions such as pregnancy, to thrombosis and venous congestion. An increase in venous pressure or arterial perfusion ultimately leads to adrenal hemorrhage. Reperfusion hemorrhage may occur when the normal pressure of arterial perfusion is restored. A single central vein drains each adrenal gland, and its thick muscular wall may contract in response to the release of catecholamines during severe stress. During pregnancy, physiologic adrenal cortical hyperplasia and hypertrophy may occur. All these factors contribute to the pathophysiology of adrenal hemorrhage during pregnancy [4].

There should be no history of trauma, use of anticoagulants, sepsis, or tumor to call the adrenal hemorrhage spontaneous and idiopathic [2]. In pregnancy, adrenal hemorrhage can often present with maternal-fetal compromise, including intrauterine fetal death (IUFD) [3]. IUFD, if undetected, comes with its own share of complications including disseminated intravascular coagulation (DIC), which can lead to fatal complications in the mother including maternal death. In cases of retention of a dead fetus or placental tissue, the onset of DIC may be insidious or chronic. There is systemic activation of coagulation which causes consumption of platelets and coagulation factors. This leads to bleeding and tissue hypoxemia, leading to shock [5]. In the present case, the patient presented with abdominal pain and ultrasound examination revealed IUFD, with adrenal hemorrhage being the probable cause of both. IUFD and retention of placental tissue further led to DIC and shock, leading to the death of the patient.

The ultrasound findings of adrenal hemorrhage are nonspecific, and hence, an MRI or CT scan is needed to confirm the diagnosis and to know the etiology of the same, if any. Radiological findings and low cortisol levels in the peripartum period establish the diagnosis of adrenal hemorrhage in pregnancy [6]. In cases where a conservative management is planned, a follow-up MRI or CT scan should be done to evaluate the resolution of hematoma or its stability. Adrenal function assessment and serial measurements of hemoglobin should be done. Causes such as TTP and antiphospholipid syndrome should be excluded [2]. Emergency cesarean section delivery is required to manage cases of adrenal hemorrhage where gross maternal-fetal compromise is identified. However, the optimal mode of delivery in cases where there is no compromise is unclear [3].

In conclusion, women presenting with abdominal pain should have a high level of suspicion during pregnancy, as adrenal hemorrhage, even though very rare and uncommon, can have a fatal outcome for both the mother and the fetus. Prompt diagnosis with radiology and appropriate management with supportive care, emergency delivery if needed, and hormone replacement can have a favorable outcome.

References

1. Mehmood KT, Sharman T. Adrenal Hemorrhage. [Updated 2020 Oct 19]. In: StatPearls [Internet]. Treasure Island (FL): StatPearls Publishing; 2021.
2. Gupta A, Minhas R, Quant H. Spontaneous adrenal hemorrhage in pregnancy: a case series. Case reports. Obstet Gynecol. 2017;2017:1–3.
3. Street S, Dekker Nitert M, Callaway LK. Successful vaginal delivery following spontaneous adrenal haemorrhage at term. BMJ Case Rep. 2016;2016:bcr2016215096.
4. Bockorny B, Posteraro A, Bilgrami S. Bilateral spontaneous adrenal hemorrhage during pregnancy. Obstet Gynecol. 2012;120(2 part 1):377–81.
5. Kumar V, Abbas A, Aster J. Robbins and Cotran pathologic basis of disease. 10th ed. p. 669–71.
6. Kadhem S, Ebrahem R, Munguti C, Mortada R. Spontaneous unilateral adrenal hemorrhage in pregnancy. Cureus. 2017;9(1):e977.

Disseminated Miliary Tuberculosis: A Classic Case of Fatality!

24

Kusum D. Jashnani, Lalita Yoganand Patil, and Rakesh R. Bhadade

24.1 Clinical History

A 24-year-old primigravida, married for 1 year with 35.6 weeks' gestation, was referred from a peripheral hospital in view of breathlessness and a BP of 160/100 mmHg. She had complaints of fever with chills for 3 days, breathlessness, cough, and cold for 10 days. There were no complaints of abdominal pain, bleeding/leaking per vaginum/ absent fetal movements. There was past history of pulmonary TB, taken antikochs treatment (AKT) for 3 months, which was stopped, and blood transfusion in 2005 and 2013 for some hematological disorder.

On examination, the general condition was fair, afebrile, pallor+. No icterus/cyanosis/clubbing/LNs. BP was 120/80 mm Hg, CVS-S1S2-N, RS-b/l rhonchi, RR-26/min. Laboratory investigations revealed LDH-2805, DCT/ICT-negative, INR-12.5, ANA+VE [1:80], homogenous pattern, dsDNA-negative, Hb varied from 11 to 3.4 g/dL, which decreased over the days, platelet count from 111,000 to 80,000/mm^3, TLC from 8700 to 1200/mm^3, PS- tear drop cells+, basophilic stippling+, cabot rings+, anisocytosis, poikilocytosis, macrocytes, toxic granules+, suggestive of megaloblastic anemia. The reticulocyte count was 5%. Bone marrow aspirate showed features of erythroid hyperplasia with megaloblastic erythropoiesis and no increase in blasts.

Biochemical and other coagulation profiles were within normal limits. RMAT, Lepto, dengue, HIV, HBsAg, and HCV tests were negative. CT thorax showed multiple nodules randomly distributed, scattered throughout bilateral lung parenchyma, suggestive of active miliary TB with enlarged multiple subcentimetric pretracheal LNs along with hepatomegaly and massive splenomegaly.

Clinical diagnosis was primigravida with 35 weeks with preeclampsia in a case of miliary TB, myelofibrosis, and hemolytic disorder.

She was transfused with 4 pints of FFP and 2 pints of packed red blood cells and started on antituberculous treatment. She was stable for 4 days with mild fever and BP varying from 140/100 to 140/80 mm Hg with fetal movements present. On the fifth day morning, she had a spontaneous vaginal preterm delivery of 1.72 kg female, who CIAB, and placenta expelled spontaneously. Postdelivery she was stable, afebrile, pallor + BP -110/70 mm Hg, P/A uterus soft well contracted, P/V no bleeding. Three hours later, she suddenly became pulseless, with BP not recordable, gasping, and succumbed in spite of all resuscitative measures. A complete autopsy was performed after taking due permission.

K. D. Jashnani (✉) · L. Y. Patil
Department of Pathology, Topiwala National Medical College and BYL Nair Charitable Hospital, Mumbai, Maharashtra, India

R. R. Bhadade
Department of Medicine (Critical Care Unit), Topiwala National Medical College and BYL Nair Charitable Hospital, Mumbai, Maharashtra, India

K. D. Jashnani (ed.), *Maternal Mortality - Lessons Learnt from Autopsy*,
https://doi.org/10.1007/978-981-19-3420-9_24

24.2 Autopsy Findings

She was well-built and well-nourished. The liver was enlarged, weighed 3 kg, and showed multiple gray white tubercles on its external and cut surface. The lungs both weighed 300 g each, pleura was thick and hazy with multiple millet like tubercles 1–2 mm all over the surface, the cut surface—similar tubercles seen all over the parenchyma (Fig. 24.1). In the kidney and the spleen (weighing 1.8 kg), there were multiple tubercles scattered on external and cut surfaces. Lymph nodes—2 × 2 to 1 × 1cm with cheesy white caseous necrotic material. The mesentery of the small intestine also showed multiple millet-size as well as confluent tubercles (Fig. 24.2). The rest of the organs were unremarkable.

On microscopy, multiple well-formed caseating and noncaseating epithelioid cell granulomas were seen in bilateral lungs and kidneys, spleen, liver, mesentery, and pituitary (Figs. 24.3 and 24.4). There was a rim of lymphocytes surrounding the epithelioid cells and occasional Langhans giant cells. The liver in addition showed multiple cirrhotic regenerating micronodules (less than 3 mm in size, which were missed on gross). Single adrenal gland and the serosa of a fallopian tube showed occasional epithelioid cell granulomas. Special stains for acid-fast bacilli (AFB) (Ziehl Neelsen stain) as well as PAS and GMS were all negative. There was no evidence of thrombi/thromboemboli in any organs. Bone marrow examination showed a hypercellular marrow with micronormoblastic and megaloblastic erythropoiesis with no evidence of ECGs. The rest of the organs including uterus, cervix and ovaries were unremarkable.

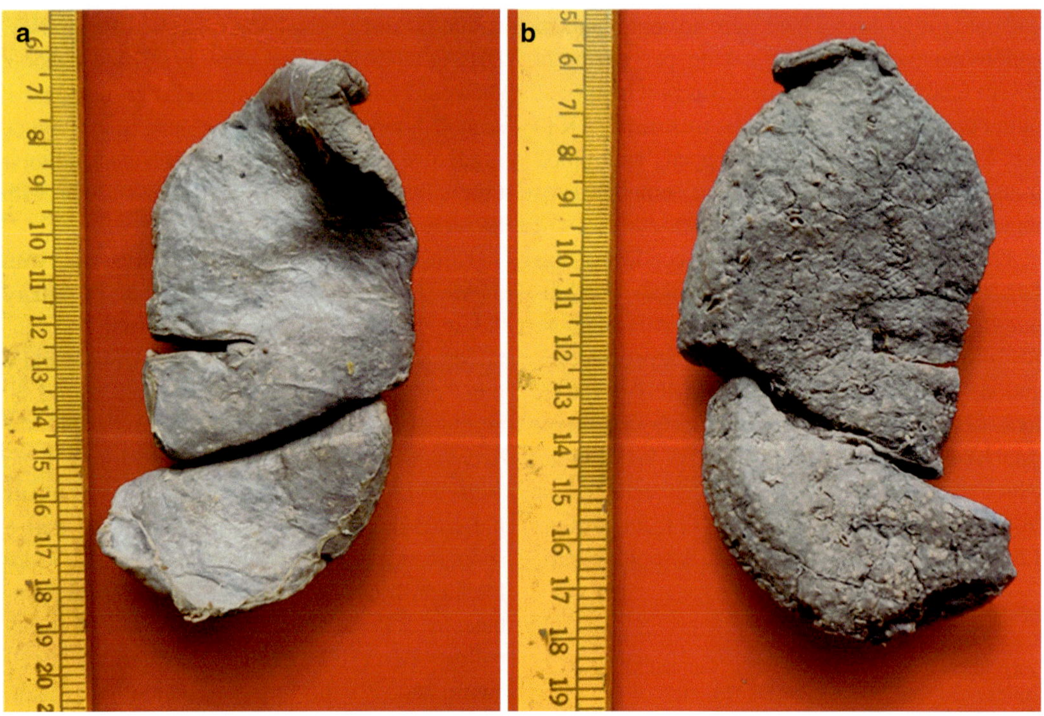

Fig. 24.1 Gross specimen of a lobe of the lung showing an opaque thick fibrinous pleura with visible millet-size gray-white tubercles all over the surface (**a**) as well as on the cut surface (**b**)

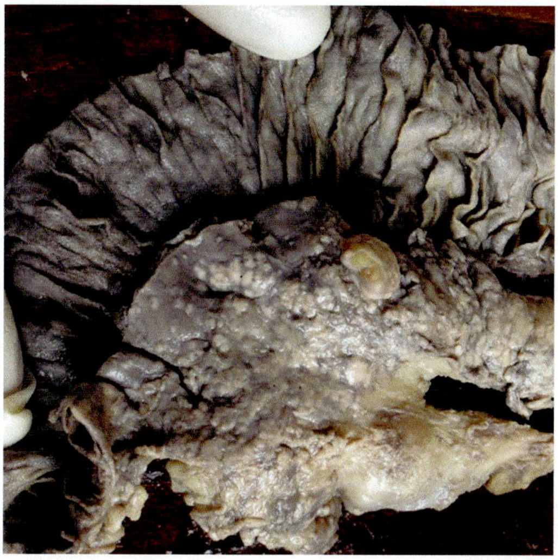

Fig. 24.2 Millet size as well as confluent tubercles on the small intestine mesentery

24.3 Final Cause of Death

Disseminated miliary tuberculosis in a postpartum female.

24.4 Clinicopathologic Discussion

Of all patients with TB, disseminated miliary tuberculosis, estimated to be present in 1.3%, is a potentially life-threatening type which occurs when a large number of bacteria travel through the blood stream and spread throughout the body [1, 2]. The term dissemination means the presence of two or more non-contiguous sites resulting from hematogenous spread of *Mycobacterium tuberculosis* occurring as a result of progressive primary infection or reactivation of a latent focus

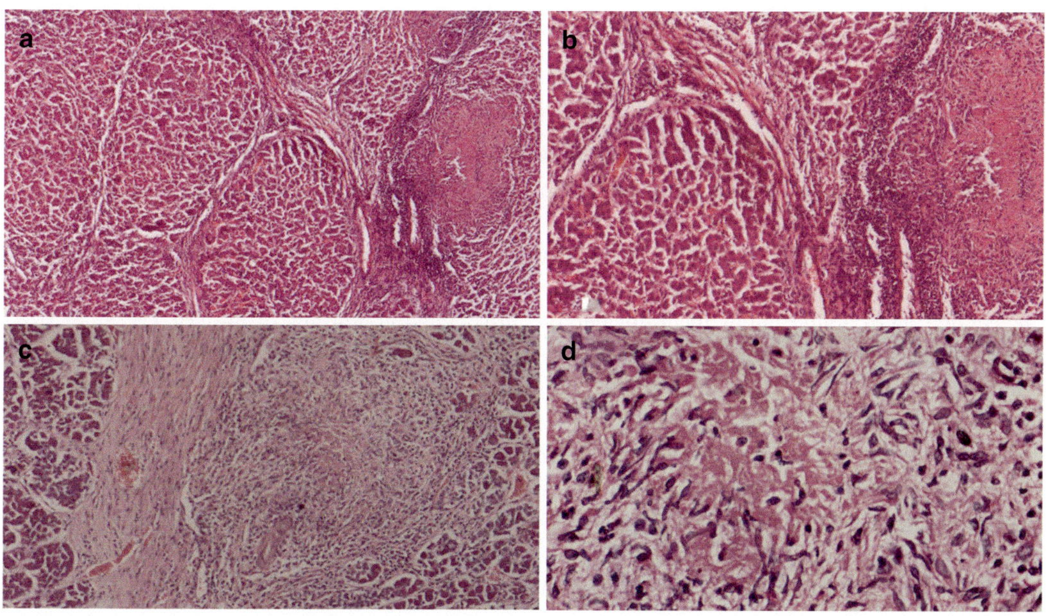

Fig. 24.3 (**a**) Caseating epithelioid cell granuloma in the background of cirrhotic liver 100× H&E. (**b**) Caseating epithelioid cell granuloma in the background of cirrhotic liver 200× H&E. (**c**) Caseating epithelioid cell granuloma in pituitary gland 200×, H&E. (**d**) Caseating epithelioid cell granuloma in pituitary gland 400×, H&E

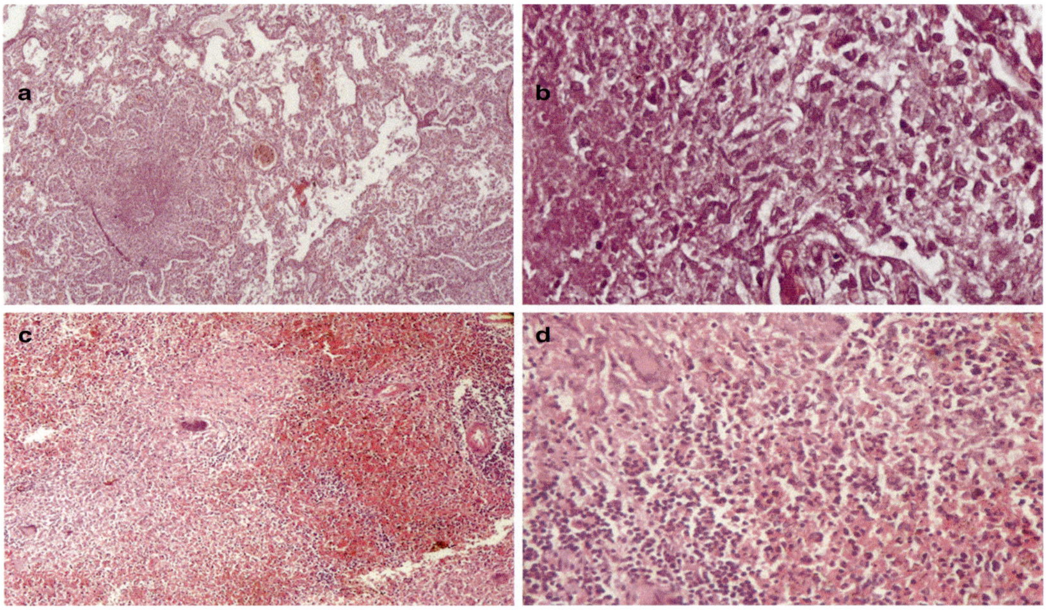

Fig. 24.4 (**a**) Caseating epithelioid cell granuloma in lung 200×, H&E. (**b**) Caseating epithelioid cell granuloma in lung 400×, H&E. (**c**) Caseating epithelioid cell granuloma along with langhans giant cells in spleen 200×, H&E. (**d**) Caseating epithelioid cell granuloma in spleen 400×, H&E

with subsequent spread. According to the World Health Organization (WHO), TB is one of the top 10 causes of death worldwide, having killed almost 1.7 million people in 2016. TB is most common in developing countries and is usually preventable and curable under the right conditions [3]. It's more common in people whose immune system isn't working right, i.e., immunocompromised.

Miliary TB got its name in 1700 from John Jacob Manget based on how it appears on an autopsy, after a patient expired [3]. Classic miliary TB is defined as millet like (1–3 mm) gray white tiny tubercles seen on gross morphology in the lung or any other organ; this term was originally a pathologic and then also a radiographic description. Pulmonary miliary tuberculosis is seen when bacilli draining through lymphatics enter the venous blood and go back to the lung via the right side of the heart. In systemic miliary tuberculosis, as seen in the present case, bacilli are spread via the systemic arterial blood supply. These two forms of miliary spread can occur independently or together. Cryptic miliary TB means the absence of fever but is characterized by progressive wasting strongly mimicking a metastatic carcinoma. TB is a common non-obstetric cause of maternal death, with pregnancy and puerperium being one of the predisposing associated conditions of miliary TB, apart from cancer, transplantation, HIV infection, malnutrition, diabetes, etc. Immunological changes during pregnancy such as downregulation of Th-1 cytokine and natural killer cell cytotoxicity and a reduction in interferon gamma production make the activation of latent TB infection or de novo infection more likely than among non-pregnant women [4]. Most patients present with nonspecific symptoms such as fever, weight loss, shortness of breath, malaise, headache, or hypotension, which mimic the physiological changes of pregnancy itself and thereby lead to diagnostic and treatment delays. However, in our case, the patient was diagnosed as pulmonary miliary TB on CT imaging and started on antituberculous treatment, yet she succumbed, indicating that timely anti-TB treatment is vital for curing TB. If untreated, the mortality associated with disseminated miliary tuberculosis is assumed to be close to 100%.

In symptomatic women and asymptomatic women with a recent tuberculosis contact, the Centers for Disease Control and Prevention (CDC) and others recommend a shielded chest radiograph, which poses minimal risk to the fetus. Other tests recommended for early diagnosis of TB in general are fundus examination for detecting choroid tubercles and other imaging modalities like CT and MRI to define the extent of organ system involvement. Examination of the sputum (three morning samples), body fluids, image-guided fine-needle aspiration cytology or needle biopsy from various enlarged organ sites, bone marrow aspiration, molecular testing (e.g., Xpert MTB/RIF), and mycobacterial culture must be carried out as appropriate and feasible. Mantoux test can be an invaluable simple test on pregnant women with induration of more than 4 mm in HIV-seropositive women, more than 9 mm in high-risk women, and more than 14 mm in low-risk women considered as evidence of current or past tuberculosis infection [5]. Basic antenatal TB screening for symptoms of cough of any duration, fever, night sweats, and weight loss should be routinely included in high burden TB/HIV resource-limited settings, and the high risk of TB in the postpartum period should also be considered in TB screening guidelines [6]. The absence of these symptoms has a negative predictive value of 90–97.7%, even in peripartum women, but poor sensitivity and positive predictive value. Some studies have not been able to demonstrate the utility of TB symptom screening questionnaires in a routine setting among HIV-infected or non-infected women [7]. Clinicians should always consider tuberculosis in the differential diagnosis of fever in pregnancy and puerperium.

Granulomas are not restricted to mycobacterial infections, being found in many different kinds of bacterial, viral, and fungal infections and even in non-infectious inflammatory diseases. Histoplasma infection can show granulomas and sometimes caseation similar to tuberculosis. The key to diagnosis is to check the surrounding tissue reaction and special stains [8]. In the present case, the histopathologic caseating epithelioid cell granulomas were classic for tuberculosis, though negative for acid-fast bacilli on Ziehl Neelsen stain. Other special stains like GMS and PAS were also negative for any fungal organisms including histoplasma. The gross miliary tubercles in the lungs and other organs were diagnostic of disseminated miliary TB, which was confirmed on histopathologic examination. Disseminated metastasis can be in the form of tubercles seen on gross morphology, which would again have a histopathologic confirmation.

References

1. Sharma SK, Mohan A, Sharma A. Miliary tuberculosis: a new look at an old foe. J Clin Tuberc Mycobact Dis. 2016;3:13–27.
2. Sharma SK, Mohan A. Miliary tuberculosis. Microbiol Spectr. 2017;5(2). https://doi.org/10.1128/microbiolspec.TNMI7-0013-2016. PMID: 28281441.
3. Miliary tuberculosis. https://www.healthline.com/health/miliary-tuberculosis#diagnosis.
4. Carmen T, Zailan LB, Singh R, Wright A. Miliary tuberculosis presenting as pyrexia of unknown origin in pregnancy. J Clin Gynec Obstet. 2019;8(4):114–7.
5. Newton ER. Tuberculosis and pregnancy. Glob Libr Women's Med. 2008. https://doi.org/10.3843/GLOWM.10186.
6. Bekker A, Schaaf HS, Draper HR, Kriel M, Hesseling AC. Tuberculosis disease during pregnancy and treatment outcomes in HIV-infected and uninfected women at a referral hospital in Cape Town. PLoS One. 2016;11(11):e0164249. https://doi.org/10.1371/journal.pone.0164249.
7. Kosgei RJ, Szkwarko D, Callens S, Gichangi P, et al. Screening for tuberculosis in pregnancy: do we need more than a symptom screen? Experience from western Kenya. Public Health Action. 2013;3(4):294–8.
8. Mukhopadhyay S, Gal AA. Granulomatous lung disease an approach to the differential diagnosis. Arch Pathol Lab Med. 2010;134(5):667–90.

25 Disseminated Miliary TB with Missing Millet Tubercles on Gross: Suspect Severe Immunocompromised State

Kusum D. Jashnani, Lalita Yoganand Patil, and Padmashree K. Haldankar

25.1 Clinical History

A 23-year-old female, married, P3L2A1 with no known comorbidity, had spontaneous abortion 15 days back (LMP was 11 weeks back). She underwent a check curettage at a private hospital for the same. Later she developed fever with chills for 15 days that was intermittent and high-grade. Nausea and vomiting for 10 days, which was non-projectile and non-bloodstained. Pain in abdomen generalized, as well as yellowish discoloration of skin and eyes for 8 days, with loose motions for 3 days, watery in consistency and breathlessness for the last 1 day. She was transferred to our hospital with these complaints. There was no history of chest pain, cough, cold, bleeding from any sites, altered sensorium, bleeding, or foul-smelling vaginal discharge. There was no history of hypertension, TB, diabetes, epilepsy, or any other medical illness. She gave history of TB infection in her sister who was on treatment.

Obstetric history: para 3, one 3-year-old male child and a second 2-year-old female child were both full-term normal deliveries. Her blood group was B Rh negative, and she had taken anti-D injections after both deliveries and the current abortion.

K. D. Jashnani (✉) · L. Y. Patil · P. K. Haldankar
Department of Pathology, Topiwala National Medical College and BYL Nair Charitable Hospital, Mumbai, Maharashtra, India

On examination, she was pale and icteric, with hepatosplenomegaly and minimal per vaginal bleeding. She was negative for HBsAg, HIV, HCV, HEV, HAV, fever profile (Widal, lepto IgM & IgG, RMAT, Dengue IgM & IgG), TRUNAAT for COVID-19, Mantoux test, and blood culture. CBC-Hb varied from 7.0 to 9.7 g/dL, TLC varied from 5900 to 6590/mm^3, and platelet count varied from 60,000 to 164,000/μL. On PS examination, schistocytes were seen; the differential count was normal.

LFT: total bili 5.5 mg/dL, D. bili 2.3 mg/dL, SGOT 254 U/L, SGPT 100 U/L, ALP 1295 U/L, T. protein/albumin varied from 5.0/2.3 to 4.6/2.1, LDH 3068 U/L. Se creatinine 0.5 mg/dl, Se amylase 22 U/L, Se haptoglobin <5.0 mg/dL, Se ferritin >16,500 mg/mL, PT INR varied from 18/1.40 to 61.3/3.7 (control for PT 14 s), fibrinogen <100 mg/mL, FDP 18.47 μg/mL, aPTT 62.3 to 180 s (control of 25 s), D-dimer >10,000 ng/mL. DCT was negative, while ICT was positive, which were compatible with the Rh-negative status of the patient.

25.1.1 Radiological Investigations

A CT scan of the thorax and abdomen showed bilateral ground glass opacities in the lung parenchyma suggestive of impending ARDS with few areas of interlobular septal thickening and multiple enlarged mediastinal lymph nodes. There was mild hepatosplenomegaly with diffuse fatty tissue

K. D. Jashnani (ed.), *Maternal Mortality - Lessons Learnt from Autopsy*,
https://doi.org/10.1007/978-981-19-3420-9_25

infiltration of the liver and mild ascites. USG showed an anteverted uterus with no retained products of conception and a cyst in the left ovary.

Clinical diagnosis was acute febrile illness and DIC with hepatic involvement with encephalopathy on Day 16 post spontaneous abortion with Rh incompatibility. Slowly her general condition deteriorated from Day 3, and she had tachycardia with pulse of 180/min, bilateral crepitations on RS examination, became unconscious, and succumbed on Day 5 of her hospital stay. A complete autopsy was performed after taking due permission.

25.2 Autopsy Findings

She was poorly built and nourished (cachexic), with the presence of pallor and icterus. There was no evidence of cyanosis, edema, or lymphadenopathy on external examination. The liver was enlarged, weighed 2.2 kg, and was greenish in color on the cut surface. The bilateral lungs weighed around 500 grams each, with a pleura that was smooth and shiny. The cut surface was rubbery to firm in consistency. At places, blood was oozing out under pressure and sink test was positive. The spleen was enlarged, weighing 420 g, and fibro-congested on the cut surface. Mediastinal lymph nodes were enlarged, matted showing yellowish cheesy necrotic material on the cut surface (Figs. 25.1 and 25.2).

25.2.1 Microscopy Findings

The lungs showed mild pleural fibrous thickening with patchy areas of intra-alveolar edema and hemorrhages. Bronchioles and blood vessels were unremarkable with no evidence of thromboemboli. Dispersed throughout the parenchyma were multiple tiny well-defined foci of granular caseous necrosis with nuclear debris without any epithelioid cells—caseating tubercles. Acid-fast bacilli were detected on Ziehl-Neelsen stain.

Lymph nodes showed large areas of caseous necrosis with nuclear debris and occasional foamy macrophages. It was loaded with AFB on ZN stain (Fig. 25.1c, d). Multiple similar caseating tubercles were seen in the liver, spleen, and adrenal glands (Fig. 25.3). Occasional ill-formed caseating tubercles with few macrophages were seen in the thyroid, bilateral kidneys, bone marrow (which was hypercellular with normoblastic erythropoiesis) (Fig. 25.2c, d), and uterine myometrium. The hallmark of all these caseating tubercles was the absence of epithelioid cells. All these organs were reexamined again grossly with naked eyes, but no millet seed-like tubercles or any other lesions were noted grossly. The rest of the organs including uterus, cervix and bilateral adnexae were unremarkable on gross and microscopy.

25.3 Final Cause of Death

Disseminated miliary tuberculosis with suspected immunocompromised status in a case of medical termination of pregnancy following first trimester abortion.

25.4 Clinicopathologic Discussion

Disseminated miliary tuberculosis (TB) is a life-threatening disease resulting from the hematogenous spread of *Mycobacterium tuberculosis*. Diagnosis is challenging owing to its subtle non-specific clinical presentation, which usually reflects the underlying organ involved. It involves many organs such as the lung, liver, spleen, bone marrow, kidney, adrenals, eyes, and thyroid. In the present case, except for the eyes (which could not be confirmed), all the above mentioned organs were affected. Numerous small, gray-to-reddish brown, punctate rounded tubercles similar to millet seeds (1–2 mm in size) should be seen over the surface of various organs. These were not present in our case even after examining

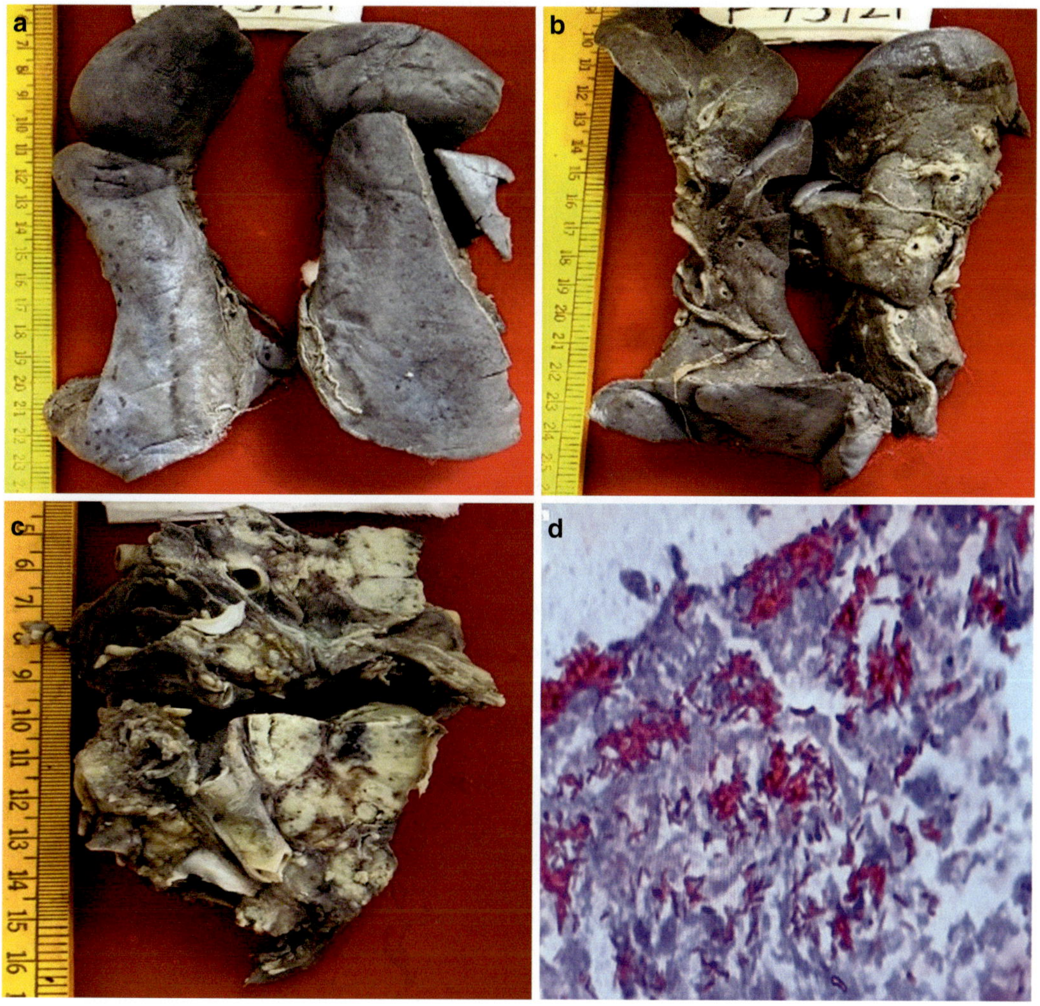

Fig. 25.1 External and cut surface of lungs is congested, firm to rubbery in consistency without any millet seed-like tubercles or any other lesions (**a**, **b**); a matted group of mediastinal enlarged lymph nodes showing yellow-white areas of cheesy caseous necrosis (**c**); ZN stain showing LN loaded with acid fast bacilli, 400× (**d**)

it very minutely with the naked eye multiple times. These tubercles show epithelioid cell granulomas with or without central caseation (for their cheesy appearance on gross examination) and few multinucleate giant cells called Langhans cells (formed by the fusion of macrophages) surrounded by T lymphocytes on microscopy [1, 2]. Epithelioid cells are activated macrophages with a shape similar to epithelial cells. A granuloma is developed by the host to contain the infection and eliminate the bacteria (host defense mechanism). Death of the infected epithelioid cells causes the formation of a necrotic zone in the center of the granuloma. These are classic granulomas, which are characteristic of tuberculosis in immunocompetent patients. Other types of granulomas may not show epithelioid cells, but instead show foamy cells. These foamy cells have lost their phagocytic and bactericidal activities and allow mycobacterial persistence in a dormant state [3]. It is generally presumed that the lipids present in these cells can serve as a source of nutrients for the bacteria, and these cells are loaded with AFB on ZN stain.

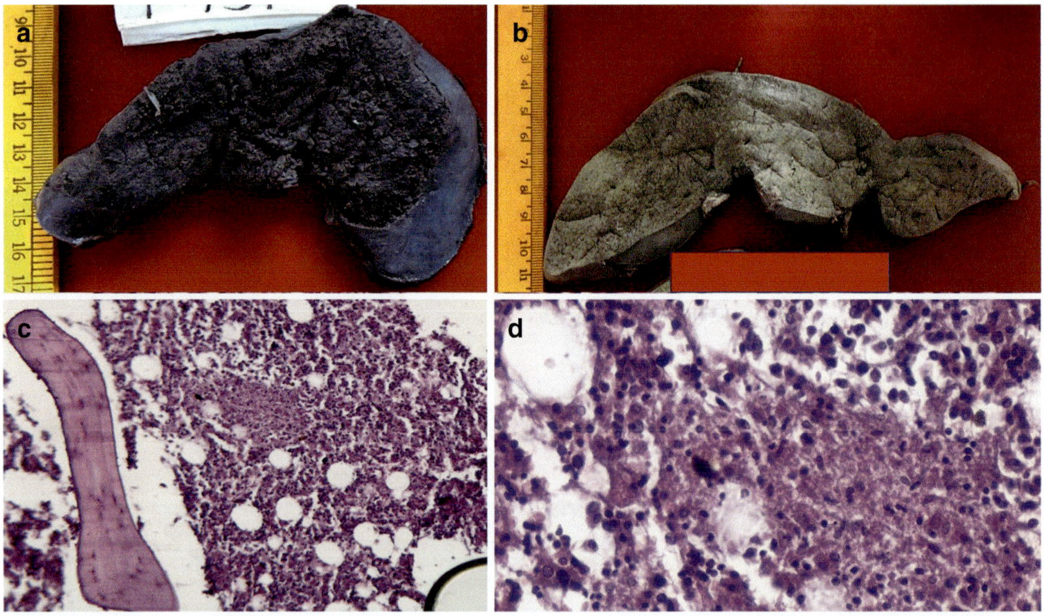

Fig. 25.2 Gross specimens of an enlarged spleen and an icteric liver with no evidence of any millet seed-like tubercles or any other lesions (**a**, **b**); histology of bone marrow showing increased marrow cellularity and presence of a single caseating tubercle with necrosis, few foamy macrophages without any epithelioid cells (**c**—H&E, 200×) (**d**—H&E, 400×)

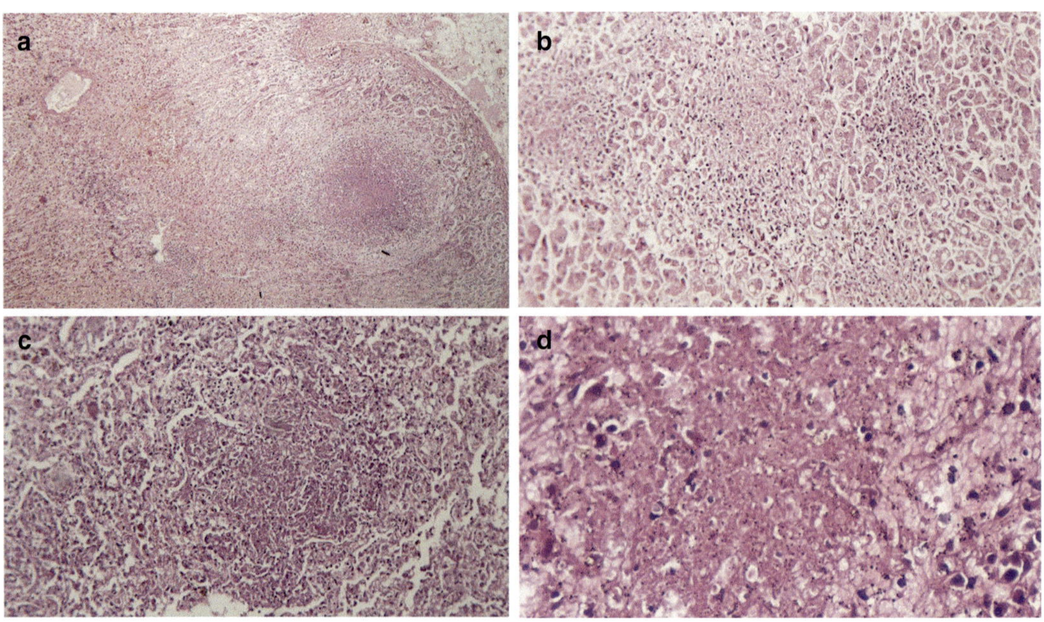

Fig. 25.3 Histology showing epithelioid cell poor caseating tubercles with necrosis and nuclear debris in the adrenal gland, liver, lung, and spleen (**a**, **b**, **c**—H&E, 200×) (**d**—H&E, 400×), respectively

Neutrophils can also be seen in granulomas, described as the first line of defense against tuberculosis. They are activated directly by *M. tuberculosis* products, such as lipoarabinomannan in particular. Our case had granulomas composed of caseous necrosis, nuclear debris, few neutrophils, and few foamy macrophages. Epithelioid cells were typically missing. The immune response to M. tuberculosis is highly dependent upon gamma interferon (IFN-y) and tumor necrosis factor (TNF) production by macrophages and antigen-specific T cells [4].

TNF deficiency plays an important role in causing accelerated necrotic death of macrophages and release of bacteria without giving them enough time to transform into epithelioid cells in immunosuppressed patients, thereby causing a stark morphological difference between the organized granulomas of TNF-sufficient mice and the disorganized, necrotic structures of TNF-deficient mice. This establishes the idea that TNF participates in granuloma formation and may explain the absence of millet tubercles on gross examination and the absence of epithelioid cells on microscopy in the present case [5].

Some studies have also shown that IFN-y and reduced vascularization/hypoxia of the lesion are involved in the caseation process. Caseation is associated with an increase in lipid metabolism. This is consistent with a role for foamy macrophages in the formation of the central necrotic zone. Based on in vitro studies, it has been proposed that apoptosis is a host strategy that kills the mycobacteria and promotes antigen presentation, thereby stimulating T cells, in contrast to necrosis of infected cells, which releases the bacteria and promotes inflammation and tissue damage.

Hematological abnormalities include anemia of different types, leukopenia, mainly lymphopenia, leukemoid reaction, high erythrocyte sedimentation rate, and disseminated intravascular coagulation. Suppression of erythropoiesis by inflammatory mediators is an important cause of anemia. Chronic inflammation results in a hyperplastic mononuclear phagocytic system and is responsible for extravascular hemolysis and also the trapping of free iron. This eventually results in decreased stainable iron in erythrocytes (hypochromia of RBC on peripheral smear). Chronic inflammation also decreases erythropoiesis, leucopoiesis, and megakaryopoiesis, ultimately leading to pancytopenia [1].

Abnormal liver function tests, usually with slight elevations in transaminases and bilirubin, and moderate to severe elevation of alkaline phosphatase are signs of infiltrative liver disease such as TB, rather than chronic active hepatitis, cirrhosis, or hepatic congestion. Similar elevations were seen in our patient. The presence of hyponatremia and anemia in our patient reflects malnutrition and chronic illness, respectively [6].

TB causes elevation of inflammatory markers like CRP, IL-1, IL-6, D-dimer, TNF alpha, and ferritin, so hyperferritinemia in our patient can be explained. Cytokines induce hepatic acute phase responses that alter levels of coagulation proteins such as fibrinogen and factor VIII. Widespread disturbances in homeostasis lead to the activation of vascular intima and render it more thrombogenic. These lead to increase in PT, INR, and aPTT (all these were observed in our patient). Hence it is characterized immunologically by an acute-phase response and hematologically by impaired fibrinolysis consistent with a hypercoagulable state. All the above lab findings can be considered as clinical clues for disseminated miliary TB, so as to raise the suspicion of the same [7].

Atypical presentations of tuberculosis in immunocompromised state include increased frequency of false negative sputum smears, false negative Mantoux test, atypical radiological findings, extrapulmonary TB, absence of characteristic epithelioid cell granulomas in tissues, and high mycobacterial load in macrophages; majority of these features were seen in our case. This patient was poorly built and nourished but HIV-negative; the definite cause of her immunosuppression could not be ascertained. This case of disseminated military TB is in contrast to the other similar case of military TB showing millet-sized tubercles on gross and characteristic caseating epithelioid cell granulomas on microscopy (Refer Chap. 24).

References

1. Khan FY. Review of literature on disseminated tuberculosis with emphasis on the focused diagnostic workup. J Family Community Med. 2019;26(2):83–91. https://doi.org/10.4103/jfcm.JFCM_106_18.
2. Miranda MS, Breiman A, Allain S, Deknuydt F, Altare F. The tuberculous granuloma: an unsuccessful host defence mechanism providing a safety shelter for the bacteria. J Immunology Research. 2012;2012:139127. 14 pages. https://doi.org/10.1155/2012/139127.
3. Peyron P, Vaubourgeix J, Poquet Y, et al. Foamy macrophages from tuberculous patients' granulomas constitute a nutrient-rich reservoir for M tuberculosis persistence. PLoS Pathog. 2008;4(11):e1000204.
4. Puissegur MP, Botanch C, Duteyrat JL, Delsol G, Caratero C, Aaltare F. An in vitro dual model of mycobacterial granulomas to investigate the molecular interactions between mycobacteria and human host cells. Cell Microbiol. 2004;6(5):423–33.
5. Ramkrishnan L. Revisiting the role of the granuloma in tuberculosis. Nat Rev Immunol. 2012;12:352–66.
6. Wang JY, Hsueh PR, Wang SK, Jan IS, et al. Disseminated tuberculosis—a 10 year experience in a medical center. Medicine. 2007;86:39–46.
7. Gonzalez RD, Prince O, Cooper A, Khader S. Cytokines and chemokines in Mycobacterium tuberculosis infection; Microbiol Spectr. 2016;4(5).

26 Mystic Hepatopathy in a Sickle Hemoglobinopathy

Shilpa Kapil Lad, Kusum D. Jashnani, and Vrinda Kiran Kulkarni

26.1 Clinical History

A 20-year-old female delivered a stillborn male fetus at home at 7 months of gestation. She was admitted for PV bleeding 1 h following delivery and had jaundice, fever with chills for 3 days. She also presented with altered behaviour. There was a history of splenectomy done 7 years ago, details of which were not available. Investigations at admission showed a hemoglobin level of 4 g/dL, a total WBC count of 50,600/mm^3, and a platelet count of 106,000/mm^3. Peripheral blood smear showed hypochromasia, microcytosis, polychromasia, anisocytosis, target cells and sickle cells with 89 nucleated RBCS/100WBCs. Liver function test revealed total bilirubin of 33 mg/dl with direct bilirubin of 13.8 mg/dl, SGOT of 10,000 U/L, SGPT of 1350 U/L, and alkaline phosphatase of 774 KA units. Prothrombin time was prolonged to 28 s (contro of 12 s) with an INR of 2.14. Viral markers for hepatitis B, C, and E were negative. She was given 3 pints of packed red cells and 3 pints of fresh frozen plasma. A sickling test done on day 2 of admission was positive. Blood sample for hemoglobin electrophoresis was sent just prior to her death which revealed HbS of 50.6%, HbA of 32.6%, HbF of 4.8%, and HbA 2 of 4.0%, suggestive of sickle beta + thalassemia. An ultra sound examination showed multiple hypoechoic lesions in the liver 13 mm × 11 mm suggestive of abscesses. The spleen was not visualised on ultrasound examination. She did not give any past history of transfusions. Her sister and mother were also subjected to the hemoglobin electrophoresis which revealed a sickle cell trait in them. Tests for leptospirosis and RMAT were negative. During her stay of 2 days, she was given broad spectrum antibiotics, vitamin K injections and supportive treatment. Her condition deteriorated and she died on the third postpartum day. She had a total hospital stay of 2 days. A complete autopsy was performed on this patient.

26.2 Autopsy Findings

All organs were normal, except the liver which was enlarged, weighed 2 kg, and showed diffusely scattered nodules on the external and cut surface. The nodules were of varying sizes ranging from 1 mm to 1.6 cm. The liver was markedly congested with the centre of these nodules

S. K. Lad · K. D. Jashnani (✉)
Department of Pathology, Topiwala National Medical College and BYL Nair Charitable Hospital, Mumbai, Maharashtra, India

V. K. Kulkarni
Department of Medicine and Clinical Hematology, Topiwala National Medical College and BYL Nair Charitable Hospital, Mumbai, Maharashtra, India

K. D. Jashnani (ed.), *Maternal Mortality - Lessons Learnt from Autopsy*,
https://doi.org/10.1007/978-981-19-3420-9_26

appearing yellow (Fig. 26.1). The lungs weighed 300 g each and were markedly congested.

Histopathologic examination of the liver showed a completely distorted architecture due to regenerating nodules separated by broad fibrous septae (Fig. 26.2). The hepatic sinusoids were severely congested and packed with sickled RBCs. The centre of the majority of nodules showed ischemic necrosis of the hepatocytes (Fig. 26.3). Within the fibrous septae, there was mild lymphocytic infiltrate and minimal canalicular cholestasis. Few regions showed the presence of bridging necrosis. Special stains like Prussian blue for iron deposits, orcein for copper and viral inclusions, and periodic acid Schiff

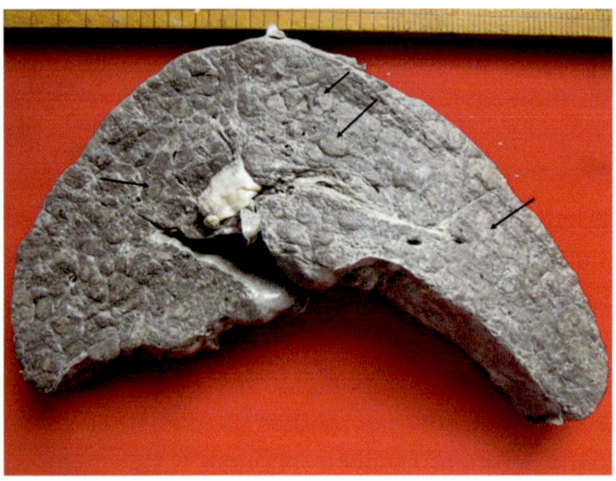

Fig. 26.1 Slice of liver showing cirrhosis composed of varying sized nodules. The entire liver is congested with the centre of nodules appearing yellow (infarction) (Black arrows)

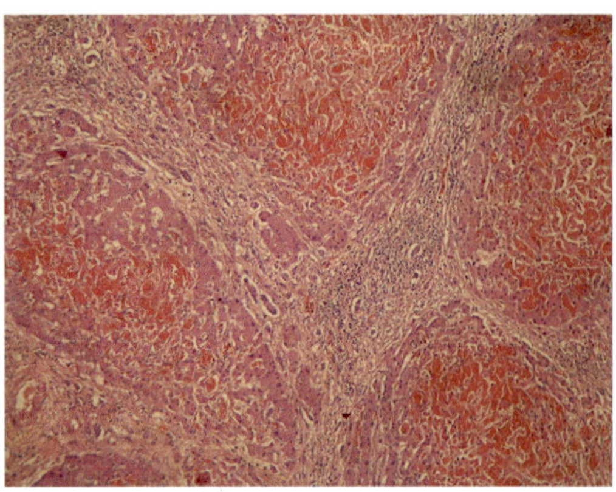

Fig. 26.2 Liver showing loss of normal liver architecture which is replaced by multiple regenerating nodules separated by fibrous septae. The centre of the nodules is showing infarction. 100×, H&E

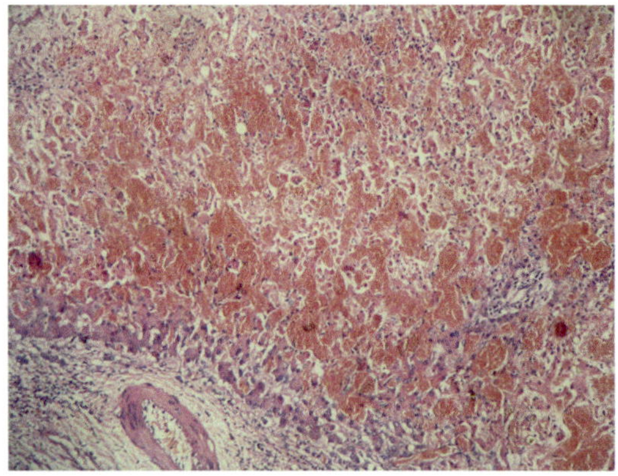

Fig. 26.3 Liver showing infarcted hepatocytes and sinusoidal plugging with sickle cells. 400×, H&E

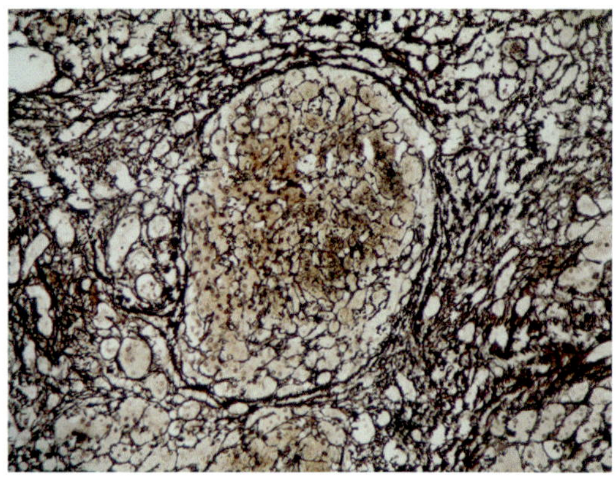

Fig. 26.4 Liver showing regenerating nodules. 100× reticulin stain

with diastase (PAS D) for alpha 1 antitrypsin were done, and all were negative. Reticulin stain was done, which showed regenerating nodules separated by fibrous septae (Fig. 26.4).

Sections of the lung showed a fibrotically thickened pleura. Alveolar septal vessels were congested and packed with sickled red blood cells. There were focal areas of pulmonary edema with few macrophages. An occasional epithelioid cell granuloma was seen. The rest of the organs were unremarkable on gross and histopathology.

26.3 Final Cause of Death

Hepatic encephalopathy following mixed nodular cirrhosis in a postpartum female with sickle beta+ thalassemia.

26.4 Clinicopathologic Discussion

Sickle cell disease is an inherited hematologic disorder. It can occur as homozygous sickle cell anemia, heterozygous sickle cell trait or in association with other hemoglobinopathies. The clinical presentation of sickle cell disease may vary from acute sickle hepatic crisis, hepatic sequestration crisis, and acute sickle intrahepatic cholestasis to cirrhosis [1, 2]. The liver histology in sickle cell disease can vary from distended Kupffer cells, sinusoidal obstruction and distension with sickle cells, focal parenchymal necrosis and cirrhosis [3].

Cirrhosis is reported in 16–29% of patients with sickle cell disease. Cirrhosis is defined as a chronic and diffuse process with the replacement of normal liver architecture by regenerating nodules separated by irregular fibrous bands. It is an end stage disease due to multiple causes. The most frequent are post viral cirrhosis, alcoholic and non-alcoholic steatohepatitis. Rare causes include autoimmune diseases, biliary diseases and metabolic conditions.

However, the etiopathogenesis of cirrhosis in sickle cell disease is mainly attributed to iron overload or transfusion transmitted viral hepatitis, rather than the hematologic process itself. Sickle beta + thalassemia is usually a very mild disease with mild anemia, microcytosis and hypochromasia on peripheral smear examination. There are only very few case reports of liver involvement in patients with sickle beta + thalassemia.

Our case was a young female in the postpartum stage with an acute hepatic presentation of a chronic liver disease. We tried to rule out the possible etiologic factors for cirrhosis based on history, serum viral markers and special stains. This case represents a case of cryptogenic cirrhosis occurring in a sickle beta+ thalassemia. Our patient was in a stage of compensated cirrhosis hence did not suffer from any complications of cirrhosis or portal hypertension like hematemesis from esophageal varices, ascites, hepatorenal syndrome, etc., as these patients are usually asymptomatic. They should be screened regularly for future decompensation. If possible, these patients can be treated for their underlying disease to slow down the disease progression and avoid/delay the need for liver transplantation. The median survival observed for patients with compensated cirrhosis and decompensated stage is 9–12 years and 2 years, respectively.

There are three case reports published in the literature till date on the occurrence of cirrhosis in sickle beta+ thalassemia. One is a young Mediterranean man with sickle beta+ thalassemia with cirrhosis with negative viral markers and second degree siderosis [4]. The other case report was a Ghanaian man with Sβ^+ thalassemia who was asymptomatic for liver disease until adulthood. He presented with features of subacute liver failure and cirrhosis with superimposed cholestasis and necrosis [5].

The third case was a Sicilian woman with Sβ^+ thalassemia with cryptogenic cirrhosis. She developed allograft dysfunction and was positive for anti-nuclear antibodies (1/160). The presence of concomitant autoimmune hepatitis as a possible cause of cryptogenic cirrhosis was suggested [6].

In this case, the patient had an acute presentation due to ischemic necrosis of the hepatocytes due to sinusoidal plugging with sickle cells, which was well reflected in the markedly elevated levels of transaminases. Her bilirubin levels were significantly elevated which are commonly seen with acute sickle intrahepatic cholestasis. She had severe anemia and coagulopathy along with her hepatic manifestations. The etiologic diagnosis of cirrhosis could not be ascertained in this case. We therefore conclude that this is a case of cryptogenic cirrhosis occurring in a young female patient with sickle beta + thalassemia with acute hepatic presentation.

References

1. Mahera MM, Mansour AH. Study of chronic hepatopathy in patients with sickle cell disease. Gastroenterology Res. 2009;2:338–43.
2. Banerjee S, Owen C, Chopra S. Sickle cell hepatopathy. Hepatology. 2001;33:1021–8.

3. Bauer TW, Moore GW, Hutchins GM. The liver in sickle cell disease: a clinicopathologic study of 70 patients. Am J Med. 1980;69:833–7.
4. Santi L, Montanari G, Berardi S, Patti C, Frigerio M, Sama C, et al. Liver cirrhosis in a patient with sickle cell trait (Hb Sβ^+ thalassemia) without other known causes of hepatic disease. Case Rep Gastroenterol. 2009;3:275–9.
5. Cross TJS, Berry PA, Akbar N, Wendon J, Thein SL, Harrison PM. Sickle liver disease. An unusual presentation in a compound heterozygote for HbS and a novel B-thalassemia mutation. Am J Hematol. 2007;82:852–4.
6. Lerut JP, Clayes N, Laterre PF, Lavenne-Pardonge E, Ciccarelli O, Cavallaro S, et al. Hepatic sickling: an unusual case of liver allograft dysfunction. Transplantation. 1999;67:65–8.

27 Acute Hemorrhagic Pancreatitis and Sepsis: A Cause for Maternal Death

Sushama A. Chandekar, Kusum D. Jashnani, and Asha R. Dalal

27.1 Clinical History

A 19-year-old primigravida postpartum day 3, not registered for ANC, presented to our tertiary care hospital as a referral from a peripheral hospital with a sudden onset of generalised abdominal pain and vomiting. She had history of low-grade fever, anorexia, weight loss and recurrent vomiting since the onset of pregnancy. There was no per vaginal bleeding, hematemesis, diarrhoea or constipation or syncopal attack. She had past history of tuberculosis (details not known) at the age of 5 years and had taken treatment. She was presently also taking treatment for the same.

At the time of admission to the peripheral hospital, she had 7 months of amenorrhea with severe vomiting and pain in the abdomen. There she delivered a male child by vaginal delivery, but the baby died soon thereafter in the NICU. After delivery, the patient had continuous vomiting, anorexia, fever, poor oral intake, started lethargic, and laboured breathing which gradually increased. Due to her deteriorating condition, she was transferred to our hospital on postpartum day 3.

Clinical examination revealed patient in gasping condition with poor general condition. She was febrile, with pallor ++ and icterus ++, with ascites and pedal edema. Cardiovascular examination showed muffled heart sounds. Respiratory examination was clear. Central nervous system examination showed a deeply unconscious patient who was not responding to deep painful stimuli. Per abdomen showed gross ascites.

Hematological investigations showed a WBC of 32,000/mm^3, hemoglobin of 11.5 g/dL, and a platelet count of 1.50 lakhs/mm^3. Biochemical investigations showed blood urea nitrogen of 33 mg/dL, serum creatinine of 2.4 mg/dL. Liver function tests showed total bilirubin of 5.7 mg/dL, SGOT/SGPT of 68/37 U/L. Arterial blood gas was pH 6.8, PaO_2 30.9 mmHg. Lepto, Dengue, RMAT, peripheral smear for malarial parasite were negative. VDRL, HIV, HCV, and HBsAg were non-reactive. Clinical impression was sepsis with septic shock with acute renal failure with hepatic involvement postpartum day 3. The cause of sepsis was considered puerperal sepsis or UTI or disseminated TB. The clinical condition of the patient deteriorated, and the patient was declared dead within 7 h of admission. A complete autopsy was performed.

S. A. Chandekar · K. D. Jashnani (✉)
Department of Pathology, Topiwala National Medical College and BYL Nair Charitable Hospital, Mumbai, Maharashtra, India

A. R. Dalal
Sir H N Reliance Foundation Hospital, Mumbai, Maharashtra, India

K. D. Jashnani (ed.), *Maternal Mortality - Lessons Learnt from Autopsy*, https://doi.org/10.1007/978-981-19-3420-9_27

27.2 Autopsy Findings

She was poorly built and poorly nourished, with ++ pallor and icterus with pedal edema up to the ankle. The abdomen was distended and revealed 500 cc of hemorrhagic ascitic fluid on opening. Bowel loops were dilated with mesenteric and omental fat, showing areas of chalky white deposits suggestive of fat necrosis. The pancreas weighed 100 g; it was hemorrhagic and edematous with areas of friable necrosis on the external and cut surface with surrounding areas of peripancreatic fat necrosis (Fig. 27.1a). Both the lungs were subcrepitant and showed occasional tiny gray white areas. Hilar lymph nodes on cut surface showed caseation necrosis.

The gall bladder was unremarkable and did not show any stones. On histopathological examination, the pancreas showed focal areas of normal viable pancreatic acini. The rest of the parenchyma showed evidence of coagulative necrosis with large areas of hemorrhage as well as neutrophilic inflammatory infiltrate (Figs. 27.1b, 27.2a–d). Interlobular fatty tissue showed fat necrosis and foci of calcification. Lungs showed occasional foci of caseous necrosis surrounded by epithelioid cells and Langhans giant cells. Hilar lymph nodes also showed extensive caseation necrosis. These findings were suggestive of focal pulmonary tuberculosis with hilar tuberculous lymphadenitis. In the liver, capsule was slightly thickened with a mild mononuclear cell infiltrate with the majority of hepatocytes showing balloon degeneration and intrahepatocytic cholestasis. Intracanalicular cholestasis was seen with portal tracts showing a moderate degree of mononuclear cell infiltrate with spillage of these cells in the liver parenchyma. The uterine endometrium showed decidual change, and physiologic changes of hypertrophy and preischaemia of myometrium on microscopy. The rest of the organs were unremarkable.

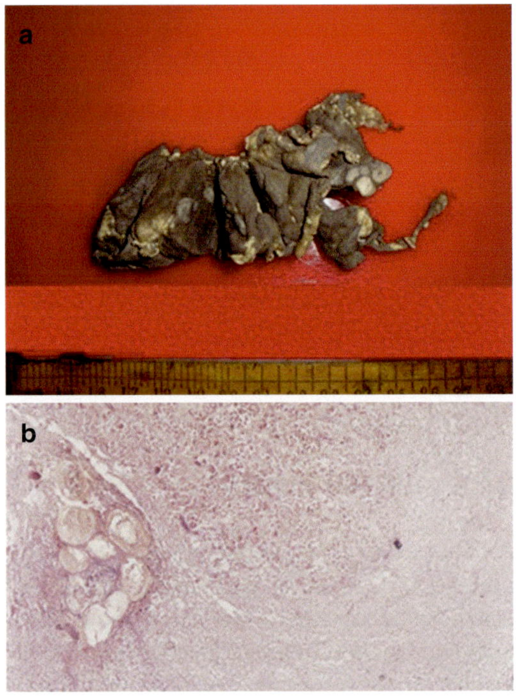

Fig. 27.1 (**a**) Gross photograph of pancreas, externally showing hemorrhagic, edematous appearance with peripancreatic fat necrosis. (**b**) Microphotograph of pancreas showing coagulative necrosis of pancreatic acini with focal areas of hemorrhages. Interlobular fatty tissue showed fat necrosis (H & E, 100×)

27.3 Final Cause of Death

Acute hemorrhagic pancreatitis and sepsis.

27.4 Clinicopathologic Discussion

Acute pancreatitis can be one of the causes of acute abdomen in pregnant women [1]. The spectrum of acute pancreatitis in pregnancy may range from mild symptoms to serious manifestations leading to necrosis, abscesses, pseudocysts, and multiple organ dysfunction syndromes causing significant morbidity and even mortality [2]. It is due to activation of pancreatic trypsinogen followed by autodigestion, which leads to cellular disruption, proteolysis, edema, hemorrhage, and necrosis.

The most common clinical presentations are abdominal pain (89.47%) and vomiting (68.42%) [3]. AP may be misdiagnosed as hyperemesis in pregnancy. Other differential diagnoses include acute fatty liver of pregnancy, HELLP

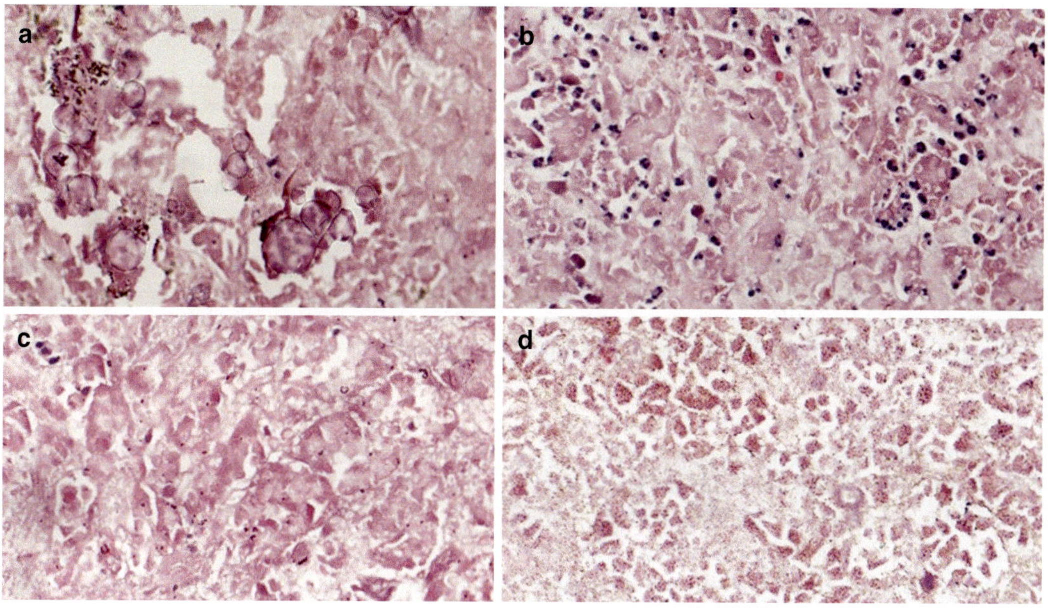

Fig. 27.2 (**a**) Microphotograph showing pancreatic calcification (H & E, 400×). (**b**) Pancreas showing coagulative necrosis of pancreatic acini with neutrophilic infiltration (H & E, 400×). (**c**) Pancreas showing coagulative necrosis of pancreatic acini (H & E, 400×). (**d**) Pancreas showing hemorrhagic area with pigment (H & E, 400×)

syndrome, acute appendicitis, biliary colic, acute cholecystitis, acute cholangitis, obstructive intestinal pathology, and postpartum intraabdominal sepsis [4, 5].

There are various factors implicated in the development of AP in pregnancy [3]. Gallstones, alcohol abuse, and hyperlipidemia are the most common causes of AP in pregnancy. During the second and third trimesters of pregnancy, there is more cholesterol secreted in the hepatic bile as compared to bile acids and phospholipids, giving rise to supersaturated bile. 10% of patients develop stones or sludge over the course of pregnancy. Hypertriglyceridemia also occurs in third trimester pregnancy, thought to represent a physiologic response to the hormonal changes (high levels of steroid hormones-estrogen and progesterone), though not sufficient to cause acute pancreatitis. In such cases, a preexisting hyperlipidemia, if present, may be a contributing factor to acute pancreatitis. In our patient, the total hospital stay was only 7 h during which not much investigations could be done. So, there are two possibilities: either a preexisting abnormality of lipid metabolism in the form of hyperlipidemia (not possible to prove in this case) or an idiopathic form of acute hemorrhagic pancreatitis in the present case.

Clinical outcomes associated with AP are quite diverse. Mortality rate is 3% with interstitial pancreatitis and 17% with pancreatic necrosis [6]. Factors like DIC, ARDS, sepsis, shock, and acute renal failure may lead to death in these cases. The diagnosis of acute pancreatitis requires two out of the three criteria: severe epigastric pain (radiating to the back), serum lipase activity (or amylase activity) at least three times higher than the upper limit of normal, and characteristic findings of AP on CT scan or MRI. There is growing body of evidence that MRI below 1.5 T is safe in pregnancy if USG fails to find out a cause of an acute abdomen.

Serial measurement of lipase and amylase is useful for the diagnosis of pancreatitis, but is neither useful to predict disease prognosis or severity nor for changing the management. The serum amylase level increases within 6–12 h of acute pancreatitis and returns to normal within 3–5 days. The serum lipase level increases within 4–8 h of the onset of symptoms, peaks at 24 h, and returns to normal within 8–14 days. The lipase elevations occur earlier and last longer as compared with elevations in amylase. Serum amylase level elevation of greater than three times the upper limit of the normal range has 67–83% sensitivity and of 85–98% of specificity, while serum lipase has a sensitivity and specificity ranging from 82 to 100%.

Hence, with regard to the high mortality rate of AP in pregnancy, early diagnosis is very important [7] and giving supportive treatment with great attention being given to rest to the pancreas, correction of fluid and electrolyte imbalance with adequate crystalloid and colloid administration until delivery of the baby. Care of the micro-circulation with vital maternal and fetal monitoring would definitely result in good maternal and perinatal outcome [8]. In conclusion, we would like to state that in cases of non-obstetric abdominal pain, one should include serum triglyceride and lipase levels in the list of laboratory investigations.

References

1. Min T, Jian-Ming X, Sha-Sha S, Diao M, Li-Jiu Z. What may cause fetus loss from acute pancreatitis in pregnancy: analysis of 54 cases. Medicine. 2018;97:7.
2. Foram PA, Aditya AM, Prashant VA. Acute necrotizing pancreatitis in a pregnant female diagnosed after caesarean delivery: a case report. Int J Reprod Contracept Obstet Gynecol. 2020;9(12):5183–6.
3. Bahiyah A, Thanikasalam KP, Lim HC, Ray JR. Severe acute pancreatitis in pregnancy. Case Rep Obstet Gynecol. 2015;2015:239068.
4. Arun S, Mohan G, Afzal A, Arvind KB. Acute pancreatitis in early postpartum period: a case report. J Obstet Anaesth Crit Care. 2013;3(2):113.
5. Satya KT, Richa P. Acute pancreatitis-rare presentation in early postpartum period. Ann Clin Case Rep Intern Med. 2019;4:1754.
6. Farzaneh F, Esmaeilzadeh A, Rezaei R. Acute pancreatitis in a pregnant women at 30–31 weeks of gestational age with complete cure. Zahedan J Res Med Sci. 2019;21(3):91408.
7. Pai PR, Shah HK, Samsi AB. Post-partum pancreatitis. J Postgrad Med. 1993;39(2):93.
8. Ducarme G, Maire F, Chatel P, Luton D, Hammel P. Acute pancreatitis during pregnancy: a review. J Perinatol. 2014;34:87–94.

Maternal Death Due to Non-Hodgkin's Lymphoma

28

Lalita Yoganand Patil, Kusum D. Jashnani, Niyati N. Sangoi, and Vrinda Kiran Kulkarni

28.1 Clinical History

A 29-year-old female, not a known case of any major illness, came with complaints of abdominal pain for 7 months and was taking treatment for the same, details of which were not available. The patient was admitted to the surgical ward at our hospital and was discovered to have right cervical, axillary, and abdominal lymphadenopathy, on further investigations. FNAC of the cervical and axillary lymph nodes revealed features suspicious of lymphoproliferative disorder and biopsy was advised. However, the patient was started on ATT and was discharged. The patient visited various hospitals as she was persistently symptomatic. She underwent medical termination of pregnancy (MTP) during her second admission to our hospital and was discharged after taking surgical opinion.

Twenty days later, the patient was re-admitted to our hospital with complaints of abdominal pain. She was found to have bilateral pleural effusion and ascites. At this time, biopsy of the axillary lymph node was performed and a diagnosis of "Non-Hodgkin's lymphoma," favoring large cell lymphoma, was given. Some days later, her condition deteriorated, and she developed breathlessness. Her oxygen saturation dropped and she was put on non-invasive ventilation with a flow rate of 6 L/min. Her chest X-ray was suggestive of left sided pleural effusion with collapse. Her CT scan of the thorax and abdomen revealed multiple, enlarged, necrotic lymph nodes in the periportal, peripancreatic, preaortic, para-aortic, mesenteric, bilateral inguinal, bilateral axillary, pre-tracheal and aortopulmonary windows with the largest lymph node measuring 3.8 × 3 cm in the left axillary region. It also showed the presence of ascites and bilateral pleural effusion (left > right). Multiple hypodense lesions in the liver and spleen were also seen suggestive of granulomas/abscesses. An intercostal chest drain (ICD) was put in view of recurrent pleural effusion. The patient was started on injection Piptaz (piperacillin and tazobactam) and injection Flagyl (metronidazole) with further treatment given as per her symptoms. Cytological examination of the pleural and ascitic fluid showed a cellular smear of reactive mesothelial cells and plenty of neoplastic lymphoid cells. Gradually her clinical condition deteriorated and she succumbed on the 22nd day of admission. A complete autopsy was performed, after due permission.

L. Y. Patil · K. D. Jashnani (✉) · N. N. Sangoi
Department of Pathology, Topiwala National Medical College and BYL Nair Charitable Hospital, Mumbai, Maharashtra, India

V. K. Kulkarni
Department of Medicine and Clinical Hematology, Topiwala National Medical College and BYL Nair Charitable Hospital, Mumbai, Maharashtra, India

K. D. Jashnani (ed.), *Maternal Mortality - Lessons Learnt from Autopsy*, https://doi.org/10.1007/978-981-19-3420-9_28

28.2 Autopsy Findings

On external examination, the deceased was pale with palpable enlarged cervical lymph nodes. Internal examination revealed the presence of approximately 200–300 mL of pale yellow colored fluid in the pleural and peritoneal cavities. The lungs weighed 200 g each and were collapsed (confirmed also on microscopy) with thickened pleura bilateral. Multiple enlarged mediastinal, mesenteric, peripancreatic, hilar, and para-aortic lymph nodes (Figs. 28.1b and 28.2a, b) were seen. On microscopy, all the lymph nodes showed similar morphology. There was complete effacement of normal lymph node architecture by large areas of individual tumor

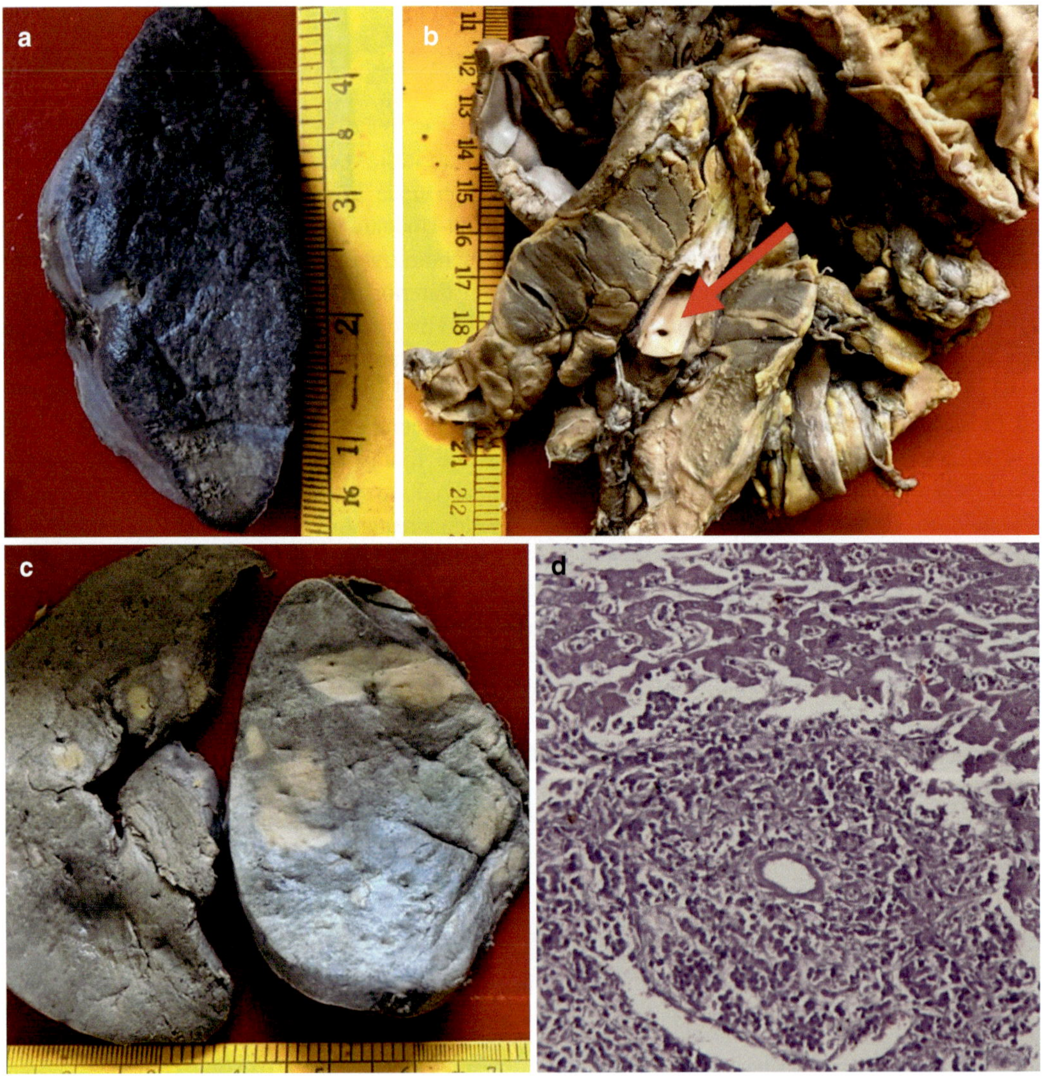

Fig. 28.1 (**a**) Gross picture of the cut surface of the spleen showing the presence of few tiny well-circumscribed, yellowish nodules (at one end). (**b**) Gross picture showing multiple enlarged abdominal para-aortic lymph nodes (red arrow indicates aorta). (**c**) Gross picture of the cut surface of the slices of liver showing the presence of multiple, well-circumscribed, yellowish, firm nodules. (**d**) Microscopy of the liver showing diffuse sheets of small, monomorphic tumor cells (H&E, 100×)

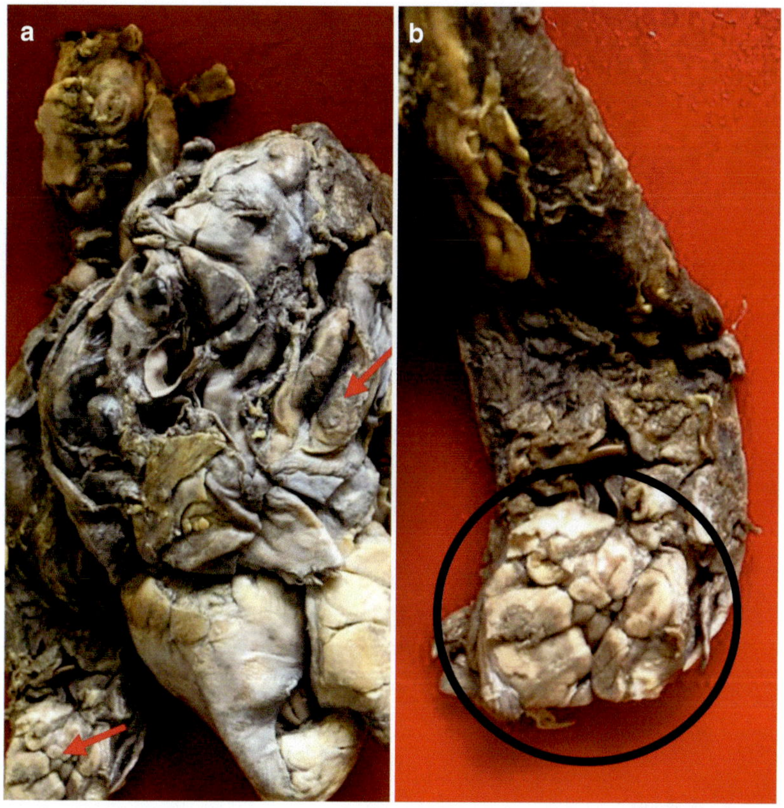

Fig. 28.2 (**a**) Gross picture showing multiple thoracic para-aortic lymph nodes (red arrows). (**b**) Gross picture showing multiple thoracic para-aortic lymph nodes (encircled in black)

cell necrosis with focally, peripherally preserved monomorphic tumor cells. Individual tumor cells were small to medium sized with scant cytoplasm, and hyperchromatic nuclei. Many mitotic figures, apoptotic bodies, and foci of hemorrhages were seen. The liver weighed 1.5 kg and showed multiple well circumscribed nodules, the largest measuring 4.5 cm × 2.5 cm and the smallest measuring 0.5 cm × 0.5 cm on the external and cut surface. These nodules were yellowish in color and firm in consistency (Fig. 28.1c). The spleen, weighing 120 g, also showed the presence of few tiny nodules on the cut surface towards one end, suggestive of metastasis (Fig. 28.1a). Microscopy of the liver (Fig. 28.1d) and spleen (Fig. 28.3a, b) showed the presence of small, monomorphic tumor cells arranged in sheets with the same histomorphologic features as seen in lymph nodes. In the liver, these tumor cells showed infiltration around the central vein and periportal region. An impression of "Non-Hodgkin's lymphoma" was given. Immunohistochemistry was done, which was positive for CD 3 and CD 45 (Fig. 28.3c, d) and negative for CD 20. These findings favored a T-cell lymphoma. Uterus with cervix measured 8 × 3 × 2 cm with the presence of copper-T IUCD in the endometrial cavity. On microscopy, endometrial stroma showed the presence of lymphocytes, plasma cells, and few multinucleated giant cells suggestive of chronic endometritis. Myometrium was unremarkable with no evidence of hypertrophy or preischemia. The gross and microscopic examination of all the other organs was unremarkable.

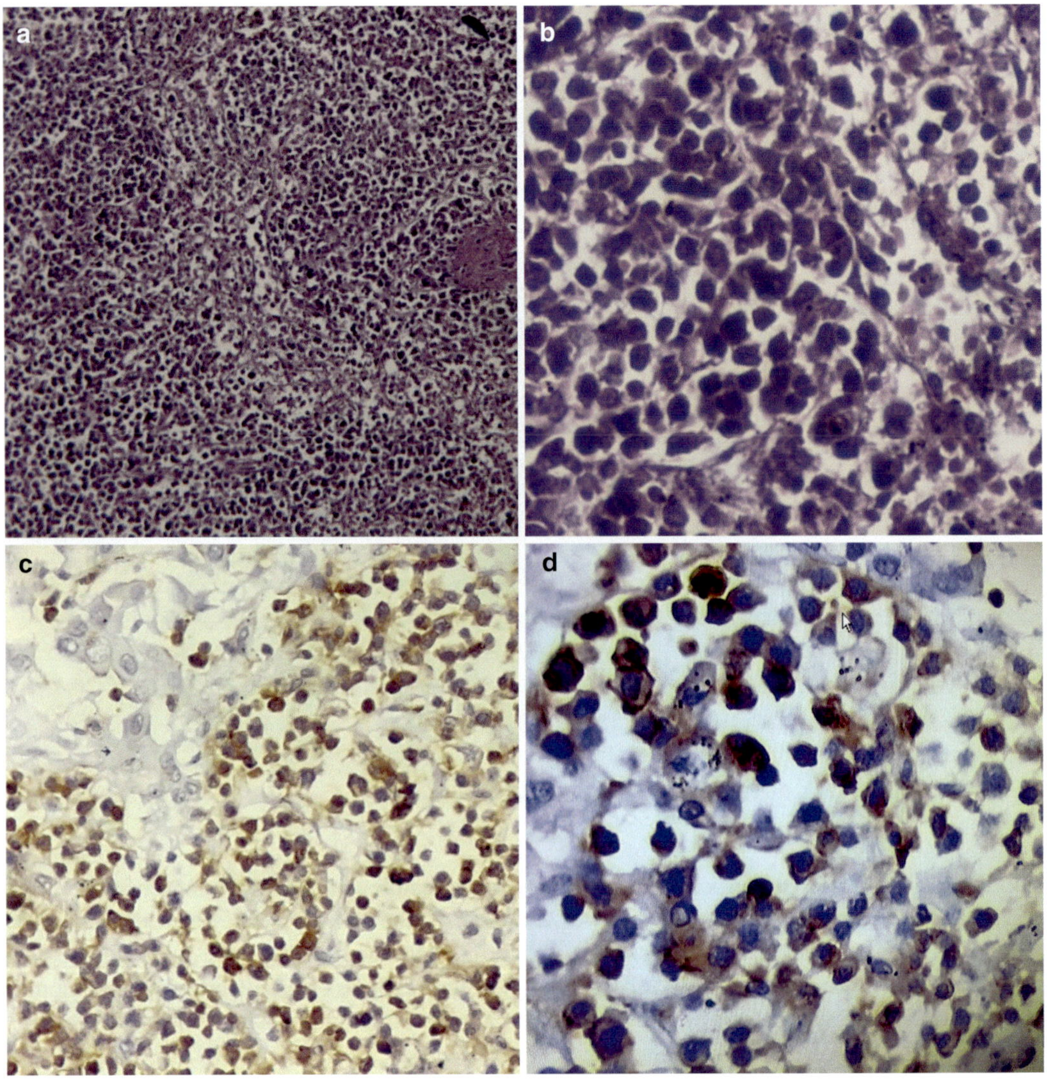

Fig. 28.3 (**a**, **b**) Microscopy of the spleen showing diffuse sheet of small, monomorphic tumor cells (H&E, 100× & 400×). (**c**) Microscopy of the lymph node showing positivity for CD3 in the tumor cells (IHC, 400×). (**d**) Microscopy of the lymph node showing positivity for CD45 in the tumor cells (IHC, 1000×)

28.3 Final Cause of Death

Disseminated Non-Hodgkin's Lymphoma with bilateral lung collapse.

28.4 Clinicopathologic Discussion

After breast cancer, hematologic malignancies represent the second most common neoplasms diagnosed during pregnancy [1]. Non-Hodgkin's Lymphoma is a neoplasm of the lymphoid tissue. It can arise from B-cell and T-cell precursors, mature B cells and T cells, and NK (natural killer) cells. It can be classified into "indolent" and "aggressive" forms. Indolent forms are slow growing, whereas aggressive forms present with rapidly increasing tumor masses and show frequent metastasis, as seen in our case. Follicular lymphoma, small lymphocytic lymphoma, and splenic marginal zone lymphoma usually have an indolent presentation, whereas Burkitt lymphoma, diffuse large B-cell lymphoma, precursor B-cell and T-cell leukemia/lymphoma, and adult T-cell leukemia/lymphoma have an aggressive course [2].

The pathogenesis of NHL includes activation of proto-oncogenes by chromosomal translocation and inactivation of tumor suppression genes by chromosomal mutation or deletion. The most common chromosomal abnormality found in NHL is t (14:18) [2].

Management of aggressive NHL during pregnancy poses a challenge to the clinician. Delayed diagnosis and treatment may lead to fatal outcomes. NHL often presents with non-specific or overlapping symptoms with those of infections like tuberculosis, including fever, weight loss, lymphadenopathy, and abdominal pain. Non-responsiveness to therapy indicated by persistence of symptoms warrants immediate attention. In the present case, even though the FNAC report of cervical and axillary lymph nodes was given as suspicious of lymphoproliferative disease and was advised biopsy, the patient was empirically started on ATT. However, she did not show any response and her condition progressively worsened, and hence, she was admitted for the third time with breathlessness caused by bilateral pleural effusion. A biopsy done during this time confirmed a diagnosis of NHL-favor DLCL on light microscopy. Immunohistochemistry (IHC) was advised to confirm and typify the diagnosis. Hence, a close follow-up of all patients started on ATT, especially on empirical basis, is necessary. Diffuse large B-cell lymphoma is the commonest large cell lymphoma, with the neoplastic cells showing B-cell marker expression (CD20/CD19/CD22/CD79a), BCL6 (60–90%), CD10 (30–60%), IRF4/MUM1 (35–65%), and variables CD45 and BCL2. IHC of our case showed CD3 and CD45 positivity with negative CD20 which favored a diagnosis of T-cell lymphoma.

Common types of T-cell lymphoma are described below:

1. Peripheral T-cell lymphoma, not otherwise specified (PTCL, NOS): Here patients usually have constitutional symptoms (i.e., fever, night sweats, and unexplained weight loss).
2. Anaplastic large cell lymphoma ALCL: This can be systemic or cutaneous. Systemic type is further classified as ALK-positive disease (common in young adults and responds well to chemotherapy) or ALK-negative disease (common in people over 60, does not respond well to chemotherapy with more chances of relapse).
3. Angioimmunoblastic T-cell lymphoma (AITL): Seen in middle-aged to elderly and diagnosed as advanced stage disease.

Adult T-cell leukemia/lymphoma, which also has blood involvement, and lymphoblastic lymphoma, which is seen in adolescents and young adults, are other uncommon types of T-cell lymphomas. Due to the limited in-house IHC panel available, it was not possible to further sub-classify T-cell lymphoma in the present case.

Serous effusions are complications of lymphoma, with pleural effusion being the most commonly observed [3]. Abdominal and pericardial effusions are relatively rare. In our case, the patient showed the presence of pleural effusion as well as ascites. Poor outcomes are observed in patients with lymphoma associated with serous effusions [3], which was seen in our case. Impaired lymphatic drainage due to obstruction in mediastinal lymph nodes or thoracic duct, pulmonary infection, venous obstruction, pleural involvement of the tumor or radiation therapy are the proposed causes for serous effusions in lymphoma [3]. In these cases, the primary treatment targets include therapeutic tapping to relieve pressure symptoms and improve quality of life.

In conclusion, lymphoma can often present with non-specific and overlapping symptoms with infections such as tuberculosis. Non-responsiveness to ATT should warrant immediate attention. A biopsy of the enlarged lymph node often aids towards the correct diagnosis. Serous effusions are a common complication of high-grade lymphomas and are associated with poor outcomes. Hematologic malignancies, although uncommon, can be encountered in pregnancy. If not correctly diagnosed early, they can lead to fatal outcomes.

References

1. Pinnix CC, Andraos TY, Milgrom S, Fanale MA. The management of lymphoma in the setting of pregnancy. Curr Hematol Malig Rep. 2017;12(3):251–6.
2. Sapkota S, Shaikh H. Non-Hodgkin lymphoma. StatPearls [Internet]. Treasure Island (FL); 2020.
3. Jiang Y, et al. An aggressive form of non-Hodgkin's lymphoma with pleural and abdominal chylous effusions: a case report and review of the literature. Oncol Lett. 2013;6(4):1120–2.

Normal Physiologic Changes of Gravid Uterus

29

Kusum D. Jashnani and Meherrituja V. Palve

29.1 Case 1

A 20-year-old female with 5 months of amenorrhoea was transferred with complaints of intermittent fever for 20 days and high coloured urine for 15 days. Her LFTs were deranged. She was found to be HEV positive. She had an intrauterine fetal death. Clinically it was diagnosed as a case of acute fulminant hepatitis with sepsis with coagulopathy and hepatic encephalopathy. The patient died within 3 h of hospital stay, and a complete autopsy was performed.

29.1.1 Autopsy Findings

Gross: The uterus with fetus weighed 500 g; the fetus alone weighed 400 g. The liver weighed 1.3 kg; capsule slightly wrinkled. The cut section was greenish-yellow, very foldable, and soft—features suggestive of submassive hepatic necrosis. The lungs weighed 500 g each. The pleura was smooth. The cut section was congested and firm rubbery in consistency.

29.1.2 Microscopy

Endometrium showed decidualisation. Myometrium showed increase in the size of each of the myometrial fibres (hypertrophy) with nuclei showing a faint blue outline (preischemic changes). Intermediate trophoblasts were seen in the decidua and superficial myometrium (Fig. 29.1d). Sections from the cervix, placenta, and umbilical cord were unremarkable. Sections from the lungs showed patchy areas of alveoli showing edema fluid and the presence of hyaline membrane along the septae suggestive of pulmonary edema and ARDS. Bronchioles and blood vessels were unremarkable. Sections from liver showed large areas of hepatic necrosis with preserved periportal hepatocytes. Hepatocytic and ductular cholestasis was seen in preserved areas.

K. D. Jashnani (✉)
Department of Pathology, Topiwala National Medical College and BYL Nair Charitable Hospital, Mumbai, Maharashtra, India

M. V. Palve
Department of Pathology, K.J Somaiya Medical College, Mumbai, Maharashtra, India

K. D. Jashnani (ed.), *Maternal Mortality - Lessons Learnt from Autopsy*,
https://doi.org/10.1007/978-981-19-3420-9_29

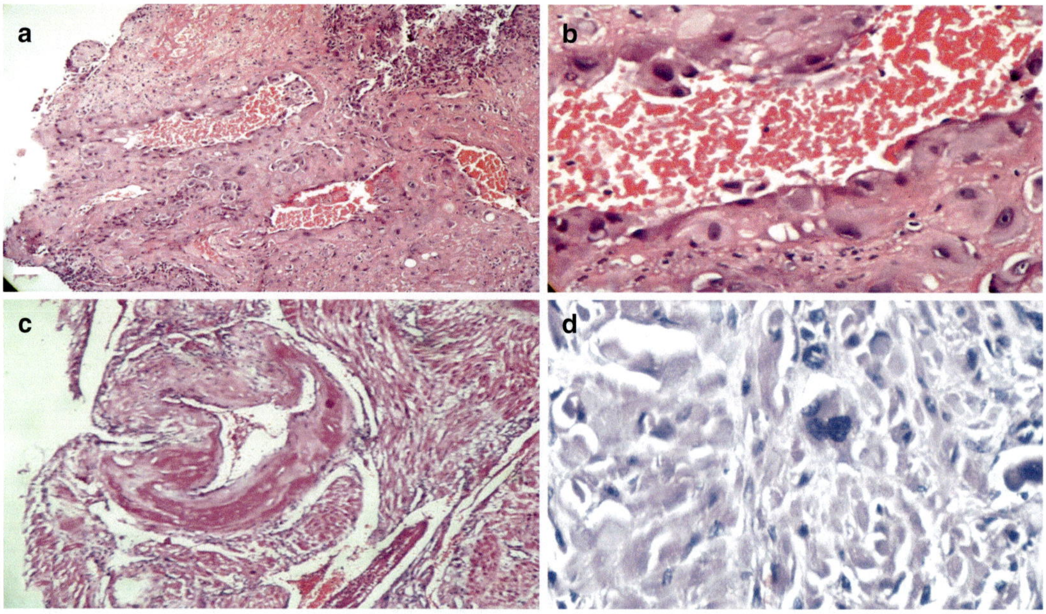

Fig. 29.1 (**a**) Vessels (3 in number) show fibrinoid material deposition with loss of muscle in the wall along with the presence of IT cells (H&E, 200×), (400×, **b**). (**c**) Fully transformed uteroplacental artery (200×). (**d**) Multinucleated IT cells in the myometrium with surrounding hypertrophied myometrial cells with preischemic change (400×)

29.1.3 Final Cause of Death

Hepatic encephalopathy following submassive hepatic necrosis and ARDS in a hepatitis E positive pregnant female.

29.2 Case 2

A 30-year-old female was referred to our hospital in view of an intracranial bleed, day fourth postpartum status with history of headache and intermittent vomiting on and off for 10 days. She had episode of generalised tonic clonic convulsion a day before. She was a known case of hypertension for 2 years. MRI brain had shown hematoma in the left temporoparietal region with a mass effect.

On examination, G.C poor, pulse, and blood pressure were not recordable. The patient was unconscious. Heart sounds were absent. The patient was intubated and CPR was given. But the patient could not be revived and was declared as brought dead.

29.2.1 Autopsy Findings

The uterus with cervix measured 10 × 7 × 5 cm (Fig. 29.2). Cut section: endometrial cavity showed blood clots with an endometrial thickness of 0.5 cm and a myometrial thickness of 2 cm. The cervix on the external and cut surface was unremarkable. The brain weighed 1.2 kg with congested meninges and marked cerebral

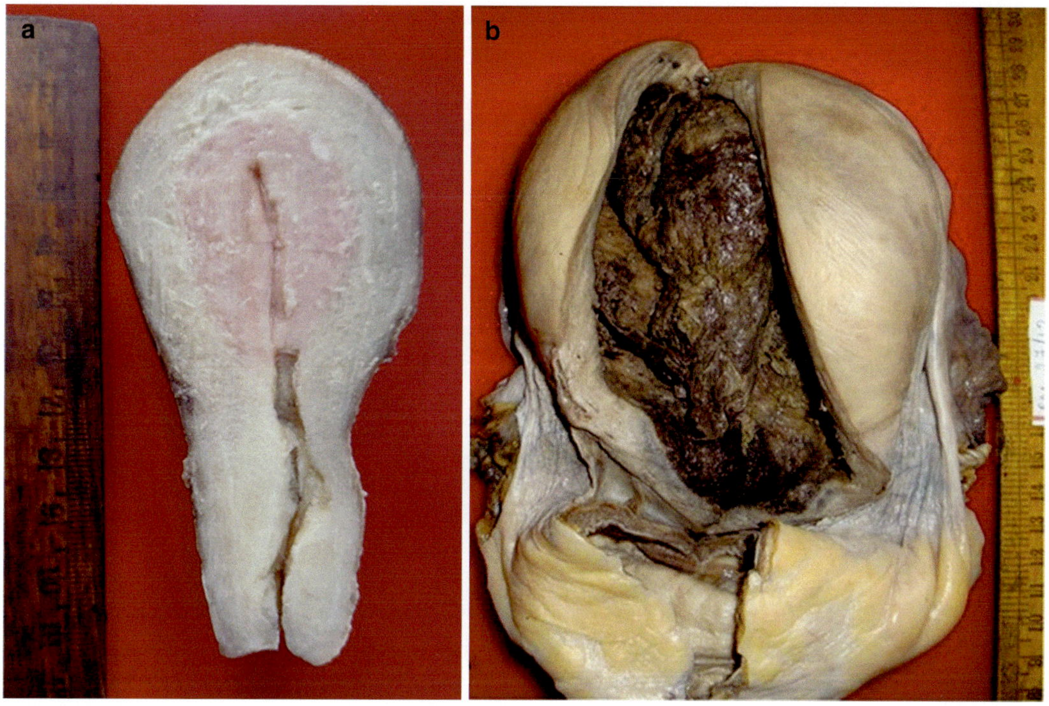

Fig. 29.2 Normal-sized uterus as seen in non-pregnant woman (**a**). Enlarged uterus in a postpartum woman (**b**)

edema. An intraparenchymal hemorrhagic lesion was present on the left temporal side measuring 3 × 2 cm along with mild tonsillar herniation. Lungs bilateral weighed 350 g each with smooth and shiny pleura. Cut section was congested, subcrepitant to rubbery in consistency. The heart weighed 300 g with the left ventricle showing concentric hypertrophy.

29.2.2 Microscopy

The endometrium showed decidual change with physiological hypertrophy and preischemia of the myometrium (Fig. 29.3a, b). Decidual and superficial myometrial vessels showed physiological changes of pregnancy in the form of vascular remodeling (Fig. 29.1a–c), and a few vessels showed fibrin thrombi. Sections from adherent clot showed a blood clot with no evidence of products of conception. Sections from the cerebrum showed features of hemorrhagic cerebral infarct and subarachnoid hemorrhage. Sections from the lungs showed features of pulmonary edema with bronchopneumonia, and a few small vessels showed thromboemboli.

29.2.3 Final Cause of Death

Raised intracranial tension due to subarachnoid hemorrhage and hemorrhagic cerebral infarct with bronchopneumonia in a hypertensive postpartum female.

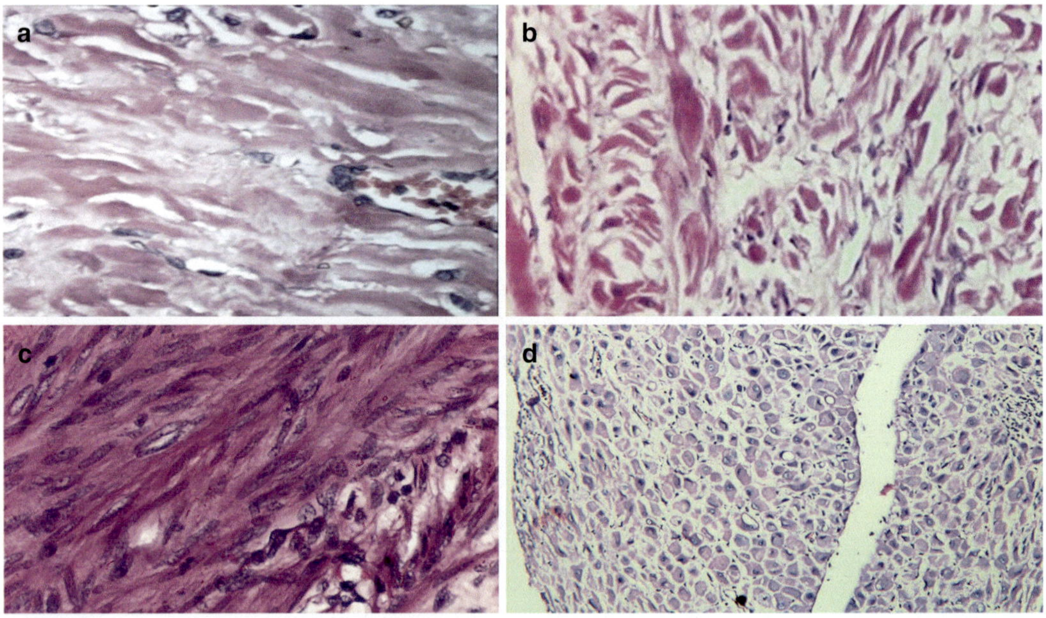

Fig. 29.3 (**a**, **b**) Hypertrophied myometrial fibres of variable degree with faint outlines of nuclei to invisible nuclei, in many cells (400×, H&E). (**c**) Normal myometrial cells in non-pregnant woman with well-defined nuclei (400×, H&E). (**d**) Decidual cells are large in size with well-defined cell borders, containing abundant pale eosinophilic cytoplasm, large vesicular nuclei with conspicuous nucleoli (400×, H&E)

29.3 Clinicopathologic Discussion

The study of physiological changes has always helped in solving the mysteries of pathological conditions. The uterus during pregnancy shows marked increase in its size from the size of a pear of 50 g to almost a football size of almost 1 kg in full-term pregnancy caused by myometrial hypertrophy and hyperplasia, in order to nurture and protect the growing fetus (Fig. 29.2a, b). Hyperplasia is an increase in the number of myometrial fibres, a change difficult to confirm on light microscopy. Myometrial hypertrophy is very well evident on light microscopy, showing moderately to markedly enlarged myometrial fibres depending on the gestational age. However, during the last few weeks of the third trimester of pregnancy, the uterine wall becomes thinner, measuring about 1.5 cm or less in thickness due to the increase in the size of the uterine cavity by the growing fetus. During this time, the myometrial fibres elongate further with decrease in their width, especially seen at term. These changes of increased uterine size are the result of hormone induced enlargement as well as a response of the uterus to the mechanical stress caused by the growing fetus, placenta, and amniotic fluid. Other physiologic changes like remodeling of uterine spiral arteries into uteroplacental arteries and decidualisation of endometrial stromal cells are changes seen also on light microscopic examination, being a visual delight for a gynecologic histopathologist. There are four types of trophoblast cells: syncytiotrophoblasts, cytotrophoblasts, and implantation-site intermediate trophoblasts and chorionic-type intermediate trophoblasts; the last two being subtypes of intermediate trophoblast (IT). The implantation site ITs have the physiologic property of invading decidua, superficial myometrium (Fig. 29.1d) as well as vascular walls, in addition to replacing the endothelial lining of these vessels. Implantation site IT cells can be mononucleated or multinucleated with a high nuclear-cytoplasmic ratio and hyperchromatic irregular nuclei with a moderate to abundant amount of eosinophilic cytoplasm. Mononucleate IT are very often mistaken for the surrounding decidual cells, the difference being- the hyperchromatic nuclei of IT versus the vesicular nuclei of decidual cells. Similarly multinucleated IT can be misidentified as syncytiotrophoblasts. Here one should remember that multinucleated syncytiotrophoblasts have multiple small round to ovoid normochromatic nuclei as against the hyperchromatic irregular nuclei of IT. Also, syncytiotrophoblasts often show vacuoles in their cytoplasm, and they do not have this property of decidual or myometrial invasion in normal physiologic conditions. Once the IT invades the vessel wall, it is characterised by the replacement of the muscular wall of the concerned artery by fibrinoid material deposition (Fig. 29.1a–c). This change results in the conversion of a thick-walled muscular artery with a taut lumen having a fixed blood flow, into a dilated funnel shaped artery with markedly increased blood flow. This way, the vascular remodeling is able to meet the ever-increasing nutritional demands of a growing fetus. Deficiency or absence of this vascular remodeling is known to be the cause of preeclampsia in women. Decidualisation in pregnancy is characterised by conversion of endometrial stromal cells into large polygonal cells (similar in size to squamous cells) with well-defined cell borders, abundant pale eosinophilic cytoplasm and large vesicular nuclei with conspicuous nucleoli (Fig. 29.3d). Deficient or absent decidualisation between the endometrium and the placental interface is characterised by abnormal adherence of the placenta to the endometrium (placenta accreta) or invasion of the placental chorionic villi into the myometrium and/or through the serosa with perforation (placental increta and percreta respectively). These conditions of placenta creta are characterised by excessive intra or postpartum hemorrhage, and may be a cause of maternal death due to hemorrhagic shock. The predecidual endometrial stromal cell change occurs in the late secretory phase on the 24th day of a normal menstrual cycle, when it develops around the prominent spiral arterioles in the endometrium. These cells are comparatively smaller in size with a moderate amount of eosinophilic cytoplasm and a slightly enlarged ovoid nucleus and ill-defined cell borders. If conception occurs, these predecidual cells transform into decidual cells of pregnancy. Pseudodecidual cells are cells of intermediate size, between predecidual cells and decidual cells, seen in the context of poorly formed spiral arterioles, inactive endometrial glands, and the polypoidal architecture of endometrium. This change of pseudodecidual cells is seen in women on exogenous progesterone, and therefore is also known as Pill endometrium [1].

Both of our cases showed a common feature of preischemia in the myometrial fibres. The hypertrophied muscle fibres showed very lightly stained to inconspicuous nuclei (Fig. 29.3a, b). These cells looked similar to those seen in tissues showing coagulative necrosis, where the cellular outlines are preserved but not the nuclei. This was in contrast to normal myometrium with well-defined nuclei in non-gravid uteri (Fig. 29.3c). There was no evidence of inflammation around the myometrial fibres. This change may be the result of the pressure effect of the growing fetus compressing the uterine spiral, arcuate, and radial arteries with reduction in their blood supply leading to ischemia like condition. It is seen in the gravid and postpartum uteri from 20 weeks of pregnancy till 16 days postpartum and should not be mistaken for coagulative necrosis by an ignorant pathologist. Ultrastructural analysis of both non-gravid and gravid myometrial fibres needs to be done in order to find a correct answer to this change of preischemia [2].

References

1. Haines M, Taylor CW, Fox H, Wells M. Chapter 39. Pathology of pregnant uterus. In: Haines and Taylor obstetrical and gynaecological pathology. 5th ed. Edinburgh: Churchill Livingstone; 2003. p. 1327–57.
2. Jashnani K, Palve M. Uterine Myometrial Preischemia: Yet Another Physiological Change of Pregnancy. J Lab Physicians. 2021. https://doi.org/10.1055/s-0041-1734016.

Lobar Pneumonia: A Fatal Non-obstetric Infection!

30

Meherrituja V. Palve, Kusum D. Jashnani, and Rakesh R. Bhadade

30.1 Clinical History

A 25-year-old P1L1 was a primi with 36 weeks' gestation and a known case of pregnancy-induced hypertension. She had complaints of laboured breathing for 10 days. The patient delivered and later developed atonic postpartum hemorrhage which was managed with pitocin and prostodin. The patient had sudden onset breathlessness and low blood pressure. The patient's blood pressure rose after the administration of DOPA. The patient was then transferred to our hospital.

On examination: the patient's general condition was moderate, she was conscious, oriented, afebrile and pale. Pulse was 88/min, low volume with blood pressure—140/100 mm Hg. Respiratory rate was 44/min and breathing was laboured with bilateral rhonchi. Per abdomen: soft, ascites +. CVS: S1S2 normal. Per vaginal: No laceration/ hematoma, episiotomy healthy. Her Hb was 7 g/dL, and platelets were reduced 50,000/cumm, Total leukocyte count- 8500/cumm. SGOT/SGPT were raised (2556 U/L and 910U/L, respectively). Total bilirubin:3.6 mg/dl, direct bilirubin: 1.2 mg/dl. She was transfused with 6 units of FFP and 2 units of packed red cells. The patient's general condition was deteriorating. She developed episiotomy wound edema a day later. Two days later, the patient became unconscious and was intubated. The patient suffered trauma to the right molar teeth and had complaints of oral and nasal bleeding. Her creatinine had risen to 5.5. She underwent dialysis twice. Ascitic fluid examination revealed protein 520 mg% and 10 degenerated WBCs. Urine examination revealed ++ albuminuria and the presence of 12–15 RBCs/hpf. Her USG abdomen revealed splenomegaly and ascites. Viral markers like HEV, HIV, and HBsAg were negative. Her total WBC count had risen to 27,200/cu mm. The patient developed metabolic acidosis and ultimately succumbed to death on the ninth day of hospital stay. A complete autopsy was performed.

M. V. Palve
K.J Somaiya Medical College, Mumbai, Maharashtra, India

K. D. Jashnani (✉)
Department of Pathology, Topiwala National Medical College and BYL Nair Charitable Hospital, Mumbai, Maharashtra, India

R. R. Bhadade
Department of Medicine (Critical Care Unit), Topiwala National Medical College and BYL Nair Charitable Hospital, Mumbai, Maharashtra, India

30.2 Autopsy Findings

The patient was pale and icteric. The patient had bilateral pedal edema, facial puffiness and 5 L of ascitic fluid. There was no evidence of lymphadenopathy.

The right lung weighed 600 g with a smooth shiny pleura, and the left lung weighed 750 g with a hazy pleura. On the cut section,

K. D. Jashnani (ed.), *Maternal Mortality - Lessons Learnt from Autopsy*,
https://doi.org/10.1007/978-981-19-3420-9_30

the left upper lobe was gray-white and firm in consistency. The left lower lobe showed similar focal gray-white firm areas (Figs. 30.1 and 30.2). There was no evidence of any enlarged lymph nodes or thromboembolism. The liver weighed 1.4 kg, enlarged. The capsule smooth. Cut section was greenish, soft, and foldable.

The uterus measured 35 × 22 × 9 cm. Endometrial cavity showed the presence of blood clots. The myometrium, cervix, bilateral ovaries and fallopian tubes appeared unremarkable. The rest of the organs were unremarkable.

Sections from the left lung-upper lobe showed all alveoli filled with fibrinosuppurative exudate with retraction of this exudate from the alveolar septae, producing a clear space between the exudate and the septae, typical of the gray hepatisation phase of lobar pneumonia (Figs. 30.3, 30.4, and 30.5) on microscopy. Sections from firm areas of the lower lobe of the left lung also showed similar histopathologic features. The right lung showed the presence of RBCs within the alveoli and eosinophilic edema fluid within the alveoli in different patchy areas. Occasional alveoli showed eosinophilic hyaline membrane along the alveolar septae suggestive of ARDS. The bronchioles and arteries were unremarkable.

Sections from the brain showed edema and congested meninges. No evidence of exudates or intracerebral hemorrhages. Sections from the liver showed focal areas of necrosis with the presence of inflammatory cells. Microvesicular fatty change in 20% of hepatocytes and intrahepatic cholestasis were present. Sections from the kidney showed patchy areas of acute tubular necrosis. Sections from the stomach showed submucosal hemorrhages and ischemic changes of the overlying mucosa. The endometrium showed decidual change. Myometrium showed physiologic changes of hypertrophy and preischemia. Decidual vessels and superficial myometrial vessels showed normal physiological changes of pregnancy. Sections from the cervix showed multiple congested blood vessels in the wall. The rest of the organs were unremarkable.

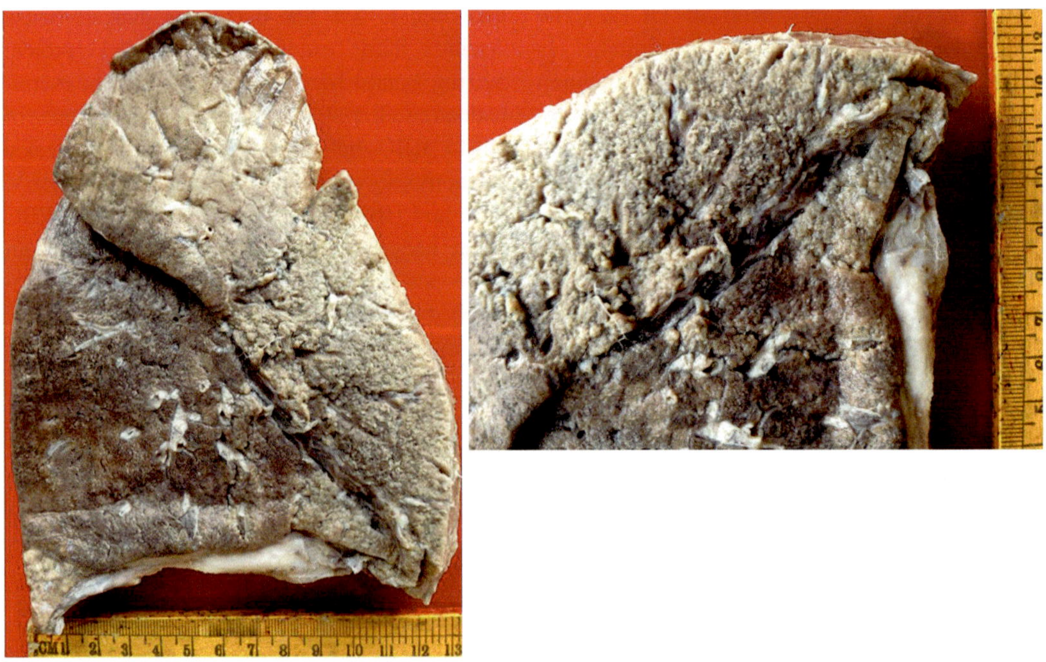

Figs. 30.1 and 30.2 Gross of the left lung: Upper lobe is gray white, consolidated, firm, and liver-like throughout. Similar tiny areas seen in lower lobe also

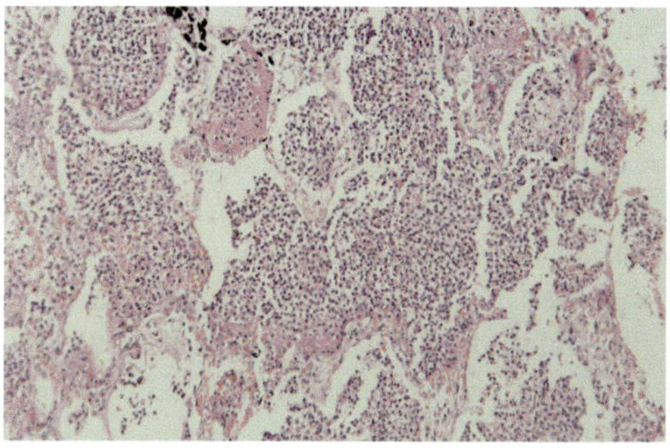

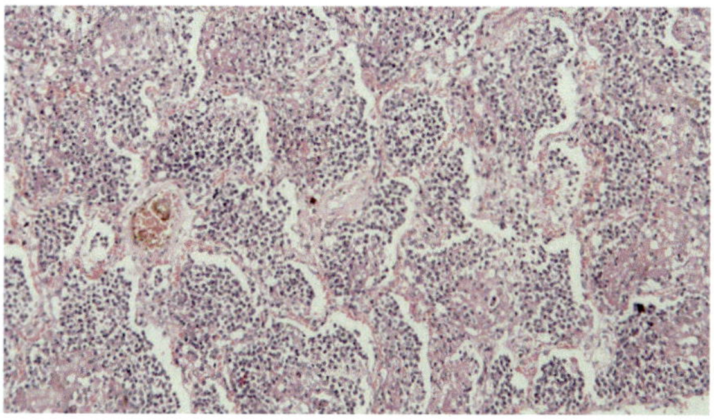

Figs. 30.3 and 30.4 Sections from the lung show alveoli filled with neutrophils, fibrin and occasional macrophages, and RBCs. There is a clear space between the fibrinosuppurative exudate and the alveolar septae. H & E, 200×

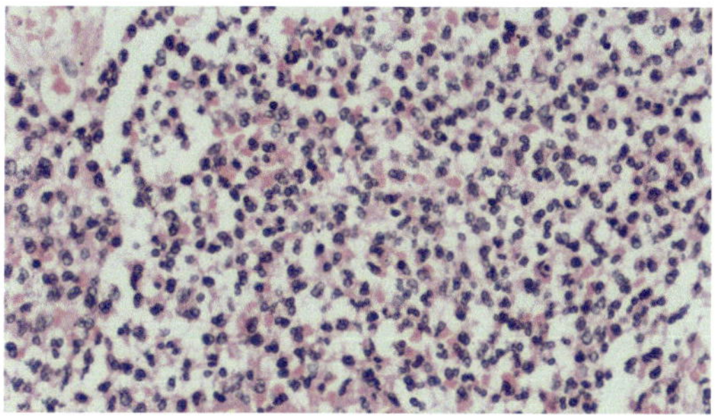

Fig. 30.5 Neutrophilic inflammatory infiltrate and few rbcs within the alveolar spaces H & E, 400×

30.3 Final Cause of Death

Lobar pneumonia and ARDS in a case of hepatitis in a postpartum female.

30.4 Clinicopathologic Discussion

The patient in our case presented mainly due to postpartum hemorrhage. She was also a known case of PIH, and that could have contributed to most of the complications. However, respiratory complaints like laboured breathing and the presence of bilateral rhonchi point towards a pulmonary pathology. Although imaging was not done, the autopsy findings in the lungs both gross and microscopically confirmed lobar pneumonia with ARDS.

Pneumonia is broadly defined as any infection of the pulmonary parenchyma. It is caused whenever there is impairment to the local and systemic defence mechanisms [1]. It occurs more commonly at the extreme of ages; however, pneumonia in young adults can be severe and fatal. Pneumonia is one of the common ailments seen in pregnant patients. Several physiological and immunological changes occur during pregnancy, which predispose pregnant women to a severe course of pneumonia. Downregulation of cell-mediated immunity, increased oxygen consumption, decreased functional residual capacity, decreased chest compliance and increased risk of aspiration make the pregnant patient more susceptible to severe respiratory infections [2–4]. Advanced gestational age has been proven to be an independent maternal risk factor for pneumonia [5]. Other risk factors are anemia, asthma, smoking, use of antepartum corticosteroids and tocolytic agents [4].

Pneumonia is classified according to the specific etiologic agent or by distinct clinical setting in which infection occurs. There are four categories: community-acquired pneumonia (CAP), hospital-acquired pneumonia (HAP), healthcare-associated pneumonia (HCAP), and ventilator-associated pneumonia (VAP) [6]. In a study by the Centres for Disease Control and Prevention, of 2500 adults with pneumonia, pathogens were identified only in 38%; 23% were viruses, 11% bacteria, both in 3% and fungi and protozoa in 1% [7]. Community acquired pneumonia (CAP) is the most common form of pneumonia in pregnancy. It refers to bacterial pneumonia occurring in otherwise healthy individuals that are acquired from a normal environment as against in a hospital. Most often, it is caused by *Streptococcus pneumoniae*, followed by Klebsiella *pneumoniae*, Haemophilus influenzae, and Pseudomonas aeruginosa.

The pulmonary defence mechanisms such as cough reflex, mucociliary clearance system, and immune response help maintain low levels of the microbiome. CAP occurs when there is a defect in normal host defence, or a virulent pathogen overwhelms the immune response or a large infectious microbial inoculum. The invasion and propagation of these virulent strains of bacteria in the lung parenchyma cause the host immune response to initiate a cascade of inflammatory response, causing pneumonia [8].

Bacterial invasion of the lung causes consolidation or solidification of the parenchyma; histologically seen as acute inflammatory exudates within the alveoli, as seen in this case. Depending on the area of the lung involved, bacterial pneumonia has two patterns of distribution: bronchopneumonia, characterised by patchy consolidation confined to one lobe or multilobar, frequently basal and bilateral, and the other is lobar pneumonia, in which the entire lobe or large part of the lobe gets consolidated, as was seen in our case. However, these anatomic patterns often overlap.

Lobar pneumonia progresses through four stages:

1. Stage of congestion: in the first 24 h in which the lungs are heavy, red, and boggy. It is microscopically characterized by alveolar septal congested vessels and intra-alveolar edema. Many bacteria and few neutrophils may be present.
2. Red hepatisation: begins 2–3 days after congestion and affected lung is red-pink, dry, granular, airless with firm liver-like consistency. Microscopically marked cellular infiltrate of neutrophils with some showing ingested bacteria, extravasation of erythrocytes, and fibrin within the alveoli are seen. The alveolar septa become less prominent because of the exudate.
3. Gray hepatisation: occurs 2–3 days following red hepatization and lung appears gray with liver-like consistency due to fibrinopurulent exudate, progressive disintegration of red blood cells, and hemosiderin. The macrophages begin to appear.
4. Resolution: The enzymatic action begins by the eighth day, which liquefies the previous solid fibrinous content and eventually restores aeration. Macrophages are the predominant cells which contain engulfed neutrophils. Lobar pneumonia can cause complications like pleural effusion, empyema, lung abscess, bacteremia, and septicaemia [1, 8].

Clinically, patients with lobar pneumonia present with cough, fever, dyspnea, sputum production, and sometimes hemoptysis and pleuritic chest pain. Constitutional symptoms such as fatigue, headache, myalgia, and arthralgias can also be seen [8]. It is difficult sometimes to distinguish between symptoms related to physiological changes of pregnancy and more menacing symptoms of pneumonia like dyspnea [4]. Chest radiography is essential for diagnosis and should be used with an abdominal shield without hesitation as the radiation exposure rarely reaches the dose associated with fetal harm. The most common radiological findings are consolidation, nodular infiltrates, cavity, and pleural effusion [9]. However, a chest x-ray cannot reliably differentiate bacterial from a non-bacterial cause.

Severe pneumonia is a common cause of ARDS during pregnancy, and such patients may need mechanical ventilation. Pneumonia is a significant cause of maternal and fetal morbidity and mortality. Pregnancy leads to increased risk of respiratory failure in pneumonia. Pneumonia can cause pregnancy complications like preterm labour [10]. Higher prevalence of preeclampsia/eclampsia has been reported too [4]. Effects on the fetus include small for gestational age, intrauterine and neonatal death [4, 11, 12].

In our case, gross and microscopy of the lung showing features of gray hepatisation point towards classic lobar pneumonia. The most common cause of lobar pneumonia is *Streptococcus pneumoniae* [8]. Other causative organisms that may cause a lobar pattern include *Klebsiella pneumoniae*, *Legionella pneumophila*, *Hemophilus influenzae*. The superimposition of reduced respiratory reserve in the setting of a PPH- and PIH-induced hepatorenal failure in this case may have contributed to the irreversible deterioration of the patient's condition.

In developing countries like ours, poor hygiene, overcrowding, malnutrition, and hesitancy to take timely and continuous medical care cause susceptibility to infectious diseases like lobar pneumonia. Prompt use of chest radiography and early medical care can help prevent the morbidity and mortality associated with pneumonia in pregnancy.

References

1. Hussain NA. The lung. In: Kumar V, Abbas KA, Aster CJ, editors. Robbins and Cotran pathologic basis of disease: South Asia edition. 9th ed. India: Reed Elsevier India Pvt. Ltd.; 2014. p. 669–726.
2. Vasudeva A, Bhat RG, Ramachandran A, Kumar P. Infection and acute respiratory distress syndrome during pregnancy: a case series of preventable maternal deaths from southern India. J Infect Public Health. 2013;6:55–7.
3. Mehta N, Chen K, Hardy E, Powrie R. Respiratory disease in pregnancy. Best Pract Res Clin Obstet Gynaecol. 2015;29:598–611.
4. Tang P, Wang J, Song Y. Characteristics and pregnancy outcomes of patients with severe pneumonia complicating pregnancy: a retrospective study of 12 cases and a literature review. BMC Pregnancy Childbirth. 2018;18(1):434. https://doi.org/10.1186/s12884-018-2070-0.
5. Graves CR. Pneumonia in pregnancy. Clin Obstet Gynecol. 2010;53:329–36.
6. Sattar SBA, Sharma S. Bacterial pneumonia. In: StatPearls [Internet]. Treasure Island, FL: StatPearls Publishing; 2021. https://www.ncbi.nlm.nih.gov/books/NBK513321/.
7. Jain S, Self WH, Wunderink RG, et al. Community-acquired pneumonia requiring hospitalization among U.S. adults. N Engl J Med. 2015;373(5):415–27. https://doi.org/10.1056/NEJMoa1500245; Epub 2015 Jul 14
8. Pahal P, Rajasurya V, Sharma S. Typical bacterial pneumonia. In: StatPearls [Internet]. Treasure Island, FL: StatPearls Publishing; 2021. https://www.ncbi.nlm.nih.gov/books/NBK534295/.
9. Durga K, Yuvarajan S. Clinical profile of pregnant women with community acquired pneumonia attending tertiary care hospital. Indian J ObstetGynecol Res. 2019;6(1):91–3.
10. Lapinsky SE. Acute respiratory failure in pregnancy. Obstet Med. 2015;8(3):126–32. https://doi.org/10.1177/1753495X15589223.
11. Romanyuk V, Raichel L, Sergienko R, Sheiner E. Pneumonia during pregnancy: radiological characteristics, predisposing factors and pregnancy outcomes. J Matern Fetal Neonatal Med. 2011;24:113–7.
12. Chen YH, Keller J, Wang IT, Lin CC, Lin HC. Pneumonia and pregnancy outcomes: a nationwide population-based study. Am J Obstet Gynecol. 2012;207(288):e1–7.

Uterine Arteriovenous Malformation

31

Rushabh Shah, Pradeep Vaideeswar, and Kusum D. Jashnani

31.1 Clinical History

Case A: A 24-year-old female with 4 months of amenorrhea presented with abdominal pain and vaginal bleeding in a private nursing home. Ultrasonography revealed 22 weeks' gestation with intrauterine fetal death. She had a spontaneous abortion followed by profuse postpartum hemorrhage. She was referred to our tertiary-care center in a state of shock. An obstetric hysterectomy was being planned but she succumbed within a day of admission.

Case B: A 24-year-old female, 22 days postpartum, was referred to the emergency services department of our institute in view of fever with vomiting and anorexia, progressive shortness of breath, anemia, an infected perineal tear with recto-vaginal fistula, jaundice, edema of feet, and altered sensorium. On examination, the general condition was extremely poor with a pulse rate of 120/min and a blood pressure of 60 mm Hg. There was pallor, icterus, and bilateral pitting pedal edema. She was conscious but disoriented. The systemic examination further revealed muffled heart sounds, bilateral lower zone crepitations, 3 cm hepatomegaly, ascites, palpable 12 weeks' size retracted uterus and perineal wound gape with sloughed rectal mucosa communicating with the wound. In view of sepsis, persistent hypotension and disseminated intravascular coagulation, therapy with antibiotics, inotropes, and blood components, respectively, were started. The patient continued to deteriorate and succumbed within 22 h of admission.

31.2 Autopsy Findings

Complete autopsies were performed in both the cases, and similar findings were noted in both uteri. The uteri measured 7 × 4.5 × 4 cm and 8 × 6 × 5 cm, respectively. The endometrial cavity in Case B was dilated and contained small blood clots. The endometrial surfaces appeared shaggy and hemorrhagic. The myometria (2–2.4 cm thick) showed the presence of multiple small and large vascular channels transmurally, giving the walls a sievelike appearance (Fig. 31.1a–d). Some contained blood clots while others had occlusive, friable, pale-brown thrombi. On histology, the thrombi

R. Shah
SRL Dr Avinash Phadke Labs, Mumbai, Maharashtra, India

P. Vaideeswar (✉)
Department of Pathology (Cardiovascular and Thoracic Division), Seth GS Medical College and KEM Hospital, Mumbai, Maharashtra, India

K. D. Jashnani
Department of Pathology, Topiwala National Medical College and BYL Nair Charitable Hospital, Mumbai, Maharashtra, India

K. D. Jashnani (ed.), *Maternal Mortality - Lessons Learnt from Autopsy*, https://doi.org/10.1007/978-981-19-3420-9_31

(Fig. 31.2) and clots were present in large vein-like channels with smooth muscle walls of varying thickness, amidst hypertrophied myometrial smooth muscle fibers. Similar channels were also seen in the upper part of the cervix. Other organs in the first case were normal. Mural ventricular thrombi (Fig. 31.3a), pulmonary thromboemboli (Fig. 31.3b), and focal hepatocytic hemorrhagic necroses (Fig. 31.3c) were seen in the second case.

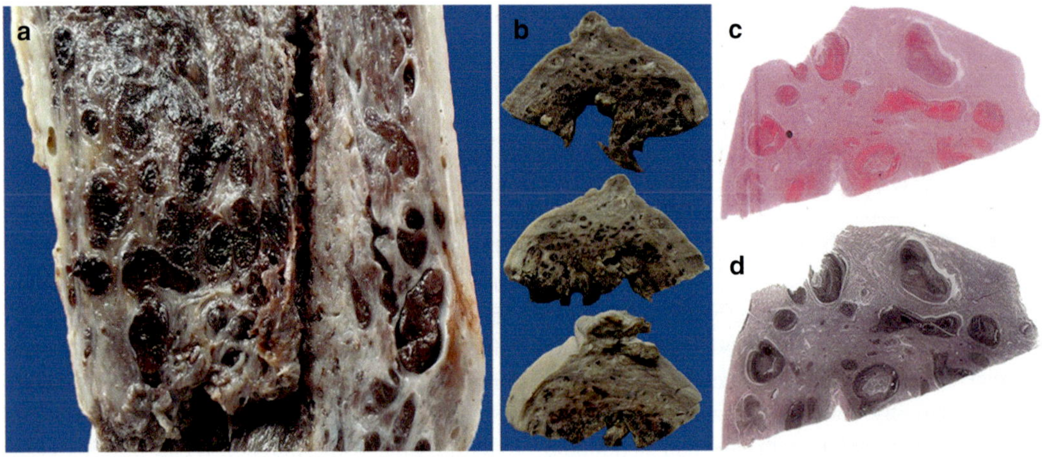

Fig. 31.1 Sievelike appearance of the entire wall of the uterus produced by small and large vascular channels as seen on gross examination. (**a**) Bisected uterus in Case A and (**b**) Serial transverse slices in Case B; a similar appearance is seen in the scanned sections of the uterus of Case B stained by (**c**) H&E and (**d**) Elastic van Gieson

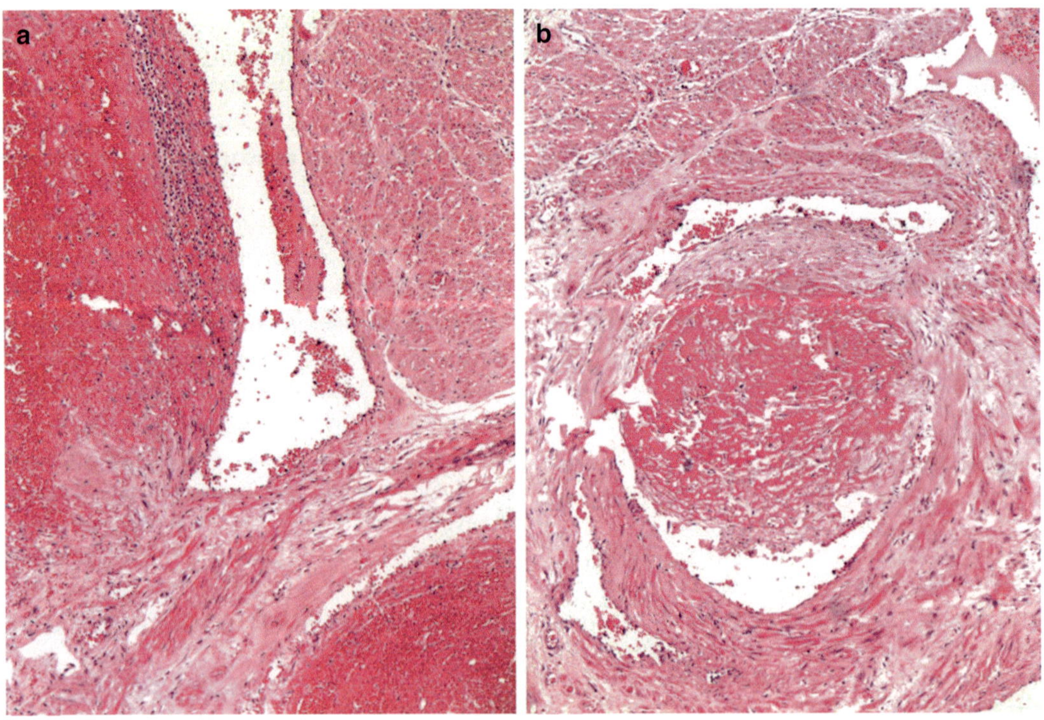

Fig. 31.2 (**a**) and (**b**) show the presence of occlusive fresh thrombi in the uterine vascular channels in Case A (H&E × 200)

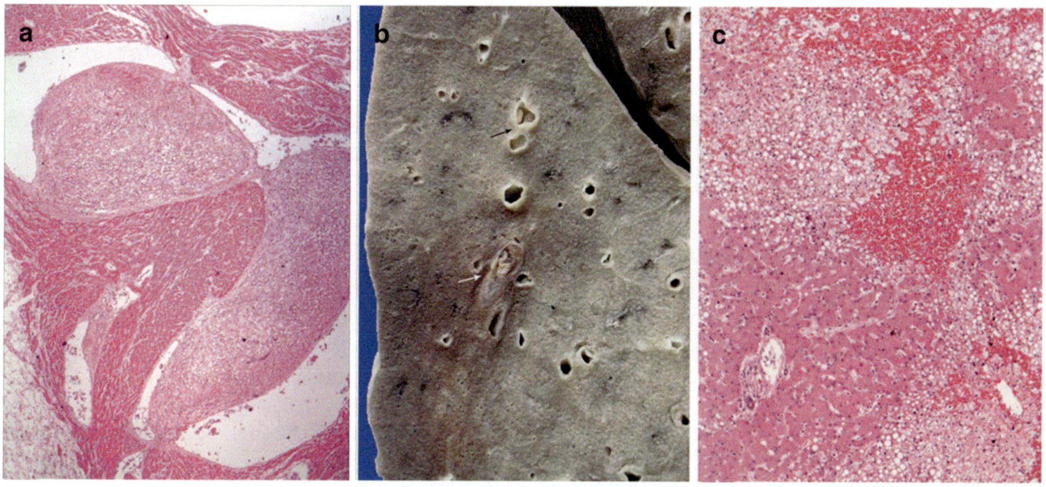

Fig. 31.3 (**a**) Mural right ventricular fresh and organizing thrombi (H&E x 200); (**b**) Close-up of the lung showing presence of arterial occlusive thromboemboli; (**c**) Hemorrhagic necroses in the liver amidst changes of passive venous congestion (H&E × 200)

31.3 Final Cause of Death

Case A: Hypovolemic shock due to post-partum hemorrhage.

Case B: Septicemia with acute myocarditis and pulmonary arterial thromboembolism.

31.4 Clinicopathologic Discussion

Despite being one of the most common soft tissue lesions, vascular anomalies are prone to incorrect nomenclature and misdiagnosis. On the basis of clinical examination, histomorphology, clinical behavior, and cellular kinetics, these anomalies are currently divided into two distinct categories of vascular tumors associated with endothelial proliferation and vascular malformations with underlying mesenchymal and/or angiogenetic disorder [1]. Such UVAs are uncommonly located in the female genital tract. In both the cases presented, large vascular channels with occlusive thrombi distributed in the entire myometrium had imparted a distinct honey-comb-like appearance to the uterine wall, and this appearance suggested a vascular malformation. Such malformations are uncommonly located in the female genital tract and are seen as venous ('cavernous hemangiomas') or AVMs [2]. Some of them are indeed congenital and thought to arise from embryonic sequestration of mesodermal rests or arrested vascular embryological development and failure in differentiation. The histological feature of thick- and thin-walled blood vessels without clear-cut arterial or venous morphology was suggestive of AVM. Majority of AVMs are acquired lesions that develop following uterine trauma (that includes operative procedures), infections, retained products of conception, trophoblastic and non-trophoblastic uterine tumors, and hormonal therapy [2, 3]. The clinical symptomatology of these vascular anomalies is varied. They are frequently asymptomatic; some patients may have abdominal pain, dysfunctional uterine bleeding, or infertility.

In exceptional circumstances, these vascular malformations may be associated with pregnancy with maternal and/or fetal morbidity and mortality. Both our patients did not have any significant past history and were pregnant for the first time. In pregnancy, which is associated with hormonal changes and uterine architectural alterations, the histo-morphological features may have features of both venous malformation or AVMs [4, 5] and these have often led to descriptive diagnosis such as "massive multicystic dilatation of the uterine wall" [6]. As per model proposed by Sun et al.

[7], elevated estrogen levels influence vasculogenesis by increasing the mitotic rate in the capillary endothelial cells via increased endothelial progenitor cells, and on angiogenesis via an indirect pathway of angiogenic factors from increased release of matrix metalloproteinase, vascular endothelial growth factor, nitric oxide, and other related factors. All of this, in turn, promotes the growth of pre-existing vascular lesions, if any. The myometrial fibers undergo hypertrophy and hyperplasia with a criss-cross arrangement, which permits occlusion of the uterine vessels during delivery and involution. However, this physiological process may be affected by the hormone-related overgrowth of the pre-existing vascular proliferation, leading to imperfect, uncoordinated uterine involution and persistence of the cavern-like vascular spaces. Importantly, this was seen to affect the uterine myometrium in its entirety [8]. The end result would be the development of uterine atony and post-abortal or postpartum hemorrhage [9], as was seen in the first case. Additionally, disturbed venous drainage leads to a large volume of blood collection in the uterine wall. Blood stasis, platelet trapping in the pre-existing vascular spaces, and recurrent trauma to fragile vessels promote thrombosis. Hypercoagulable state of pregnancy (the second case had right ventricular mural thrombi) can further complicate the whole scenario, ultimately triggering fatal complications like DIC and pulmonary thromboembolism [10]; the latter was present in the second patient.

Antenatal diagnosis of such rare anomalies is difficult and requires a multidisciplinary approach involving gynecologists, pathologists, and radiologists. Traditional and gold standard for definitive diagnosis is histological examination of a hysterectomy specimen, which is not always possible, and hence a better option is the use of various imaging modalities. Though some lesions can spontaneously regress, the management in the remaining cases depends upon age, desire for future pregnancy, hemodynamic status, and severity of bleeding. Conservative treatment may not always be possible in refractory lesions and life-threatening situations. The diagnosis of UVA was not considered in both our patients. Timely diagnosis is of significance to give prompt treatment and prevent fatal outcomes.

References

1. Sadick M, Muller-Wille R, Wildgruber M, Wohlegemuth WA. Vascular anomalies (part I): classification and diagnostics of vascular anomalies. Rofo. 2018;190:825–35.
2. Szpera-Goździewicz A, Gruca-Stryjak K, Bręborowicz GH, Ropacka-Lesiak M. Uterine arteriovenous malformation - diagnosis and management. Ginekol Pol. 2018;89:276–9.
3. Giurazza F, Corvino F, Silvestre M, Cavaglia E, Amodio F, Cangiano G, et al. Uterine arteriovenous malformations. Semin Ultrasound CT MR. 2021;42:37–45.
4. Aka KE, Horo GA, Fomba M, Kouyate S, Koffi AK, Konan S, et al. A rare case of important and recurrent abnormal uterine bleeding in a post partum woman caused by cavernous hemangioma: a case report and review of literature. Pan Afr Med J. 2017;28:130.
5. Knight P, Robertson M, Paoletti D. Uterine cavernous haemangioma in pregnancy. Australas J Ultrasound Med. 2016;19:37–41.
6. Uotila J, Dastidar P, Martikainen P, Kirkinen P. Massive multicystic dilatation of the uterine wall with myometrial venous thrombosis during pregnancy. Ultrasound Obstet Gynecol. 2004;24:461–3.
7. Sun ZY, Yang L, Yi CG, et al. Possibilities and potential roles of estrogen in the pathogenesis of proliferation emangiomas formation. Med Hypotheses. 2008;71:286–92.
8. Capmas P, Levaillant JM, Teig B, Fernandez H. Uterine arteriovenous malformation involving the whole myometrium P. Ultrasound Obstet Gynecol. 2013;41:715–7.
9. Stiepel HR 3rd, Burke CT, Stewart JK. Embolization of uterine arteriovenous malformation causing postpartum hemorrhage using n-butyl cyanoacrylate: a case report. Radiol Case Rep. 2021;16:1188–90.
10. Bhavsar T, Wurzel J, Duker N. Myometrial cavernous hemangioma with pulmonary thromboembolism in a post-partum woman: a case report and review of the literature. J Med Case Rep. 2012;6:397.

32 Herpes Simplex Pneumonitis

Heena Desai and Pradeep Vaideeswar

32.1 Clinical History

A 22-year-old woman had complained of headache for the past 2 days, followed by vomiting and 3 episodes of generalized tonic-clonic convulsions and unconsciousness. She was admitted to a rural hospital, where she was found to have gestational hypertension (blood pressure of 140/100 mm Hg). With a clinical diagnosis and treatment for eclampsia, an emergency cesarean section was performed (female baby, 2.16 kg). She was then referred to our tertiary-care center on the second postpartum day in an unconscious state for further management. On examination, the patient was unconscious in a poor general condition with poor reflexes, no demonstrable motor power and bilateral crepitations. Investigations revealed anemia (hemoglobin ranging from 83 to 101 g/L), neutrophilic leukocytosis (counts ranging from 22 to 35.9 x 10^9/L), hepatic dysfunction (SGOT 316 IU/L, SGPT 113 IU/L, and alkaline phosphatase 250 IU/L), an altered coagulation profile that suggested disseminated intravascular coagulation, and lymphocytic meningitis (cerebrospinal fluid proteins of 241 mg/dl and lymphocytes of 240/cmm). She received antibiotics, anticonvulsants, and intracranial tension lowering agents. A magnetic resonance imaging performed on the eighth day of admission also revealed meningitis with ventriculitis. The patient continued to be unconscious and succumbed after 12 days of admission.

32.2 Autopsy Findings

A complete autopsy was performed. Remarkable findings were present in the lungs. The visceral pleurae were patchily covered by granular grayish-white fibrinous exudates. The trachea and the main bronchi (Fig. 32.1a) had a shaggy mucosal lining with yellowish-white pseudomembranes. The lungs were heavy and had a firm consistency in most places. There were bilateral large geographic areas of yellowish-white, granular consolidation (Fig. 32.1a, b). Similar mucosal changes were seen in the intrapulmonary airways, some of which also appeared occluded (Fig. 32.1b). On microscopy, many of the bronchi showed ulceration of the lining epithelium with transmural destruc-

H. Desai
Department of Pathology, Topiwala National Medical College and BYL Nair Charitable Hospital, Mumbai, Maharashtra, India

P. Vaideeswar (✉)
Department of Pathology (Cardiovascular and Thoracic Division), Seth GS Medical College and KEM Hospital, Mumbai, Maharashtra, India

K. D. Jashnani (ed.), *Maternal Mortality - Lessons Learnt from Autopsy*,
https://doi.org/10.1007/978-981-19-3420-9_32

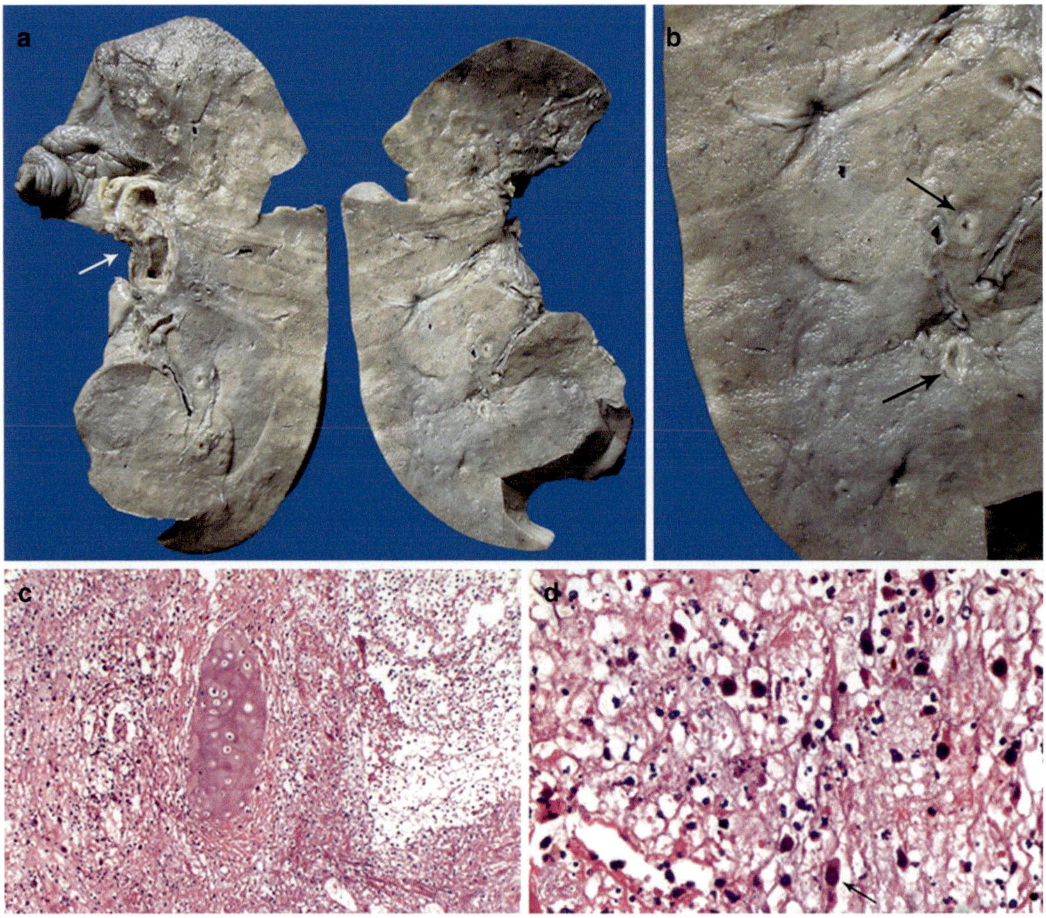

Fig. 32.1 (**a**) Bisected halves of the right lung which has been sliced through the hilum. The bronchi are covered by shaggy whitish exudates (arrow). There is almost a complete consolidation of the lung; (**b**) Close up of the right lower lobe shows geographic white areas of consolidation with obliteration of the bronchi by exudates (arrows); (**c**) Extensive destruction of a bronchus, identified only by the cartilaginous plate (H&E × 200); (**d**) The nuclei of the columnar cells amidst the necrosis and inflammation show small pink intranuclear inclusions (arrow, H&E × 400)

tion of their walls (Fig. 32.1c) with scattered mixed inflammatory inf iltrate amidst fibrin. Some of the epithelial cells amidst the necrotic tissue had small intranuclear eosinophilic inclusions (Fig. 32.1d), suggesting the cytopathic effects of HSV infection. Necrotizing consolidation with extensive hyaline membrane formations and abundant nuclear debris (Fig. 32.2a, b) were seen in the lung parenchyma. Some of the alveolar epithelial cells also showed HSV inclusions (Fig. 32.2c). Other findings at autopsy included chronic lymphocytic meningitis, focal hepatic and adrenal necrosis with demonstrable HSV inclusions (Fig. 32.2d, e). There was no involvement of the upper aerodigestive tract.

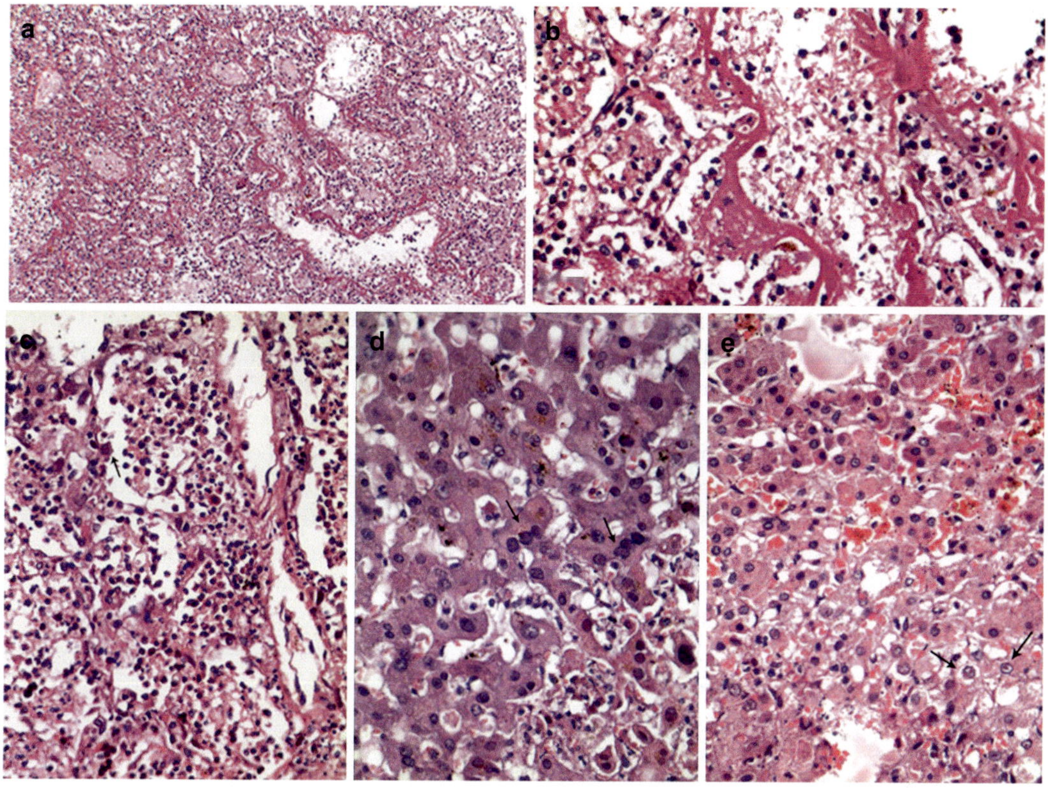

Fig. 32.2 Necrotizing pneumonia with abundant hyaline membrane formations (**a**) H&E × 200 and (**b**) H&E × 400; Characteristic intranuclear HSV inclusions in the (**c**) Alveolar epithelial cells, (**d**) Hepatocytes and (**e**) Adrenocortical cells (H&E × 400)

32.3 Final Cause of Death

Acute respiratory distress syndrome in a case of disseminated HSV infection.

32.4 Clinicopathologic Discussion

Multi-organ HSV infection and bilateral confluent consolidation were responsible for morbidity and mortality in this young mother. Though pregnancy is considered as a physiological condition, it is associated with a series of sequential changes in various organ systems with the sole goal of fetal growth and protection. Since the fetus is unfortunately perceived as a collection of "foreign" antigens by the mother's immune system, various alterations take place in the cell-mediated and humoral immunity in the second and third trimesters [1], and hence pregnancy is an immunomodulated state, rather than being immunesuppressed. These immunological changes can at times prove detrimental to the mother, predisposing her to infections by various pathogens ranging from bacteria to viruses. However, with maternal viral infections, the major focus of concern and management is directed mainly towards prevention of vertical transmission [2].

The attenuated immune adaptation is accompanied by changes in the respiratory system (especially decreased chest compliance and functional residual capacity) [3], which leads to an increased susceptibility to the development of pneumonia, a common non-obstetric infection [4]. Pneumonic consolidation is often caused by bacteria or mycobacteria. The cause in our case was *H. simplex*, which is a double stranded DNA virus of the family *Herpesviridae*. The two types, HSV 1 and HSV 2, are identified on the basis of the presence of specific glycoproteins; moreover, they are responsible for upper aerodigestive tract and genital lesions, respectively. The disease manifests in immunocompromised and even in immunocompetent individuals as a de novo infection or an infection following reactivation of the virus lying dormant in the sensory ganglia. A similar modus operandi occurs in pregnant women as well [5]. The involvement of the lower respiratory tract is produced mainly by HSV 1 through contiguous spread, aspiration (a common problem in pregnancy) of infected contents or viral shedding [6] and manifests as ulcerative tracheobronchitis, bronchial and bronchiolar-centered necrotizing consolidation, interstitial pneumonitis and DAD [7]. In this case, there was disseminated maternal disease with involvement of the meninges, liver, and adrenals; surprisingly, there was no involvement of the esophagus, oral cavity, or larynx.

The question that arises is "Are there any clinical or pathological criteria to diagnose viral pneumonias in pregnancy?" In general, the diagnosis of HSV pneumonia is problematic as the clinical manifestations, laboratory findings, and imaging characteristics are not specific. Awareness of the condition with a high index of suspicion is often a key to the diagnosis. Clinically viral pneumonias should be suspected when a pregnant lady is not responding to antibiotics and presents with fever, skin lesions with single organ or systemic disease. The diagnostic difficulty is further highlighted in our case as she did not show the usual skin or upper aerodigestive tract involvement. The diagnosis depends mainly on the identification of the classic cytopathic changes in the form of multinucleation, ground-glass nuclear opacity, and intranuclear inclusions. These pink inclusions have a glassy appearance, may be large, and are surrounded by a halo and a rim of marginated chromatin [7]. These are identified usually at the edge of the necrotic lesions on histopathology and can also be demonstrated in cytoplogical preparations. Since DAD can occur as a non-specific reaction to many types of lung injury, the co-existence of DAD with bronchiolitis should alert the pathologist for a careful search for viral inclusions. Immunohistochemical stains and/or in situ hybridization techniques can be helpful to identify the HSV infected cells in tissue or in lavage specimens [7]. Serological testing for detection of HSV antibodies can be performed. Since there always remains a difficulty in reaching a diagnosis, prophylactic acyclovir could be considered.

References

1. Morelli SS, Mandal M, Goldsmith LT, Kashani BN, Ponzio NM. The maternal immune system during pregnancy and its influence on fetal development. Res Rep Biol. 2015;6:171–89.
2. Silasi M, Cardenas I, Racicot K, Kwon JY, Aldo P, Mor G. Viral infections during pregnancy. Am J Reprod Immunol. 2015;73:199–213.
3. Mehta N, Chen K, Hardy E, Powrie R. Respiratory disease in pregnancy. Best Pract Res Clin Obstet Gynaecol. 2015;29:598–611.
4. Tang P, Wang J, Song Y. Characteristics and pregnancy outcomes of patients with severe pneumonia complicating pregnancy: a retrospective study of 12 cases and a literature review. BMC Pregnancy Childbirth. 2018;18:434.
5. Stephenson-Famy A, Gardella C. Herpes simplex infection during pregnancy. Obstet Gynaecol Clin North Am. 2014;41:601–14.
6. Odani K, Tachibana M, Tamashima R, Tsutsumi Y. Herpes simplex virus pneumonia: Importance of aspiration etiology. Case Rep Pathol. 2019;2019:7623576, 3 pages
7. Pritt BS, Aubry MC. Histopathology of viral infections of the lung. Semin Diagn Pathol. 2017;34:510–7.

Renal Cortical Necrosis in Pregnancy: Still a Sad Reality in Developing Countries

33

Kanchan Dilip Trichal, Kusum D. Jashnani, and Rakesh R. Bhadade

33.1 Clinical History

We present a case of a 20-year-old primigravida in the third trimester of pregnancy who was taken to a private hospital around midnight with abdominal pain and altered sensorium. There was no known history of any major illness in the past. She underwent normal delivery and gave birth to a healthy baby within few hours of admission. However, sometime later, she started talking irrelevantly and was getting aggressive. Reduced urine output was also noted. A decision was made to shift her to another hospital in the same city. She arrived there with altered sensorium, and they clinically suspected HELLP syndrome with acute renal failure. Two cycles of hemodialysis were given in the next 2 days. She was also transfused with 8 pints of RDP and 4 pints of FFP. She continued to have reduced urine output and also developed dyspnea on exertion grade 3–4, which was gradually increasing. She also had yellow discolouration of the sclera, bilateral pedal edema, amnesia and constipation.

On day 5 of postpartum, the patient was shifted to our hospital. Clinically, there were low GCS, pallor, fever, low blood pressure and bilateral crepitations in the patient.

Blood investigations revealed dropping levels of hemoglobin (falling up to 5.7g/dL) and total leucocyte count; blood urea nitrogen and serum creatinine levels were raised (84 mg/dl and 6.7 mg/dl, respectively), so were bilirubin levels (8 mg/dl – 5.7 mg/dl). SGOT and SGPT levels were mildly raised (118 U/L and 86 U/L). Fever profile was negative. PT-INR and fibrinogen levels were in the normal range.

The CT thorax reported bilateral pleural effusion and collapse consolidation of lung parenchyma; few areas of mosaic attenuations in bilateral lungs were noted. Ultrasound reported a bilateral bright kidney, which indicates medical renal disease.

After all possible measures, the patient could not be saved and expired on day 4 of hospital admission. An autopsy was performed after due consent.

K. D. Trichal
University Hospital of North Durham, County Durham and Darlington NHS Foundation Trust, Durham, UK

K. D. Jashnani (✉)
Department of Pathology, Topiwala National Medical College and BYL Nair Charitable Hospital, Mumbai, Maharashtra, India

R. R. Bhadade
Department of Medicine (Critical Care Unit), Topiwala National Medical College and BYL Nair Charitable Hospital, Mumbai, Maharashtra, India

K. D. Jashnani (ed.), *Maternal Mortality - Lessons Learnt from Autopsy*,
https://doi.org/10.1007/978-981-19-3420-9_33

33.2 Autopsy Findings

33.2.1 Gross Examination

Kidneys: The external surface was very pale with scattered yellowish and congested areas. On the cut surface, the corticomedullary differentiation and ratio were maintained with whitish-yellow geographic necrotic areas involving cortex extensively bilateral (Figs. 33.1 and 33.2).

Bilateral lungs were boggy and voluminous, on cut surface they had angry red appearance.

Rest of the organs were unremarkable.

33.2.2 Microscopy

Kidney: The subcapsular thin rim of renal parenchyma was preserved; however it showed a dense neutrophilic infiltrate. Below this, the entire cortex showed coagulative necrosis (Fig. 33.3). The underlying medulla was preserved with an intervening zone of neutrophilic infiltrate and vascular proliferation in between the infarcted cortex and the preserved medulla. Few glomerular capillaries showed fibrin thrombi.

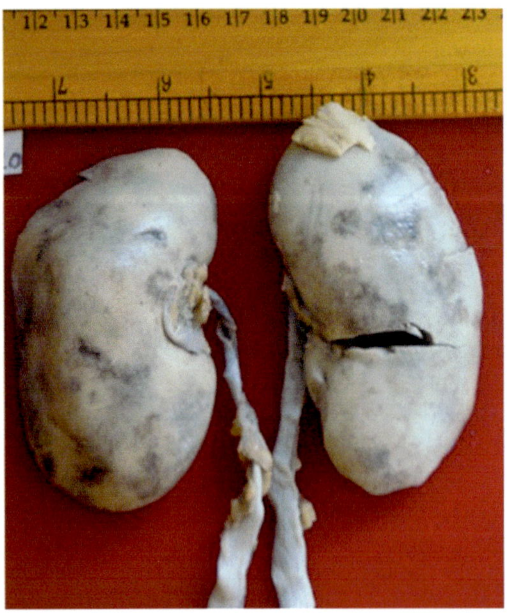

Fig. 33.1 External surface was very pale with scattered yellowish and congested areas

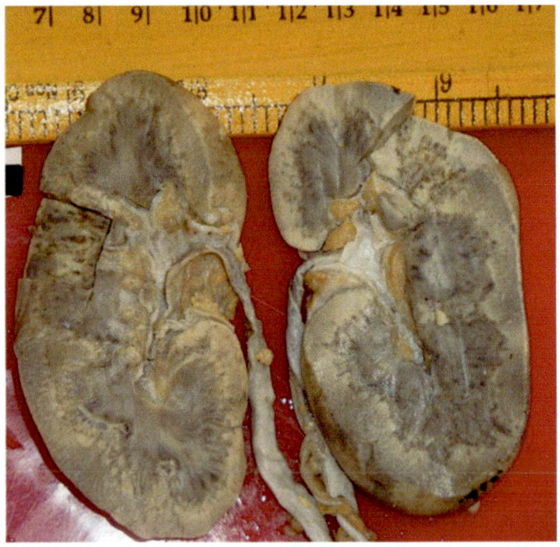

Fig. 33.2 On cut surface the corticomedullary differentiation and ratio was maintained with whitish-yellow geographic necrotic areas involving cortex extensively bilateral

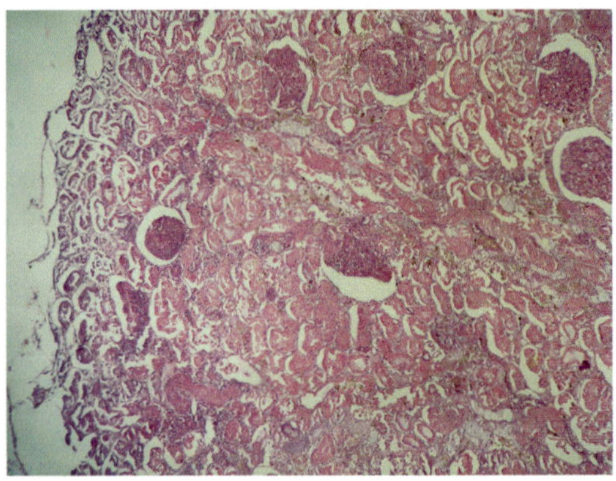

Fig. 33.3 Renal cortex showing presence of extensive coagulative necrosis with preserved thin rim of subcapsular tissue. (H&E, 200×)

Lungs: Multiple patchy areas of intra-alveolar hemorrhage, edema and neutrophilic infiltrate. Some of the alveolar septae were lined by an eosinophilic hyaline membrane. Some bronchioles showed ulceration of the lining epithelium with the presence of fibrin and neutrophils in their lumina. Few small and medium-sized blood vessels showed the presence of fibrin thrombi.

Uterus: Endometrium showed decidual changes, with the presence of few intermediate trophoblasts. Myometrium showed physiologic hypertrophy and preischemia. The blood clot collected from the uterus showed only red blood cells without any evidence of chorionic villi.

Rest of the organs were unremarkable on gross and histopathology.

33.3 Final Cause of Death

Acute respiratory distress syndrome and bilateral renal cortical necrosis in a postpartum female.

33.4 Clinicopathologic Discussion

Renal cortical necrosis (RCN) is a serious complication of acute kidney injury (AKI) that can lead to chronic renal failure and the need for chronic dialysis. RCN is a potentially fatal condition with poor renal outcomes. The following two types of cortical necrosis have been identified on the basis of renal histology: (1) *Diffuse cortical necrosis*: Confluent global cortical destruction extends into the columns of bertin. Thin rim of subcapsular and juxtamedullary tissue is preserved. Irreversible renal failure leading to end stage renal disease (ESRD) is the final outcome of diffuse cortical necrosis, and (2) *patchy cortical necrosis*: contiguous area of cortical necrosis involves up to one-third to half of the entire cortical tissue. Partial recovery of renal function is known to occur in patchy cortical necrosis. However, diffuse variety of cortical necrosis usually leads to irreversible lesion with total loss of kidney function and end stage kidney failure. *In our case, histopathology confirmed diffuse cortical necrosis, which required dialysis, but treatment could not restore the renal functions.*

We found multiple studies concluding that the incidence of RCN is much higher in obstetrical AKI (10–30%) as compared to other causes of this condition (5%) and that obstetric causes are overall the most dominant causes for RCN (56–61% of cases) [1, 2].

Septic abortion, abruptio placenta, puerperal sepsis, eclampsia, obstetric hemorrhage, intrauterine death, and thrombotic microangiopathy of pregnancy (P-TMA) are the common causes of RCN in a pregnant woman [3].

The usual presenting symptoms of acute RCN are absolute anuria (urine output nil in 24 h) or anuria (urine output <100 mL/24 h). In our case also, the patient presented with reduced urine output which kept worsening despite dialysis. Prolonged anuria in the clinical setting of hemorrhage, sepsis, shock or disseminated intravascular coagulation suggests the clinical diagnosis of RCN. A similar picture was seen in our case following anuria.

Additionally, in our case, the patient also developed ARDS. Incidence of mortality, length of intensive care unit stay and complexity of management is known to increase drastically in the setting where AKI and ARDS overlap [4]. Acute respiratory distress syndrome (ARDS) is a life-threatening condition characterized by severe hypoxemia due to respiratory failure. With literature search, we found studies suggesting AKI in conjunction with ARDS increases mortality drastically.

A recent study published in Society of Critical Care Medicine found that hospital mortality increased from 31% in acute respiratory distress syndrome patients with no acute kidney injury to 50% in mild-moderate acute kidney injury (serum creatinine 132–354 μmol/L) and 58% in severe acute kidney injury (serum creatinine >354 μmol/L). Similarly, another study by Darmon et al. showed that the mortality in patients who had ARDS and AKI was 42.3%, while that in patients without AKI was 20% [5].

Experimental studies suggest that AKI may increase the risk of lung injury, chiefly via the activation of proinflammatory and proapoptotic pathways because of renal ischemia/reperfusion [5]. Conversely, modalities for treatment of ARDS like mechanical ventilation and liberal amounts of fluids has shown to be detrimental for the renal functions [6–8]. Also, a recent meta-analysis suggested that both ARDS and mechanical ventilation were associated with a threefold increase in the risk of AKI [7].

In our case, we had clinical as well as histopathological evidence of diffuse RCN and ARDS, which as established above does not end well for the patients. Increasing deleterious effects of lung dysfunction, its treatment strategies, and subsequent kidney injury explain the natural progression to multi-organ failure. Unfortunately, we lost the patient even after all the possible efforts to revive her.

Nevertheless, on a positive note, we found studies indicating that incidence of obstetric RCN is reducing in developing countries, most likely due to better aseptic precautions, timely delivery, and also availability of dialysis and advanced medical care [1, 4].

33.5 Conclusion

- Because of the catastrophic sequelae of RCN, its prevention and aggressive management should always be important for the better renal outcome and prognosis of the patients.
- The development of acute kidney injury, even mild-moderate in severity, is associated with a substantial increase in mortality in patients with acute respiratory distress syndrome.
- There is a decreasing trend in the incidence of RCN in patients with ARF in recent years, which is associated with increased patient survival and better renal prognosis.

References

1. Prakash J, Singh VP. Changing picture of renal cortical necrosis in acute kidney injury in developing country. World J Nephrol. 2015;4(5):480. https://doi.org/10.5527/wjn.v4.i5.480.
2. Bhaduaria D, Kaul A, Lal H, Mishra P, Jain M, Prasad N, et al. Acute cortical necrosis in pregnancy still an important cause for end-stage renal disease in developing countries. Saudi J Kidney Dis Transpl. 2019;30(2):325–33. https://www.sjkdt.org/article.asp?issn=1319-2442;year=2019;volume=30;issue=2;spage=325;epage=333;aulast=Bhaduaria
3. Siribamrungwong M, Chinudomwong P. Relation between acute kidney injury and pregnancy-related factors. J Acute Dis. 2016;5(1):22–8.
4. Upadhyaya VD, Shariff MZ, Mathew RO, Hossain MA, Asif A, Vachharajani TJ. Management of acute kidney injury in the setting of acute respiratory distress syndrome: review focusing on ventilation and fluid management strategies. J Clin Med Res. 2020;12(1):1–5. https://doi.org/10.14740/jocmr3938.
5. Darmon M, Clec'h C, Adrie C, Argaud L, Allaouchiche B, Azoulay E, et al. Acute respiratory distress syndrome and risk of AKI among critically ill patients. Clin J Am Soc Nephrol. 2014;9(8):1347–53. https://doi.org/10.2215/CJN.08300813.
6. Panitchote A, Mehkri O, Hasting A, Hanane T, Demirjian S, Torbic H, et al. Factors associated with acute kidney injury in acute respiratory distress syndrome. Ann Intensive Care. 2019;9(1):74. https://doi.org/10.1186/s13613-019-0552-5.
7. van den Akker JPC, Egal M, Groeneveld JAB. Invasive mechanical ventilation as a risk factor for acute kidney injury in the critically ill: a systematic review and meta-analysis. Crit Care. 2013;17(3):R98. https://doi.org/10.1186/cc12743.
8. Rush B, Martinka P, McDermid RC, Boyd JH, Celi LA. Acute respiratory distress syndrome in pregnant women. Obstet Gynecol. 2017;129(3):530–5. https://doi.org/10.1097/AOG.0000000000001907.

Severe Anemia and Pregnancy

34

Sushama A. Chandekar, Kusum D. Jashnani, and Girish Rajadhyaksha

34.1 Clinical History

Our patient was 22 year old, primigravida with 8 months of amenorrhea (her antenatal visits were not regular), who presented to the referral hospital with pedal edema for last 2 months. She had history of cough with expectoration in the last 1 month and breathlessness for 15 days, which had increased from Grade III to Grade IV for the last 2 days for which she was referred to our hospital. Ultrasonography revealed intrauterine fetal death. There was no history of fever, abdominal pain, bleeding from any site, or hemoptysis. She had no past history of hypertension, diabetes mellitus, tuberculosis, or asthma.

Clinical examination revealed an unconscious patient in poor general condition at the initial examination. She was afebrile, with pallor +++, and bilateral pedal edema up to the ankles. Blood pressure and pulse were unrecordable. The patient was put on a portable ventilator. Respiratory examination showed bilateral harsh breath sounds. Cardiovascular examination showed muffled heart sounds. Central nervous system examination showed a deeply unconscious patient who was not responding to deep painful stimuli. Per abdomen, the uterus corresponded to 30 weeks of size. Hematological investigations showed hemoglobin of 4.9 g/dL with anisocytosis, poikilocytosis, hypochromasia, and microcytosis. Clinical impression was intrauterine fetal death with severe anemia. The clinical condition of the patient deteriorated, and the patient was declared dead within 2 h of admission. A complete autopsy was performed.

34.2 Autopsy Findings

She was averagely built and nourished, with +++ pallor and bilateral pedal edema. All organs were markedly pale in appearance (Figs. 34.1a–d and 34.2a). The heart showed biventricular dilatation. The pleura was smooth and shiny with frothy fluid oozing out on pressure from the lungs on the cut surface. Bilateral kidneys were pale. The cut section showed medullary congestion. The cerebrum and stomach showed few petechial hemorrhages in addition to marked pallor. The liver showed changes of chronic passive congestion on gross (nutmeg appearance) as well as on microscopy. The uterus was of

S. A. Chandekar · K. D. Jashnani (✉)
Department of Pathology, Topiwala National Medical College and BYL Nair Charitable Hospital, Mumbai, Maharashtra, India

G. Rajadhyaksha
Department of Medicine, Topiwala National Medical College and BYL Nair Charitable Hospital, Mumbai, Maharashtra, India

K. D. Jashnani (ed.), *Maternal Mortality - Lessons Learnt from Autopsy*,
https://doi.org/10.1007/978-981-19-3420-9_34

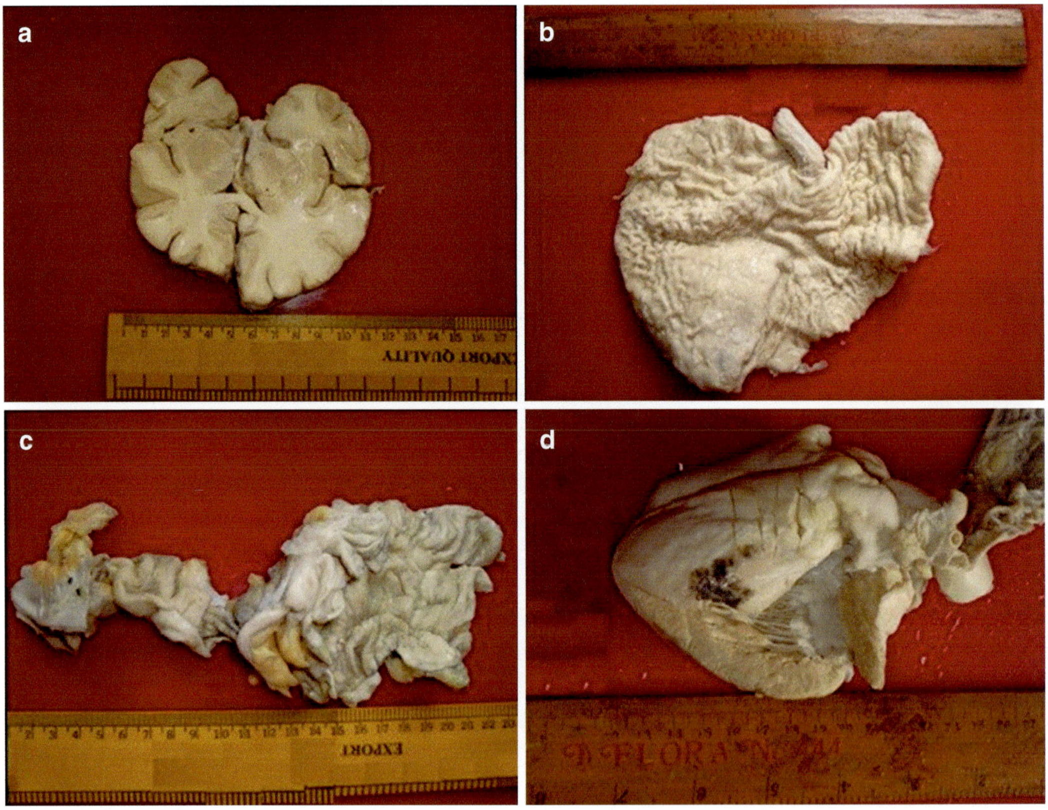

Fig. 34.1 Gross photograph of the pale appearance of (**a**) the cerebrum, (**b**) stomach (esophageal cardiac junction), (**c**) intestine (ileocecal junction), and (**d**) heart

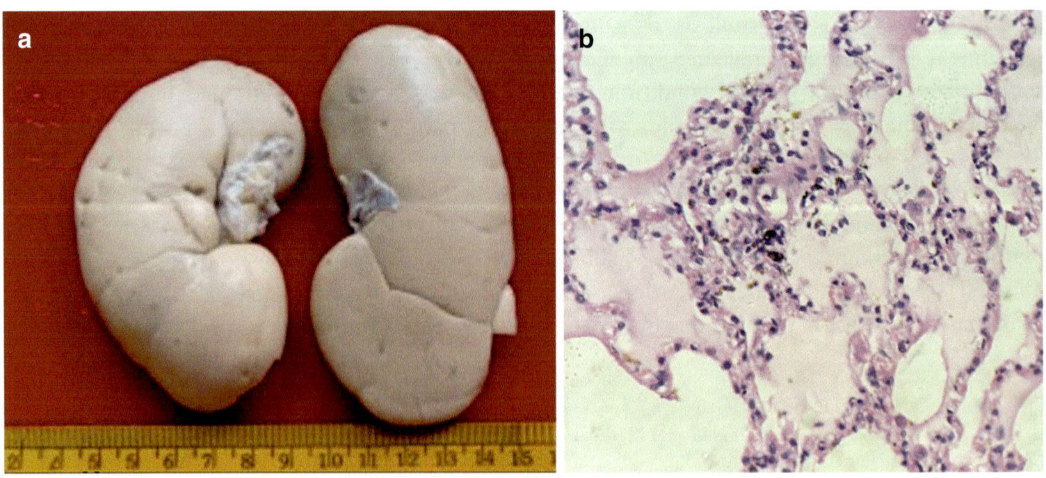

Fig. 34.2 Gross photograph of the pale appearance of the kidneys (**a**), intra-alveolar pale eosinophilic edema fluid (**b**-H&E, 200×)

weight 550 g, placenta was attached fundoanteriorily and fetus of weight 1000 g. Histopathologic examination of lungs showed intra-alveolar pale eosinophilic edema fluid with congested alveolar septal capillaries (Fig. 34.2b). Bone marrow examination revealed a hypercellular marrow with micronormoblastic erythropoiesis with normal myeloid and megakaryocytic series. There was no increase in blasts.

34.3 Final Cause of Death

Congestive cardiac failure due to severe anemia in an 8-month pregnant female with intrauterine fetal death.

34.4 Clinicopathologic Discussion

In pregnant women, anemia is defined as blood hemoglobin level < 11 g/dL as per WHO criteria. It is further categorized as mild (10.0–10.9 g/dL), moderate (7.0–9.9 g/dL), and severe anemia (<7.0 g/dL). Iron- and folate-deficiency anemias are common in developing countries with multifactorial etiology. The former is related to nutritional deficiency and intestinal helminthic infections and the latter to poor intake and chronic hemolytic states [1]. Other causes of iron-deficiency anemia in women are excessive blood loss during their menses and higher blood supply demands during pregnancy.

Iron deficiency anemia is common during pregnancy and more prevalent especially in low socio-economic group because of improper nutrition, living in unhygienic condition, high infection rate, lack of health care facilities, lack of education, early marriage, repeated childbearing with no birth spacing, no knowledge of antenatal care and exposure to domestic violence [2]. In the present case, peripheral smear examination was consistent with iron deficiency anemia. Bone marrow examination on autopsy revealed hypercellular marrow with micronormoblastic erythropoiesis. The risk of anemia increases as the number of pregnancies increases from 3–5 pregnancies. The iron demand increases in this period, and the frequency of antepartum hemorrhage is also higher. Additionally, helminth infection and malaria are also found to be important causes of anemia. A milder form of anemia has silent presentation without symptoms. A severe form of anemia presents with symptoms like fatigue, weakness, loss of normal colour in the skin, lips, tongue, and nails, dizziness, drowsiness, and dyspnea.

Anemia is an independent risk factor for cardiovascular complications. Anemia causes hypoxia due to decreased hemoglobin levels. Cardiovascular compensatory consequences of anemia are tachycardia, arrhythmia, increased cardiac output, a hyperdynamic state due to reduced blood viscosity, and vasodilation enabling tissue perfusion. Certain criteria have to be fulfilled before we say that heart disease is caused by anemia, namely (1) the presence of severe anemia, and (2) disturbance of cardiac function. Cardiovascular complications of anemia are due to worsening of the hyperdynamic state, volume overload, cardiac dilatation, valvular failure, and heart failure with increased cardiac output. In anemia, the heart must pump more blood to make up for the lack of oxygen in the blood, which can lead to an enlarged heart or heart failure [3].

There are some mechanisms operating in the anemic patient which may increase the supply of oxygen to the tissues when the oxygen carrying capacity of the blood is reduced. Under conditions of rest, a rapid velocity flow and tachycardia with an increase in minute volume of cardiac output is the first response to anemia. Production of the hormone erythropoietin by the kidney to increase erythropoiesis in the bone marrow is another response to anemia.

A milder form of anemia has a silent presentation without symptoms. A severe form of anemia presents with symptoms like fatigue, weakness, loss of normal colour in the skin, lips, tongue, and nails, dizziness, drowsiness, and dyspnea.

When the Hb concentration is <80 g/L, compensatory mechanisms fail, lactic acid accumulates, and patients become breathless at rest [4]. Cardiac failure may occur when Hb is <40 g/L, especially with twin pregnancies or splenomegaly and when anemia is not the primary cause of death, it may frequently be a contributory factor. A low number of RBCs reduces systemic vascular resistance by decreasing blood viscosity, and low Hb increases nitricoxide-mediated vasodilatation. Thus, arterial blood pressure decreases, which causes baroreceptor-mediated neurohumoral activation identical to that seen in low-output heart failure. Increased sympathetic and renin-angiotensin activity decreases renal blood flow and GFR, resulting in salt and water retention and expansion of ECF and plasma volumes. Thus, severe anemia itself may cause high-output heart failure in subjects with normal left ventricular function [5, 6]. In the present case, there was no information on the duration of anemia, as she had not been having regular ANC visits, and by the time she was referred to our hospital, she was in a clinical state of rapid cardiac decompensation with resulting cardiac failure.

There are many national programs undergoing for reducing the maternal death. But the main cause of mortality due to anemia in rural areas is the unawareness of these programs. This could have been easily prevented by doing regular antenatal check-ups. To have good healthy mothers with minimum complications, intensive efforts with proper health education need to be made in these areas to reduce the maternal mortality in developing countries like India [7].

References

1. Amatare D, G Olutoyin OE, Olaejirinde O, Donatus S, Akinwumi OK et al. Autopsy-certified maternal mortality at Ile-Ife, Nigeria. Int J Womens Health. 2014;6:41–46.
2. Jahnavi D, Javier Z, Borja MF, Joshua V, Olufemi TO et al. Risk of maternal mortality in women with severe anaemia during pregnancy and post-partum: a multilevel analysis. Lancet Glob Health 2018;6(5):e548–e554.
3. Sujan G, Haju M, Heenyun K, Hyoung-Sun J. Determining factors for the prevalence of anemia in women of reproductive age in Nepal: Evidence from recent national survey data. PloS One. 2019;14(6):e0218288.
4. Aparna MK, Anita AC, Nilam SJ, Ravindra VR, Leena AN Clinico-Pathological Co-Relation of Maternal Deaths in a Tertiary Care Centre, Southern Maharashtra. Natl J Community Med. 2016;7(4):343–47.
5. Anand IS, Gupta P. Anemia and Iron Deficiency in Heart Failure: Current Concepts and Emerging Therapies: Circulation. 2018;138:80–98.
6. Smith C, Teng F, Branch E, Chu S, Joseph KS. Maternal and Perinatal Morbidity and Mortality Associated with Anemia in Pregnancy. Obstet Gynecol. 2019;134(6):1234–244.
7. Sandhya VP, Rekha NP, Waman KR. Pathological Study of Maternal Deaths - Experience from a Tertiary Care Centre in Central India Pathology. Int J Contemp Med Res. 2020;7(2):2454.

35 Hypertrophic Cardiomyopathy as an Incidental Finding

Pradeep Vaideeswar

35.1 Clinical History

A 32-year-old woman (15 days postpartum) presented with a sudden onset of numbness and weakness of the left upper extremity, which was followed by weakness of the entire left side of her body with a deviation of the angle of her mouth. There was deterioration of consciousness, for which she was admitted to our tertiary-care center for further management. The patient had regular antenatal care visits with normal blood pressure recordings and no other antenatal complaints.

On examination, the general condition was poor with response only to painful stimuli. She was afebrile with a pulse rate of 64 per minute (regular and good volume) and a blood pressure of 80/60 mm Hg. Systemic examination of the central nervous system revealed left hemiplegia; other system examinations were normal. The routine hematological and biochemical investigations were normal. There was derangement of her coagulation profiles—prothrombin time 19.6 s (control of 13.7 s), fibrinogen 480 mg/dL (reference value 200–400 mg/dL), fibrin degradation products of greater than 160 µg/mL (reference value <20 µg/mL) and D-dimer greater than 10 mg/L (reference value in third trimester <1.70 mg/L). The computed tomography of the brain showed right cerebral acute hemorrhagic infarction. The patient was administered intra-cranial tension lowering agents, antibiotics, steroids, and anticonvulsants. She expired after 51 h of admission.

P. Vaideeswar (✉)
Department of Pathology (Cardiovascular and Thoracic Division), Seth GS Medical College and KEM Hospital, Mumbai, Maharashtra, India

35.2 Autopsy Findings

The heart weighed 350 g and was mildly enlarged in size due to mild LVH. However, serial transverse sections through the myocardium revealed asymmetric hypertrophy involving the posterior one third of the septum and posterior/lateral walls (1.8–2.0 cm in width, Fig. 35.1a); the anterior wall was 0.9 cm in thickness. Foci of scarring were also seen in the lateral wall. On histology, the myocardial hypertrophy was accompanied by very prominent areas of cardiomyocyte disarray—features of HCM (Fig. 35.1b, c) with small areas of replacement fibrosis. Smaller subendocardial scars were also seen in the right ventricular myocardium. The right coronary artery had a dominant distribution; all coronary arteries were patent. Intramural coronary arteries were also normal. The atria and valves were unremarkable. The other important finding was superior sagittal sinus and cortical venous thrombosis with right cerebral hemorrhagic infarction.

K. D. Jashnani (ed.), *Maternal Mortality - Lessons Learnt from Autopsy*,
https://doi.org/10.1007/978-981-19-3420-9_35

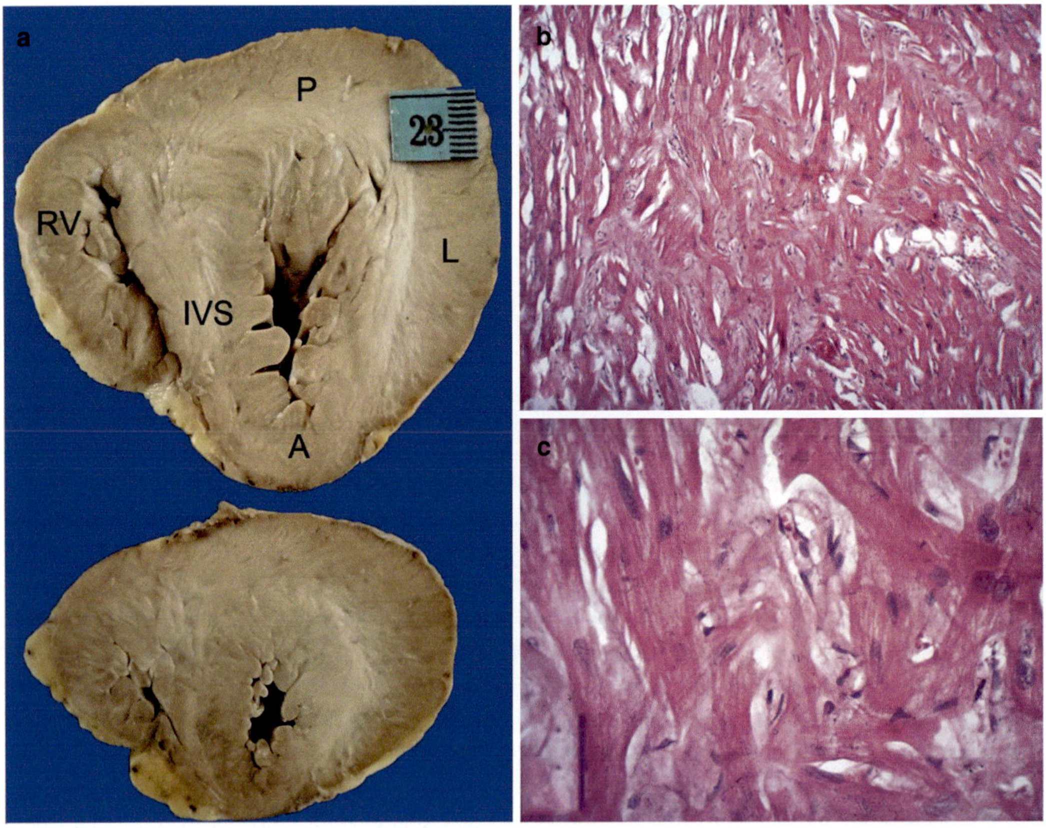

Fig. 35.1 (**a**) Serial transverse section through the ventricular myocardium reveals asymmetric hypertrophy of the posterior wall P and the adjoining interventricular septum IVS and lateral wall L. Note right ventricular RV hypertrophy (A anterior wall, LV left ventricle); microscopy revealed cardiomyocyte hypertrophy with haphazard arrangement—disarray and inter-fiber scarring (**b**) H&E × 200 and (**c**) H&E × 400

35.3 Final Cause of Death

Raised intracranial pressure due to cerebral hemorrhagic venous infarctions.

35.4 Clinicopathologic Discussion

HCM was seen surprisingly as an incidental finding in a postpartum patient who had developed intracranial venous thrombosis and hemorrhagic infarction. It is an example of cardiomyopathy, which is "a heterogeneous group of diseases of the myocardium associated with mechanical and/or electrical dysfunction that usually (but not invariably) exhibit inappropriate ventricular hypertrophy or dilatation and are due to the variety of causes that are frequently genetic" [1]. Such nonischemic myocardial disorders are often uncommonly described or well elucidated in pregnancy [2], though peripartum cardiomyopathy has been well characterized (see Chap. 10).

HCM, with a prevalence of 1 in 500, is the most common inherited cardiomyopathy; the prevalence during pregnancy is 1 in 1000. It is seen often as an autosomal dominant disease. Several mutations in the sarcomeric proteins with varied penetrance and expressivity result in the most obvious expression of the disease in the form of LVH (>15 mm as measured on imaging) at the expense of the LV cavity size; the ejection fraction may be normal or increased [3]. It is also important to rule out the more frequent causes of LVH such as hypertension, which is seen in various pregnancy-related disorders. In the case illustrated, gestational hypertension had not been documented. On examining the heart, the maximum thickness of the left ventricular myocardium was 2 cm and was found in the posterior and its adjoining walls, extending from the base to the apical portion. Such an asymmetric hypertrophy is seen in the majority of the cases of HCM and can lead to dynamic obstruction of the LV outflow tract (obstructive HCM) [4]. In histology, apart from cardiomyocyte hypertrophy, a classic feature to be noted is myocyte disarray [4], which can sometimes be seen even without hypertrophy. Marked hypertrophy and prominent disarray in the index case were also associated with areas of replacement fibrosis, though intramural coronary arteries did not show stenosis or obliteration [4].

The clinical presentation of HCM varies from person-to-person, manifesting in all age groups. Some individuals can remain asymptomatic, while in few others, the disease unfolds as adverse events in the form of cardiac failure or sudden cardiac death. Such calamities occur at similar rates in nonpregnant women and pregnant women [5]. Exertional dyspnea, angina, and syncope are the most frequent symptoms, related to diastolic LV dysfunction, sub-aortic obstruction, myocardial ischemia, and arrhythmias. Despite this, HCM is well tolerated by women in pregnancy and is rarely a contraindication for conception [6]. Normal vaginal delivery is usually advocated, and a cesarean section is performed for obstetric reasons or cardiac complications, all under the supervision of a multidisciplinary team. The development of morbidity and mortality in pregnancy is mainly related to the pregestational degree of cardiac dysfunction, outflow tract obstruction, and presence of arrhythmias in a background of strong family history [5, 6]. These parameters would also serve as contraindications for pregnancy itself. However, asymptomatic patients with HCM do have a small risk of cardiac complications in pregnancy especially during labor and in the postpartum period. Our patient had an uneventful pregnancy and delivery. HCM with significant asymmetric hypertrophy and fibrosis was detected at autopsy, yet the cause of death was not related to this disease; HCM remained an incidental finding, indicating that in some cases, it may go unrecognized [7].

References

1. McKenna WJ, Maron BJ, Thiene G. Classification, epidemiology, and global burden of cardiomyopathies. Circ Res. 2017;121:722–30.
2. Schaufelberger M. Cardiomyopathy and pregnancy. Heart. 2019;105:1543–51.
3. Geske JB, Ommen SR, Gersh BJ. Hypertrophic cardiomyopathy: clinical update. JACC Heart Fail. 2018;6:364–75.
4. Kocovski L, Fernandes J. Sudden cardiac death: a modern pathology approach to hypertrophic cardiomyopathy. Arch Pathol Lab Med. 2015;139:413–6.
5. Briller J, Vaught AJ. Cardiomyopathies in pregnancy: etiologies and management strategies. Clin Obstet Gynecol. 2020;63:893–909.
6. Saberi S. Hypertrophic cardiomyopathy in pregnancy. Cardiol Clin. 2021;39:143–50.
7. Sikka P, Suri V, Aggarwal N, Chopra S, Bahl A, Vijayverghia R. Are we missing hypertrophic cardiomyopathy in pregnancy? Experience of a tertiary care hospital. J Clin Diagn Res. 2014;8:OC13–5.

Gastrointestinal Candidiasis: An Unusual Accompaniment

36

Manjusha Karegar and Pradeep Vaideeswar

36.1 Clinical History

A 33-year-old primigravida with 30 weeks of amenorrhea was admitted to a private nursing home with complaints of abdominal pain and loose motions for a week, which was followed by bleeding per vaginum, decreasing urine output, and exertional dyspnea for 3 days. The clinical examination revealed hypertension (180/110 mm of Hg), proteinuria (urine proteins 4+), and the absence of fetal heart sounds. With a clinical diagnosis of severe preeclampsia and abruptio placentae, she underwent an emergency lower segment cesarean section, where moderate ascites and a 250 g retro-placental blood clot were noted. Subsequently, she developed right-sided pleural effusion, anuria, anasarca, and altered sensorium. The patient was transferred to our hospital on ionotropic support and in a poor general condition. Investigations revealed anemia (Hb 74 g/L), neutrophilia (total leukocyte count 24 x 10^9/L with band forms and toxic granules), thrombocytopenia (platelet count 20 x 10^9/L), azotemia (blood urea nitrogen 49 mg/dL, creatinine 2.9 mg/dL), deranged liver function tests (total bilirubin 14.8 mg/dL, direct bilirubin 7.8 mg/dL, SGOT 2507 U/L and SGPT 684 U/L), and deranged coagulation profile (prothrombin time 66 seconds (control 13 s), international normalized ratio 5.06, activated partial thromboplastin time 101.3 s (control 22–34 s), fibrinogen (50.4 mg/dL)). Despite appropriate therapy and ventilator support, the condition deteriorated and she expired within 2 days of the hospital stay.

36.2 Autopsy Findings

A complete autopsy was performed. The external examination revealed icterus and bilateral pedal edema. The stomach, the ileum, and the proximal portions of the colon showed multiple mucosal hemorrhagic lesions, ranging in size from 0.1 to 1 cm (Fig. 36.1). On histological examination, the lesions of the gastrointestinal tract revealed ischemic necrosis of the mucosa with foci of submucosal hemorrhages (Fig. 36.2). Amidst this necrotic mucosa (Fig. 36.2) and within the submucosal vessels (Fig. 36.3a, b) were seen plenty of pseudohyphae and few yeast forms, which were suggestive of *Candida* species; these were confirmed on special stains (Fig. 36.3c). Focally, the necroinflammatory infiltrate extended into the underlying muscularis propria and the subserosal regions; there was no perforation. The liver showed hydropic degeneration of the hepatocytes and geographic areas of coagulative necrosis (Fig. 36.4), while cortical necrosis was seen in both kidneys. The uterus was contracted and showed fibrinosuppurative exudate and hemorrhages on the

M. Karegar · P. Vaideeswar (✉)
Department of Pathology, Seth GS Medical College and KEM Hospital, Mumbai, Maharashtra, India

K. D. Jashnani (ed.), *Maternal Mortality - Lessons Learnt from Autopsy*,
https://doi.org/10.1007/978-981-19-3420-9_36

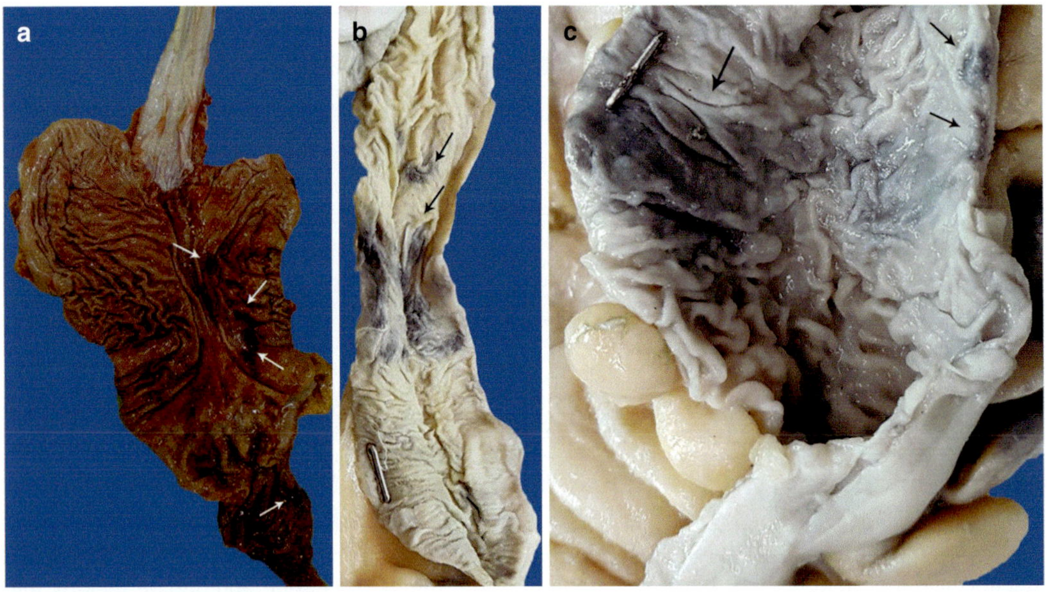

Fig. 36.1 Small and large foci of congestion and hemorrhage (arrows) in the (**a**) Stomach, (**b**) small intestine, and (**c**) large intestine

endometrial surface with thrombus-filled dilated myometrial sinuses. There was a persistent left superior vena cava draining into the coronary sinus. The lungs and other organs were normal.

36.3 Final Cause of Death

Disseminated intravascular coagulation with gastrointestinal candidiasis in a case of abruptio placentae.

36.4 Clinicopathologic Discussion

Candida species are yeasts that colonize the surface epithelium of the alimentary canal and urogenital systems of healthy humans as part of normal flora. The vagina is colonized in at least 20% of all women, rising to 30% in pregnancy. The term candidiasis is used to designate mucocutaneous and deep-seated organ infections caused by different species of *Candida* whenever commensalism is converted to opportunism. Breach in the mucocutaneous barriers, long-term use of broad-spectrum antibiotics and impairment of local or systemic immune response leads to candidial overgrowth, leading to candidiasis [1]. Invasive candidiasis, comprising bloodstream infection or candidemia and deep-seated tissue involvement, is the fourth most common infection among hospitalized patients [1, 2]. Deep-seated candidiasis arises from either hematogenous dissemination or direct inoculation of *Candida* species into a sterile site [2]. The most commonly infected organs are the lungs, kidneys, brain, heart, and eyes. More than 15 distinct *Candida* species of varying virulence can cause diseases; the most common ones are *C. albicans*, *C. glabrata*, and *C. tropicalis*, which are more virulent than *C. parapsilosis* and *C. krusei*. *C. albicans* had previously been the dominating pathogen, but in today's scenario, the non-*albicans* species have an upper hand in causing infections. Many of them have an inherent resistance to antifungal drugs with a consequent mortality rate of almost 40% in patients with invasive candidiasis.

The female genital tract is one of the most common mucocutaneous sites for candidial infection. Most episodes of symptomatic vulvovaginal candidiasis [3] occur during the second and third trimesters and are attributed to pregnancy-related factors, such as immunologic alterations, increased estrogen levels, and

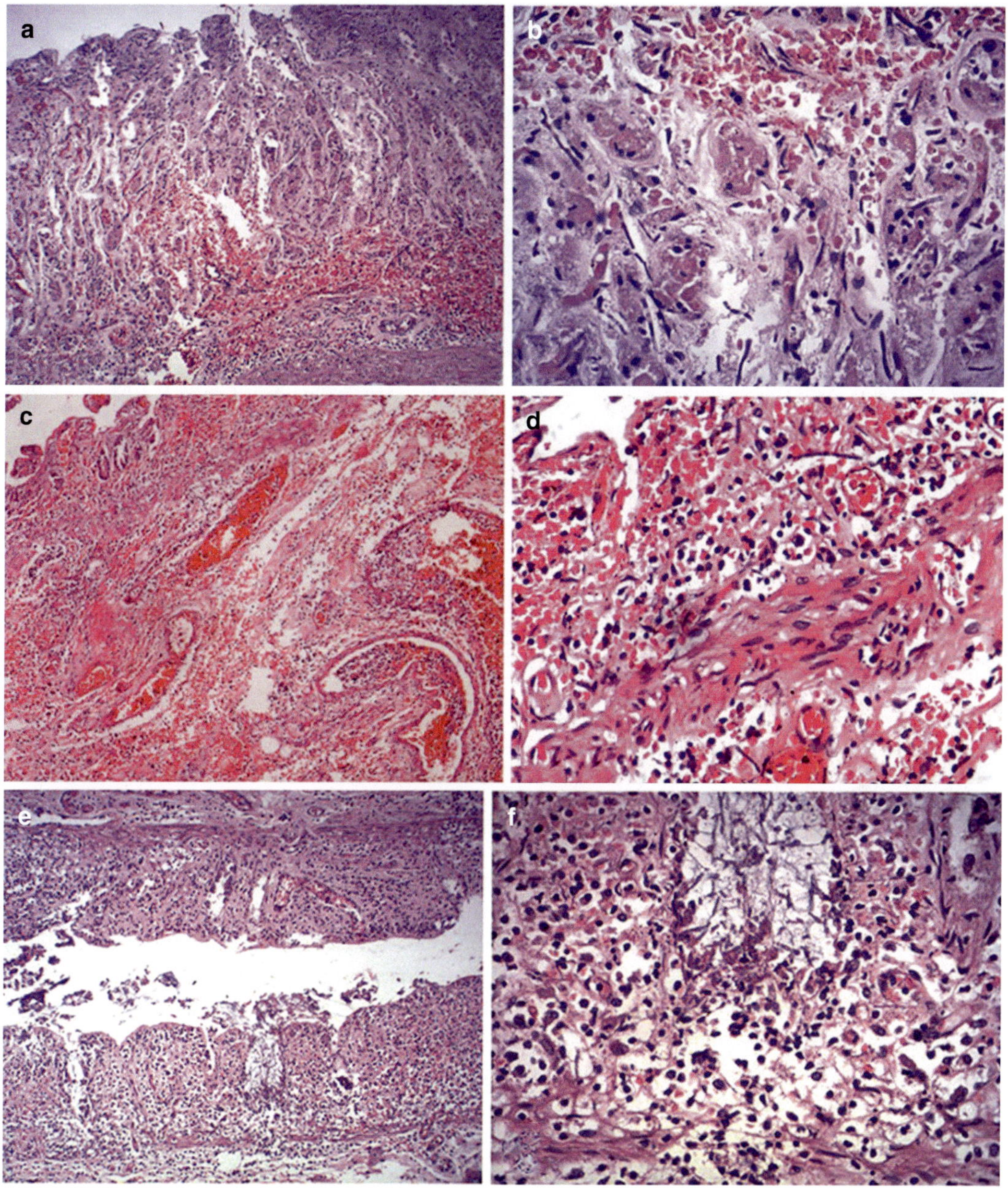

Fig. 36.2 Erosions and/or mucosal and submucosal hemorrhages in the stomach (**a**) H&E × 200 and (**b**) H&E × 400, small intestine (**c**) H&E × 200 and (**d**) H&E × 400 and large intestine (**e**) H&E × 200 and (**f**) H&E × 400. The higher powers of all sections show the presence of yeasts and pseudohyphae suggestive of *Candida* species amidst neutrophilic infiltrate

increased vaginal glycogen production [3]. Although evidence is incomplete, there is some emerging data which suggests that candidiasis in pregnancy may be associated with increased risk of pregnancy complications such as premature rupture of membranes, preterm labor, chorioamnionitis, and neonatal congenital cutaneous candidiasis [3].

In the gastrointestinal tract, the esophagus is the most common site followed by the stomach and colon [4, 5]. Candidial colonization is frequently observed in gastric ulcers and inflamma-

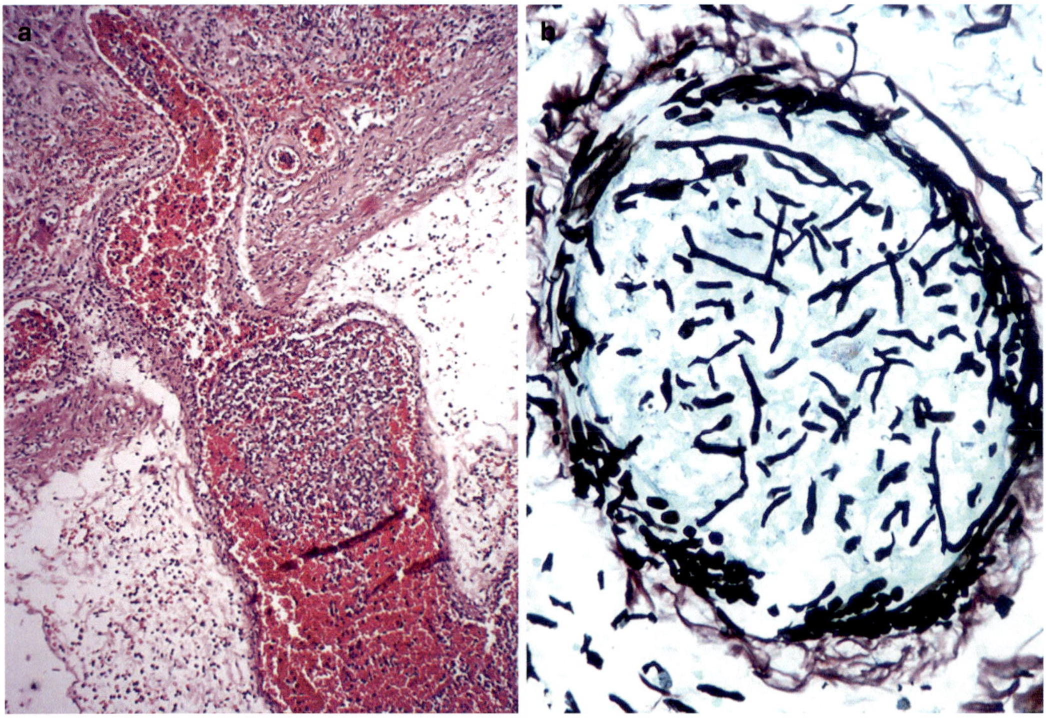

Fig. 36.3 (**a**) A serosal artery is seen to enter the wall of the small intestine. It is surrounded, infiltrated and contains large number of neutrophils (H&E × 100); (**b**) Yeasts and pseudo-hyphae demonstrated by the Gomori methenamine silver stain (×400)

tory bowel diseases like ulcerative colitis and Crohn's disease, as a result of proton pump inhibitors, or immune-modulators. The additional risk factors include smoking, old age, malnutrition, trauma, burns, surgical operations, parenteral nutrition, and immunocompromised states. Patients with three or more risk factors are considered vulnerable to infection, although there are some reports in the literature of patients with one or even no risk factors [6]. The patients present with dysphagia, vomiting, diarrhea, melena, abdominal pain, and fever [7]. Grossly, the lesions may be single, multiple, segmental, or diffuse with erosions, ulcerations, or pseudomembrane formations. The associated inflammatory response ranges from minimal to marked, with prominent neutrophilic infiltrates, abscess formation, and necrosis; granulomas are occasionally present as well. Invasion of mucosal and submucosal blood vessels is sometimes a prominent feature, and the affected segment may appear gangrenous. In between the necro-inflammatory lesions are mixtures of budding yeast forms, pseudo-hyphae or even slender hyphae, produced by all species except *C. glabrata*, which exists as tiny budding yeast forms (similar to those of *Histoplasma*) [1].

Invasive candidiasis exclusively involving the stomach, ileum, and colon without involvement of the esophagus was a surprisingly uncommon finding at autopsy and was clinically not suspected. The patient's first clinical symptom of loose motions was due to candidiasis. This patient did not have any common risk factors. Though, pregnant women are susceptible for disseminated infection as the immunological changes during pregnancy suppress T-cell-mediated immunity, which is crucial in mucosal defense. Thus, GI candidial lesions remain difficult to diagnose because of the prevalence of

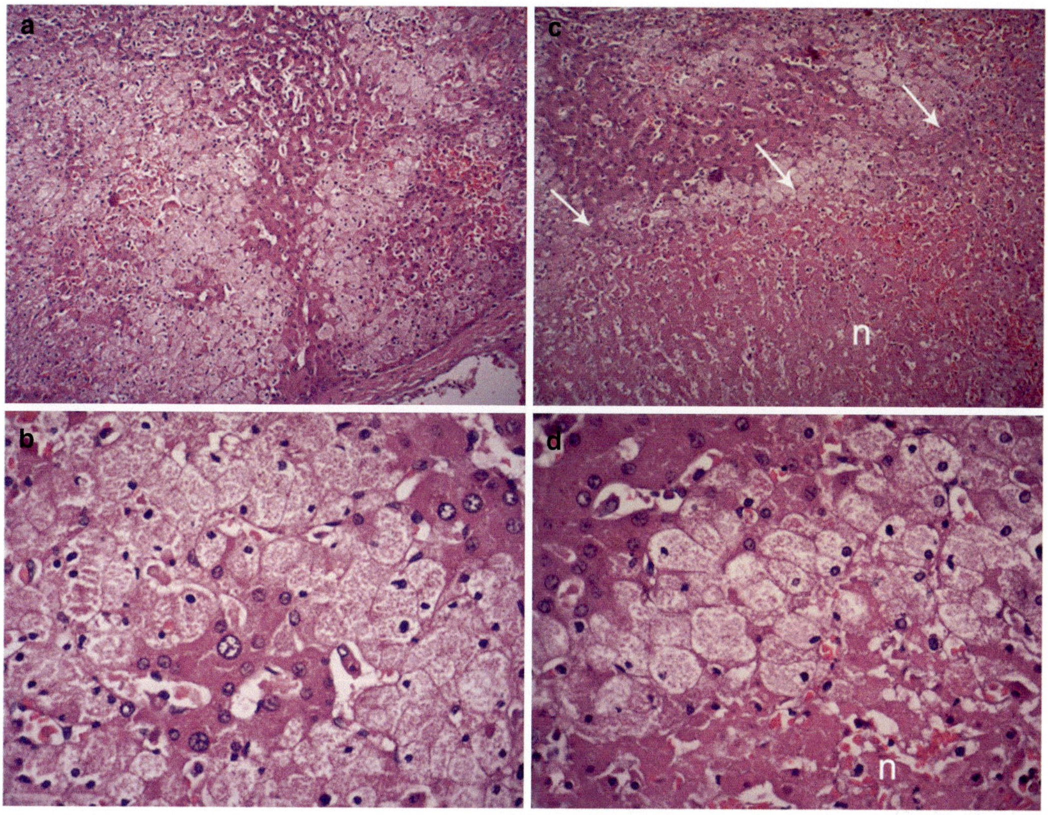

Fig. 36.4 Sections of the liver showing prominent hydropic change (**a**) H&E × 200 and (**b**) H&E × 400, along with foci of coagulative necroses n (**c**) H&E × 200 (arrows) and (**d**) H&E × 400

colonization without accompanying infection, nonspecific symptoms, and variable presentation.

References

1. Pappas PG, Lionakis MS, Arendrup MC, Ostrosky-Zeichner L, Kullberg BJ. Invasive candidiasis. Nat Rev Dis Primers. 2018;4:18026.
2. Kullberg BJ, Arendrup MC. Invasive candidiasis. N Engl J Med. 2015;373:1445–56.
3. Aguin TJ, Sobel JD. Vulvovaginal candidiasis in pregnancy. Curr Infect Dis Rep. 2015;17:30.
4. Mohamed AA, Lu X-l, Mounmin FA. Diagnosis and treatment of esophageal candidiasis: current updates. Can J Gastroenterol Hepatol. 2019;2019:3585136.
5. Praneenararat S. Fungal infection of the colon. Clin Exp Gastroenterol. 2014;7:415–26.
6. Branco SC, Ferreira AT, Saraiva S, Silva MJ, Garcia T. Fungal Gastroduodenitis. Eur J Case Rep Intern Med. 2017;4(7):000628.
7. Lamps LW, Lai KK, Milner DA Jr. Fungal infections of the gastrointestinal tract in the immunocompromised host: an update. Adv Anat Pathol. 2014;21(4):217–27.

Plugging of Visceral Blood Vessels by Atypical Cells: Clue to Leukemia!

37

Kusum D. Jashnani, Sangeeta Kini, and Rosemarie de Souza

37.1 Clinical History

A 28-year-old woman P2L2G3 with a day 3 postpartum state came with chief complaints of one episode of moderate to high grade fever and vomiting. She also had complaints of altered sensorium with drowsiness. She had a full-term normal vaginal delivery conducted at home by a midwife (Dai). She delivered a normal live male child; details of the neonate were not available. The patient was transferred from the primary health center (PHC) to our tertiary care center with a clinical impression of severe anemia with congestive cardiac failure with ongoing blood transfusion.

On examination, the patient was unconscious, had severe pallor, tachycardia, and sluggish breathing, and so was immediately intubated and transferred to the intensive care unit (ICU). Investigations done at PHC sent along with transfer notes were the following: Hb 2 g/dL, total WBC count 7000/cmm, and platelet count 37,000/cmm suggestive of bicytopenia. Peripheral smear-shift to the left with promyelocytes 5%, myelocytes 1%, metamyelocytes 2%, band forms 2%, lymphocytes 12%, and polymorphs 78%.

Biochemical profile: Glucose 99 mg/dl, BUN 44 mg/dl, S.cr 1.63 mg/dl, Na 144 mEq/L, and K 4.68 meq/L.

Obstetric clinical diagnosis was puerperal sepsis with septic encephalopathy with severe anemia on day 3 postpartum. A differential diagnosis of postpartum hemorrhage with anemia, hemolytic anemia, and complicated malaria were suggested.

Despite acute management, patient's condition deteriorated and she succumbed within 5 h of hospital stay. A complete postmortem was performed after due consent for the same.

37.2 Autopsy Findings

On external examination: Patient was well built and well nourished with marked pallor.

In situ examination: Most of the organs appeared markedly pale.

Internal examination: The liver weighed 1.4 kg, and the cut surface showed features of chronic passive congestion. Microscopy showed dilated sinusoids plugged with few neutrophils and many atypical cells. Hepatocytes showed micro and macro vesicular steatosis.

Bilateral lungs weighed 200 g each and showed subpleural petechial hemorrhages. They

K. D. Jashnani (✉) · S. Kini
Department of Pathology, Topiwala National Medical College and BYL Nair Charitable Hospital, Mumbai, Maharashtra, India

R. de Souza
Department of Medicine, Topiwala National Medical College and BYL Nair Charitable Hospital, Mumbai, Maharashtra, India

K. D. Jashnani (ed.), *Maternal Mortality - Lessons Learnt from Autopsy*, https://doi.org/10.1007/978-981-19-3420-9_37

were subcrepitant with minimal pulmonary edema. Microscopy showed fibrotic thickening of the pleura with subpleural hemorrhages. Alveolar septae showed thickening with chronic inflammatory infiltrate and few small sized vessels were plugged with similar atypical cells (Fig. 37.1a, b).

Bilateral kidneys appeared swollen, enlarged and showed subcapsular hemorrhages. On microscopy, tubules showed cloudy change with focal areas showing acute tubular necrosis and hyaline casts within the lumen.

The spleen was enlarged weighing 250 g, and the cut surface appeared congested. Microscopy showed similar atypical cells within the congested red pulp sinuses. White pulp was unremarkable.

The uterus weighed 1.5 kg and showed features of physiological hypertrophy of pregnancy with endometrial cavity containing approximately 30 cc of blood clot, consistent with postpartum status. On microscopy, apart from decidual change in endometrial stroma and physiological hypertrophy of myometrium with preischemia; the intermyometrial and even the cervical wall vessels showed plugging by atypical mononuclear cells suggestive of blast cells (Fig. 37.2a–d).

The heart weighing 400 g showed left ventricular hypertrophy with dilatation.

Bone marrow examination revealed hypercellular marrow with an increased myeloid-to-erythroid ratio and more than 40% blast cells, the majority having pale indented to kidney-shaped nucleus with moderate eosinophilic cytoplasm (Fig. 37.3a–c). These features were suggestive of acute myeloid leukemia (myelomonocytic variant).

37.3 Final Cause of Death

Severe anemia with congestive cardiac failure due to acute (myeloid) leukemia in a day 3 postpartum state.

37.4 Clinicopathologic Discussion

The combination of acute leukemia and pregnancy is rare and is estimated to be one in 75,000–100,000 pregnancies [1]. Two-thirds of pregnancy associated acute leukemia cases are acute myeloid leukemia. Diagnosis is generally made during the second and third trimester with an estimate of 23% in the first trimester, 37% in the second trimester, and 40% in the third trimester.

Most of the times, the clinical manifestations of acute leukemia are very nonspecific. Thus, clinical signs and symptoms of acute leukemia such as fatigue, weakness, dyspnea, and pallor are usually attributed to physiological and metabolic changes during pregnancy. The physiological changes associated with pregnancy can also mask certain laboratory abnormalities that are typically pres-

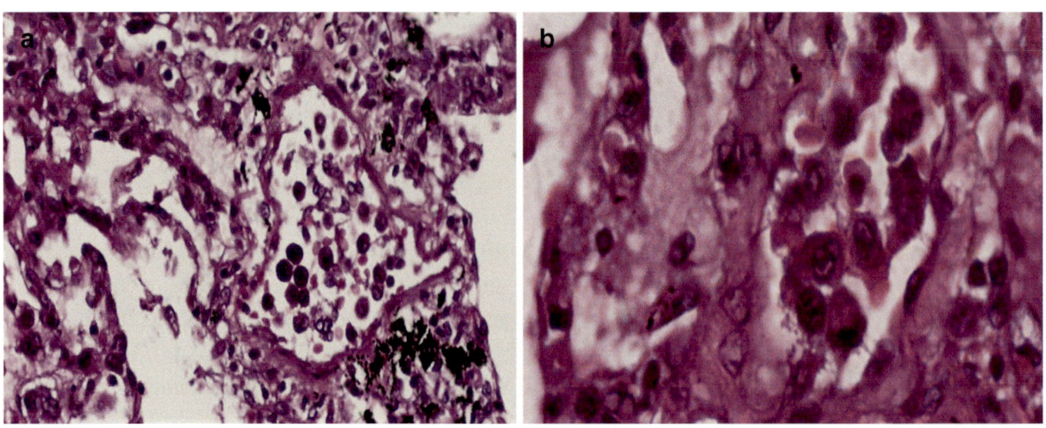

Fig. 37.1 Photomicrograph showing lung parenchymal alveolar septal vessels plugged with atypical cells resembling blasts. (**a**) H&E 400×, (**b**) H&E 1000×

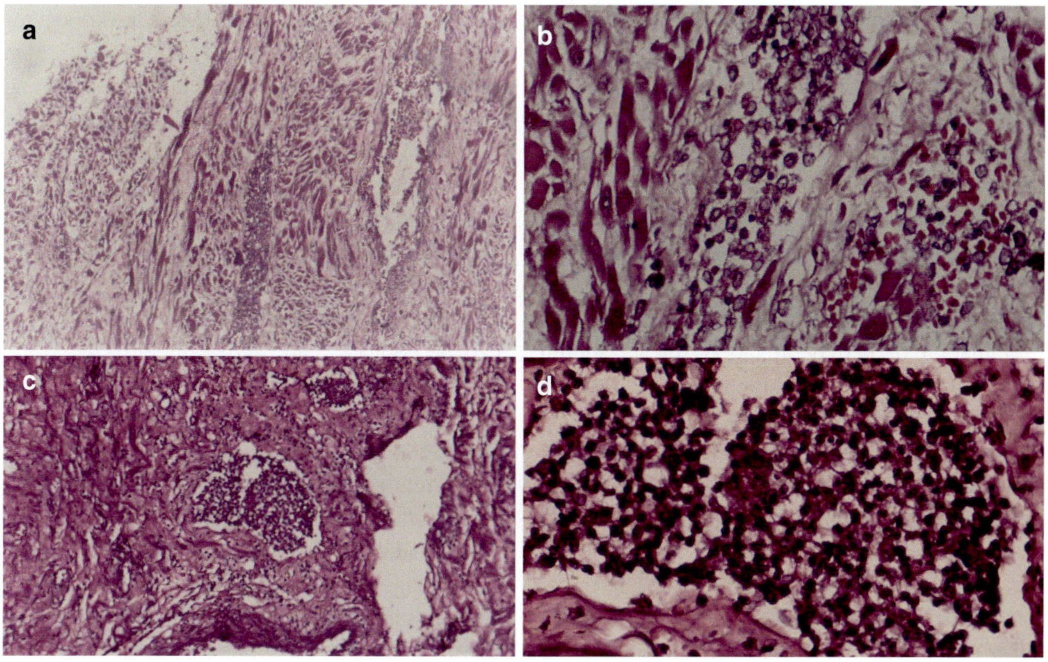

Fig. 37.2 Photomicrograph showing uterine myometrial & cervical wall vessels plugged with atypical cells resembling blasts. (**a**, **b**) Uterine myometrial vessels. H&E 200×, H&E 400×. (**c**, **d**) Cervical stromal vessels. H&E 200× & 400×

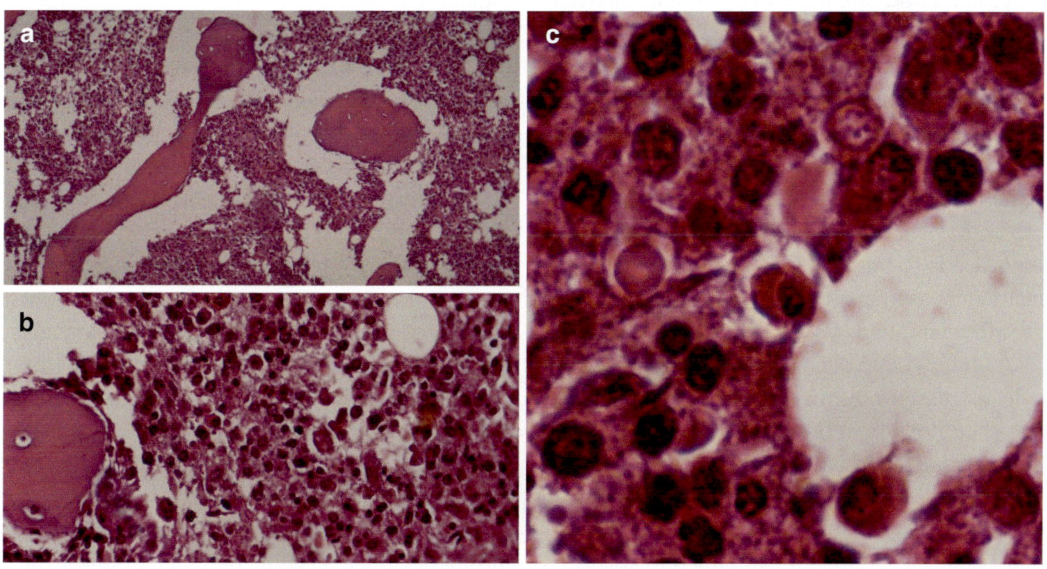

Fig. 37.3 Photomicrograph showing hypercellular bone marrow with increased myeloid series & comprising of blasts having indented/kidney shaped nucleus and moderate amount of cytoplasm resembling blasts of acute myelomonocytic leukemia. (**a**) H&E 200×, (**b**) H&E 400×, (**c**) H&E 1000×

ent in acute myeloid leukemia; such as anemia of pregnancy (due to increased demand), leukocytosis, or thrombocytopenia (gestation induced autoimmune phenomenon or eclampsia, etc.). Recurrent infections and bleeding can reflect bone marrow failure [2]. Hence diagnosis of acute leukemia during pregnancy can often get overlooked or delayed, as observed in the index case where the patient presented with severe anemia leading to congestive cardiac failure. Usually, careful examination of peripheral blood smears should be able to suspect or identify blasts and thereby be confirmed on bone marrow examination. The diagnostic approach is the same as in the general population including bone marrow aspiration for morphological examination, immunophenotyping, cytogenetics, and molecular studies. The CBC report available in the index case with the transfer notes did not mention any abnormality, which either could be a form of aleukemic leukemia or a non-reliable hematology report.

Among leukemias, acute promyelocytic leukemia (APL) is a subtype of acute myeloid leukemia (AML) with unique molecular pathogenesis, clinical manifestations, and treatment. As it is associated with coagulopathy, it may often present with a DIC- like clinical situation or with postpartum hemorrhage, thus contributing to maternal death and the diagnosis of leukemia being missed [2, 3]. Maternal death could also occur due to leukemic blast crisis/tumor lysis/sepsis. In such events, careful examination of the fetus needs to be done with complete anthropometric measurements to identify intrauterine growth retardation.

At autopsy, the diagnosis of leukemia is difficult just based on gross morphology. However, one should always consider the very rare possibility of leukemias mimicking physiologic and metabolic gestational changes. Presence of hepatosplenomegaly, multiple sites of visceral hemorrhages, and severe pallor can clinch to suspect a leukemic etiology on gross morphology during autopsy. Hence it's imperative to make peripheral blood smears/bone marrow smears as part of postmortem investigations in all cases of maternal death due to severe anemia and thrombocytopenia, coagulopathy, and infections. On microscopy of maternal deaths due to anemia and thrombocytopenia, small sized blood vessels of all viscera should be diligently seen to identify plugging of vessel lumens by atypical cells resembling blasts as observed in the present case. Autopsy bone marrow examination helps in further confirmation of leukemic etiology of maternal death. A myeloperoxidase stain on bone marrow smears can assist in differentiating myeloid from lymphoid leukemia.

Treatment of acute leukemia in pregnancy is always a clinical dilemma. In general, initiation of chemotherapy as early as possible may increase the complete remission (CR) rate. For patients who are diagnosed in the first trimester or late stage of pregnancy (>30 weeks), elective medical termination of pregnancy or induced delivery before starting chemotherapy may be a good choice for better maternal (and fetal) outcome [4, 5]. If acute leukemia treatment is taken during the antepartum period, then external congenital abnormalities in the newborn should be looked for in view of the known teratogenic effects of cytotoxic drugs [6]. Further, although maternal cells do reach the fetus, vertical transmission of malignant cells is exceptionally rare as it is limited by the placental barrier and the fetal immune system. Though the placenta possesses very effective protective mechanisms against circulating malignant cells, it is still not an absolute barrier and leukemic cells can pass from mother to fetus. Acute leukemia represented the second most frequent malignancy with malignant cells localizations in the placenta after malignant melanoma [7]. Hence, the placenta should be systematically analyzed histopathologically in the event of ante partum maternal death due to acute leukemia. Close follow-up and monitoring of patients with anemia/infection/thrombocytopenia with peripheral smear and bone marrow examination may aid in early diagnosis and deciding on a multidisciplinary team approach for the therapeutic challenge of leukemia with pregnancy.

References

1. Brenner B, Avivi I, Lishner M. Haematological cancers in pregnancy. Lancet. 2012;379:580–8.
2. Abadi U, Koren G, Lishner M. Leukemia and lymphoma in pregnancy. Hematol Oncol Clin North Am. 2011;25:277–91.
3. Horowitz NA, Henig I, Henig O, et al. Acute myeloid leukemia during pregnancy: a systematic review and meta-analysis. Leuk Lymphoma. 2018;59(3):610–6. https://doi.org/10.1080/10428194.2017.1347651.
4. Zhu D, Tang D, Chai X, Zhang G, Wang Y. Acute leukemia in pregnancy: a single institutional experience with 21 cases at 10 years and a review of the literature. Ann Med. 2021;53(1):567–75.
5. Farhadfar N, Cerquozzi S, Hessenauer MR, et al. Acute leukemia in pregnancy: a single institution experience with 23 patients. Leuk Lymphoma. 2017;58(5):1052–60.
6. Fracchiolla NS, Sciume M, Dambrosi F, et al. Acute myeloid leukemia & pregnancy, clinical experience from a single center and a review of the literature. BMC Cancer. 2017;17:442.
7. Greaves M, Hughes W. Cancer cell transmission via the placenta. Evol Med Public Health. 2018;2018(1):106–15.

Chronic Kidney Disease Masquerading as Pregnancy Induced Hypertension

38

Kusum D. Jashnani, Sushama A. Chandekar, and Rosemarie de Souza

38.1 Clinical History

A 25-year-old female with 22 weeks of gestation was transferred from a private hospital with complaints of generalized anasarca-pitting type, pallor, severe PIH, and anemia. Other history available was hypoalbuminaemia. The patient also had complaints of breathlessness with pink frothy sputum. RS—bilateral creps suggestive of pulmonary edema in the PHC. T WBC—12,000/cumm, Hb of 5.5 g/dL, creatinine of 2.2 mg/dl, T protein of 5.1 mg/dl, and albumin of 2.1 mg/dl were the investigations available in the transfer notes. She was transferred to our MICU. Investigations done in our tertiary care center revealed a urine field full of pus cells, Hb of 11.4 g/dL, INR of 1, and ABG showing metabolic acidosis. LFT in the form of T bilirubin, SGPT/SGOT were normal. The patient aborted on day 1 of admission after 3 h. It was a female child with a birth weight of 540 g, macerated bluish, and a placental weight of 185 g. Her BP varied from 150/100 to 120/70 mmHg; her urine output always remained very low throughout her hospital stay. Clinical impression was UTI with ARF with PIH with 6 months' amenorrhea. She was treated with antihypertensives and diuretics. Her condition deteriorated 2 days later; she was put on mechanical ventilation. As hemodialysis could not be done, peritoneal dialysis was done. Input was in the range of 2500 to 3000, but output remained zero. She continued to be in poor general condition (GC), was unconscious in the last 2 days, and could not be revived and was declared dead on day 8 of total hospital stay. A complete autopsy was performed after proper consent.

38.2 Autopsy Findings

She was very pale, with pitting edema up to her ankle. The peritoneal cavity contained 500 cc^3 of clear serous fluid. The liver was enlarged, weighed 2 kg, and showed alternate light and dark areas on the cut surface suggestive of the nutmeg appearance of chronic passive congestion (CPC) (Fig. 38.1a). Lungs weighed around 450–500 g each, showed multiple patchy firm raised

K. D. Jashnani (✉) · S. A. Chandekar
Department of Pathology, Topiwala National Medical College & BYL Nair Charitable Hospital, Mumbai, Maharashtra, India

R. de Souza
Department of Medicine, Topiwala National Medical College & BYL Nair Ch. Hospital, Mumbai, Maharashtra, India

K. D. Jashnani (ed.), *Maternal Mortality - Lessons Learnt from Autopsy*, https://doi.org/10.1007/978-981-19-3420-9_38

gray white areas of bronchopneumonia (Fig. 38.1b). Each kidney weighed 150 g with capsule easily stripped off, smooth external surface, cut surface revealed thin cortex with normal pelvicalyceal system (Fig. 38.2a, b). The uterus with cervix weighed 350 g, with blood clots in the endometrial cavity.

On histopathology, the lungs showed multiple patchy areas of intraalveolar neutrophilic infiltrate, few areas of intraalveolar hemorrhage and edema with many alveolar septae lined by eosinophilic hyaline membrane suggestive of bronchopneumonia and ARDS. The liver showed CPC changes. Bilateral kidneys showed cellular crescents in almost 65% of glomeruli along with endothelial and mesangial proliferation (Fig. 38.2c, d). Tubules showed hyaline and pus casts. Interstitium showed foci of mixed inflammatory infiltrate and blood vessels were unremarkable. It was a case of rapidly progressive glomerulonephritis/crescentic glomerulonephritis (GN) with acute tubulointerstitial nephritis. The rest of the organs were unremarkable.

38.3 Final Cause of Death

Bronchopneumonia with ARDS and renal failure due to rapidly progressive (crescentic) glomerulonephritis in a case of abortion.

38.4 Clinicopathologic Discussion

Chronic hypertension, gestational hypertension, preeclampsia-eclampsia, and chronic hypertension with superimposed preeclampsia are the 4 categories of hypertensive disorders of pregnancy. They are important causes of maternal and fetal morbidity and mortality. Chronic hypertension is defined as blood pressure exceeding 140/90 mmHg identified before pregnancy or before 20 weeks' gestation. Gestational hypertension (this terminology is preferred over "pregnancy-induced hypertension," PIH) [1] refers to hypertension developing in the latter part of pregnancy (>20 weeks' gestation) without

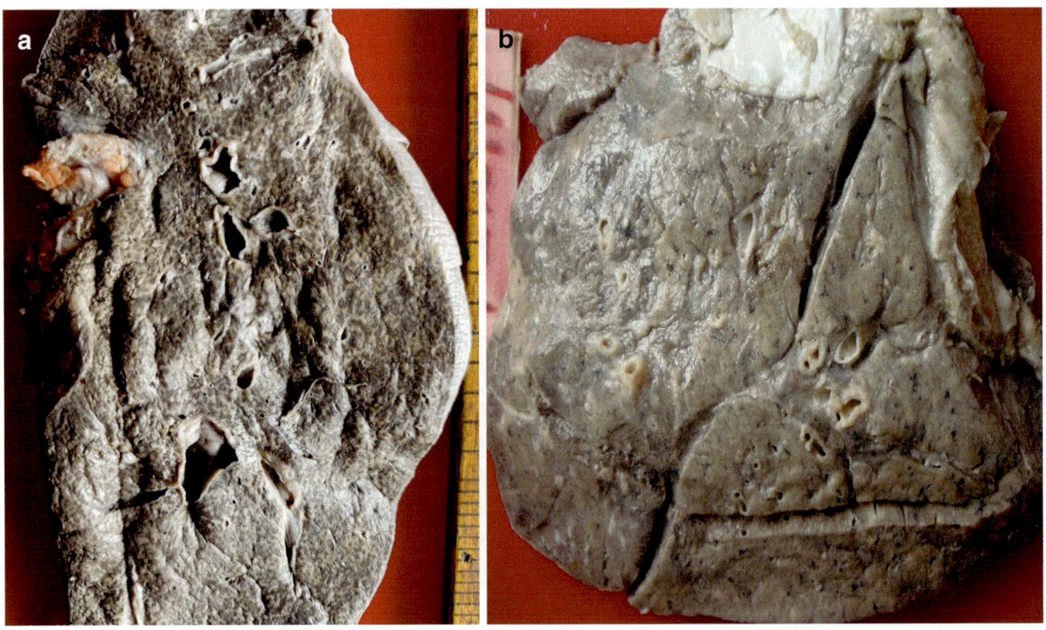

Fig. 38.1 Gross slice of liver showing alternate light and dark areas of CPC-Nutmeg appearance (**a**). Gross specimen of lung showing confluent raised gray white firm areas of bronchopneumonia (**b**)

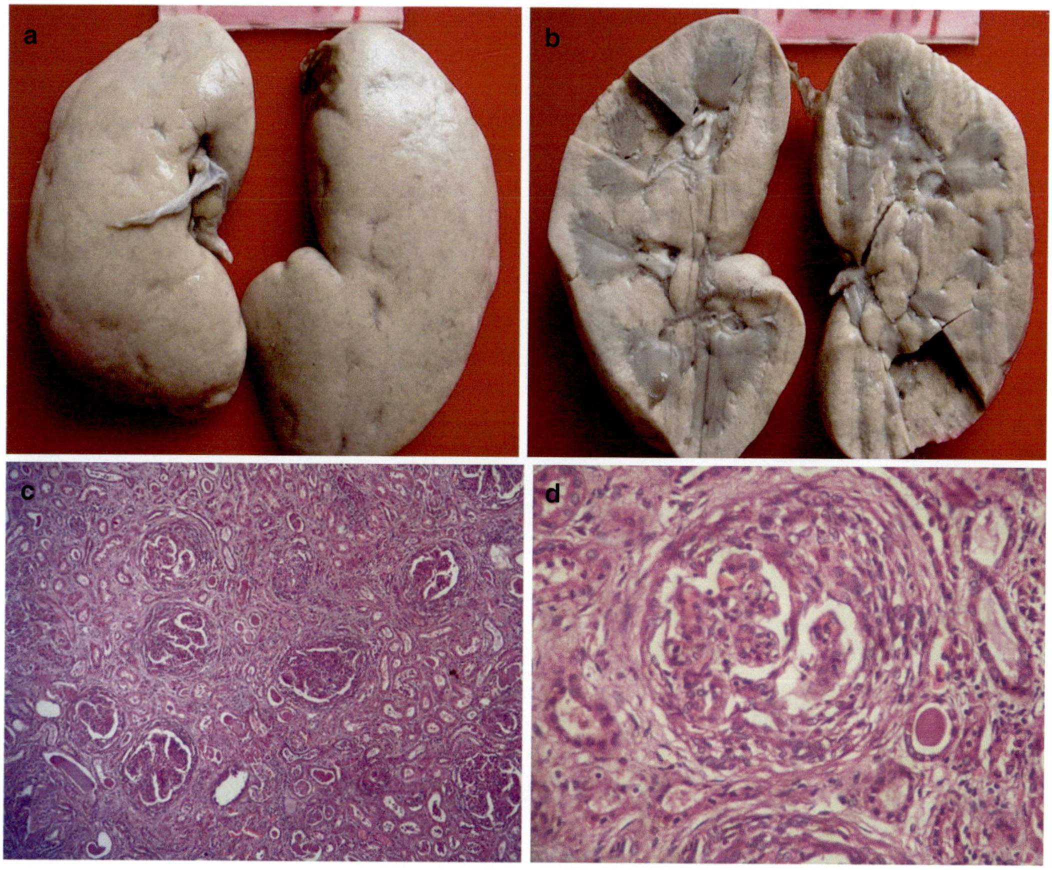

Fig. 38.2 Gross specimens of bilateral halves of the kidney showing a smooth external surface (**a**) and a thin cortex on the cut surface (**b**). Majority of the glomeruli showing cellular crescents (**c**)-H&E, 200×. (**d**)-H&E, 400×

any other features of preeclampsia, and followed by blood pressure returning to normal in the postpartum period. One third of these women develop the syndrome of preeclampsia. Gestational hypertension may also be a prelude to chronic hypertension later in life. It may sometimes be a challenge to determine whether elevated blood pressure identified during pregnancy is due to chronic hypertension or to preeclampsia, especially if blood pressure values from the first half of gestation are not available. In such circumstances, one may have to rely on history, physical examination, certain laboratory investigations [urinalysis; complete blood cell (CBC) count; and serum sodium, potassium, creatinine, glucose levels, blood urea nitrogen (BUN), albumin, calcium, uric acid, glycosylated hemoglobin, thyroid-stimulating hormone (TSH), liver enzymes, bilirubin], as well as important maternal and fetal risk factors for preeclampsia to help clarify the diagnosis. Urinalysis may be used as a screen for proteinuria wherein trace levels to +1 proteinuria are acceptable, but levels of +2 or greater are abnormal.

Preeclampsia is rare before the third trimester, and the diagnosis of severe hypertension or preeclampsia in the first or early second trimester needs exclusion of gestational trophoblastic disease. New seizures in pregnancy suggest preeclampsia-eclampsia, after excluding primary neurologic disorders [2]. Women with hypertension and suspected or established preeclampsia are admitted to the hospital for close observation and investigation. Acute severe hypertension (BP level of ≥160/110 mm Hg) in pregnancy is a medical emergency requiring treatment to lower blood pressures within 30 min of confirmation to reduce the risk of intracranial hemorrhage. Anticonvulsant therapy may be undertaken in the setting of severe preeclampsia (primary prophylaxis) or in the setting of eclamptic seizures (secondary prophylaxis). The most effective agent is IV magnesium sulfate.

Chronic kidney disease (CKD), also called chronic kidney failure, involves a gradual loss of kidney function. Diabetes, hypertension, glomerulonephritis, prolonged obstruction of the urinary tract, pyelonephritis, and polycystic kidney disease are some of the disease conditions causing CKD. Smoking, obesity, cardiovascular disease, and drug-induced kidney failure are some of the risk factors for CKD. CKD is not a barrier to reproduction in most women, but the risk of adverse pregnancy outcomes like preeclampsia, fetal growth restriction, preterm delivery, and abruptio placentae is increased in these women. This information should be made available to women with CKD. As per the guidelines offered by K Wiles et al., safe and effective contraception should be offered to women of reproductive age who are taking teratogenic medication, have active glomerulonephritis, are within one year of renal transplantation or acute graft rejection, and who do not wish to conceive. Also, women with CKD should be offered low-dose aspirin (75–150 mg) in pregnancy to reduce the risk of preeclampsia. The target blood pressure during pregnancy for women with CKD should be 135/85 mmHg or less. It is also recommended that if a histological diagnosis will change management in pregnancy, then renal biopsy can be performed in the first and early second trimester of pregnancy. The increased risk of bleeding or iatrogenic preterm delivery should be kept in mind following renal biopsy [3].

Crescentic GN is not a specific disease, but a histologic manifestation of severe glomerular damage. Crescentic glomerulonephritis is characterized by the presence of extensive glomerular crescents (usually greater than 50%) as the principal histologic finding [4]. Because it clinically presents with a rapid decline in kidney function, it is also known as rapidly progressive glomerulonephritis (RPGN). These crescents can be cellular or fibrous, circumferential or noncircumferential, and the presence of circumferential crescents in over 80% of glomeruli foretells a poor prognosis. In addition to primary RPGN, secondary RPGN due to an infectious process like poststreptococcal glomerulonephritis, infective endocarditis, or secondary to a systemic illness, systemic lupus erythematosus, Henoch-Schonlein purpura, systemic necrotizing vasculitis, malignancy; drugs such as penicillamine, rifampin, etc. can occur. It can complicate any glomerular disease like membranoproliferative glomerulonephritis type 2, membranous glomerulonephritis, or immunoglobulin A nephropathy.

The present case was an undiagnosed case of CKD with RPGN, admitted and treated as gestational hypertension (PIH), finally succumbing to renal failure and ARDS. This case highlights that every pregnant woman with raised blood pressure is not always a case of PIH, and one should also keep a high suspicion of CKD while investigating and treating such patients.

References

1. Bernheim J, Plotkin E, Bernheim J, Korzets Z. It looks like, it smells like but is it just pre-eclampsia? Nephrol. Dial. Transplant. 2005;20(2):451–2.
2. Carson MP, Gibson PS. What is the prognosis of hypertensive disorders during pregnancy? In: Springel EH, editor. Obstet Gynecol, Drugs & Diseases; 2018.
3. Wiles K, Chappell L, Clark K, et al. Clinical practice guideline on pregnancy and renal disease. BMC Nephrol. 2019;20:401.
4. Divyaveer S, Tiwari V, Patil M, et al. An unusual case of rapidly progressing glomerulonephritis in pregnancy; triple positivity or a co incidence? J Nephropathol. 2017;6(4):272–4.

Pulmonary Edema and Aspiration Pneumonia: Cause for Maternal Death

39

Kusum D. Jashnani

39.1 Clinical History

A 22-year-old female with 34 weeks of gestation, was referred from a peripheral hospital with complaints of breathlessness, with diagnosis of pregnancy-induced hypertension with chronic disseminated intravascular coagulation (DIC). Transfer notes mentioned BP of 140/90 mmHg, per vaginal bleeding^{+}, afebrile, P 102/minute, RR 40/minute, per abdomen—uterus soft, corresponding to 34 weeks' gestation, with absent fetal heart sounds (FHS). USG done showed 34 weeks' gestation, with absent cardiac activity suggestive of intrauterine fetal death (IUFD).

USG done 1 month back—single live fetus with large head, the uterus corresponded to 32 weeks of gestation, cephalic presentation. CBC: Hb 8.5 gm/dL, platelet count 37,000/cumm, T WBC count 37,000/cumm with P80, L17, Eo 03, M0.

On examination, patient was afebrile, BP was not recordable, Pulse not palpable, RS -air entry absent, heart sounds not heard, pupils dilated and fixed, not reacting to light, patient declared dead in spite of resuscitation measures, within 10 min of admission. Complete autopsy was performed after due consent.

39.2 Autopsy Findings

There was no evidence of any foreign material in the trachea and major bronchioles on gross examination. Bilateral lungs weighed 500 gms each, with smooth shiny pleura with few subpleural hemorrhages. On pressure, frothy fluid was oozing out. Microscopy showed extensive areas of intraalveolar edema fluid (Fig. 39.2b, c), with few of these alveoli as well as small bronchi and bronchioles showing vegetable fibers (Figs. 39.1 and 39.2a). There was widening of the interstitium by numerous lymphocytes and few plasma cells (Fig. 39.2d). The uterus showed the presence of a placenta and a male fetus with a weight of 1.7 kg. The liver weighed 1.5 kg showing CPC changes. The heart showed epicardial and endocardial hemorrhages. The rest of the organs were unremarkable on gross and microscopy.

K. D. Jashnani (✉)
Department of Pathology, Topiwala National Medical College & BYL Nair Charitable Hospital, Mumbai, Maharashtra, India

K. D. Jashnani (ed.), *Maternal Mortality - Lessons Learnt from Autopsy*,
https://doi.org/10.1007/978-981-19-3420-9_39

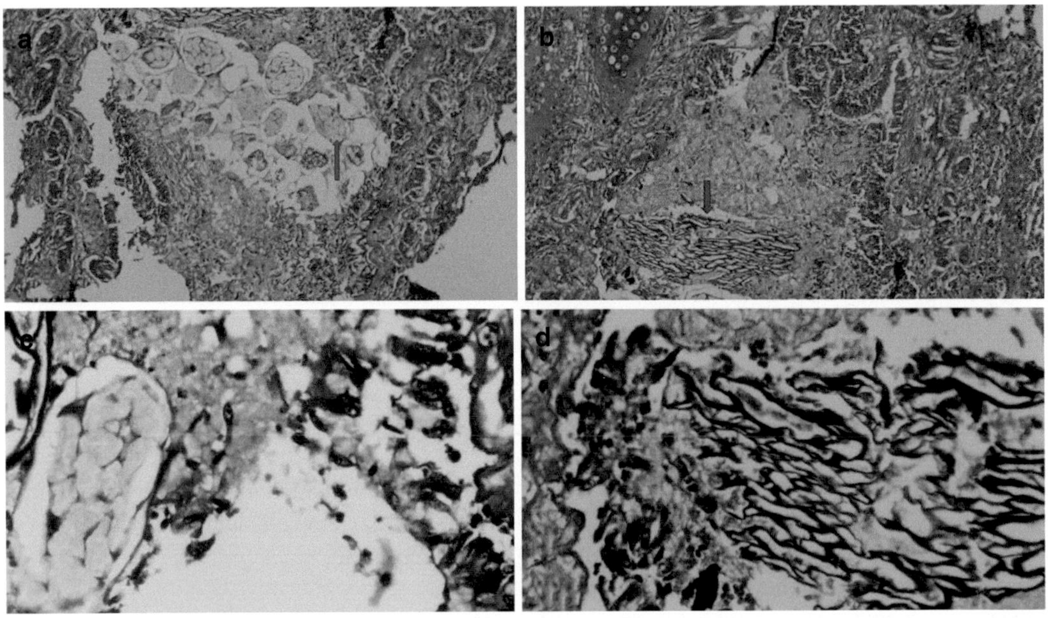

Fig. 39.1 (**a**, **b**) Show vegetable fibers within bronchi (cartilage is seen in the wall) and bronchioles H&E, 200×, (**c**, **d**) show the vegetable fibers (pointed by arrows in **a**, **b**) H&E, 400×

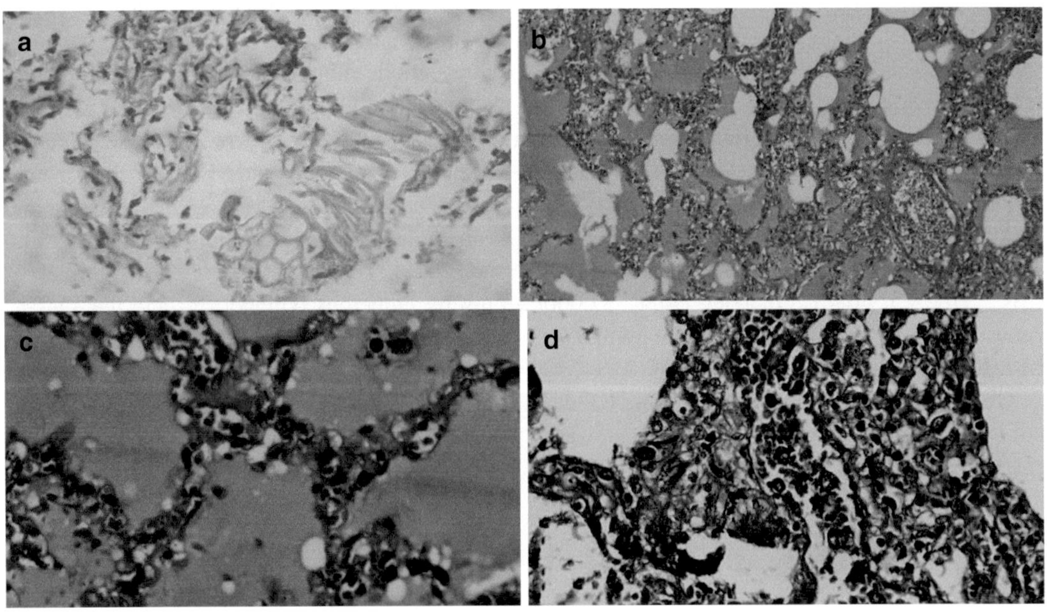

Fig. 39.2 (**a**) Shows vegetable fiber within the terminal air space, H&E, 400×. (**b**, **c**) Show the presence of intraalveolar eosinophilic edema fluid within the alveolar spaces. H&E, 200×, 400×. (**d**) Shows widened interstitial wall by chronic inflammatory cells, H&E, 400×

39.3 Final Cause of Death

Massive bilateral pulmonary edema with aspiration pneumonia in a case of PIH with IUFD.

39.4 Clinicopathologic Discussion

Acute pulmonary edema in pregnancy is a medical emergency, with high maternal/perinatal morbidity/mortality with an incidence of 0.08% to 1.5%. Chronic hypertension, preeclampsia, and eclampsia are the major causes, followed by fluid overload and decompensated heart disease (resulting from prior cardiovascular diseases like rheumatic heart disease (RHD) and peripartum cardiomyopathy (PPCM)). Multiple gestation and infection are other uncommon causes. Fluid overload in the form of infusion of fluids causes pulmonary edema when fluid balance is >2000 mL, leading to increase in hydrostatic pressure. There is systolic and diastolic dysfunction in sepsis, with decreased diastolic filling, thereby increasing the risk of pulmonary edema. Diagnosis of pulmonary edema is clinical, with the principal signs and symptoms being crackling rales, dyspnea, tachypnea, coughing, and wheezing. The mean age of patients is usually in the range of 20 to 35 years of age [1].

It occurs most commonly before delivery (58.0%) or postpartum (38.0%) [1]. This is probably due to cardiovascular changes like increased plasma volume and cardiac output associated with reduced colloid osmotic pressure during pregnancy [2]. Reducing myocardial contractility could also be one of the causes [1].

The diagnosis of pulmonary edema is usually made by the presence of shortness of breath (SOB), increased respiratory rate of more than 35 per minute, a fall in saturations to less than 94%, and bilateral crepitations on respiratory system examination. As soon as the clinical diagnosis is made, the treatment is started, with improvement of saturation to more than 94% and decrease in the respiratory rate to less than 35 per minute considered clinical stabilization. Maternal stabilization should be the priority over delivery of the fetus. Noninvasive ventilation (NIV), either in the form of CPAP or BiPAP, has a positive role in cardiogenic pulmonary edema, as it provides a high inspired oxygen concentration and displaces fluid from the alveoli into the pulmonary circulation. In the absence of an accurate etiological diagnosis, the initiation of specific treatment would be delayed, with profound effects on maternal/perinatal outcomes [3].

Aspiration, a life-threatening medical emergency, is characterized by the entry of either oropharyngeal food, drink, vomit, saliva, or gastric contents into the lungs. Volume of aspirate and the presence of contaminants determine the mortality, which can be as high as 70 percent. Four types of aspiration syndromes are known based on the quantity and nature of the aspirated material as well as the host factors responsible for aspiration. Aspiration of gastric acid causes a chemical pneumonitis; aspiration of bacteria from oropharyngeal areas causes aspiration pneumonia. Aspiration of oil (mineral/vegetable) causes exogenous lipoid pneumonia, while aspiration of a foreign body may cause an acute respiratory emergency. Risk factors for aspiration are impaired gag reflex due to brain injury or swallowing problem, or excessive use of alcohol or drugs or other neurologic disorders like dementia or any other cognitive disability. Enteral feeding through gastrostomy and nasogastric tubes also increases the risk of aspiration. Complications of aspiration include acute respiratory failure, acute respiratory distress syndrome (ARDS), and bacterial pneumonia.

Aspiration can be silent or overt, wherein silent aspiration has no symptoms and tends to occur in people with impaired senses. Overt aspiration usually causes sudden, noticeable symptoms like coughing, wheezing, or breathlessness. Overt aspiration can present as a medical emergency due to choking and hypoxia, especially if a large volume is aspirated. Promptly clearing the airway by the use of the right suction machine is critically important, for which the patient needs to be hospitalized with continuous monitoring.

As per S Mukhopadhyay et al., foreign material including most commonly vegetable or food remnants (54 cases), and less often talc or microcrystalline cellulose (7), crospovidone (4), and kayexalate (2) were identified in cases of particulate matter aspiration pneumonia. This occurs in the background of multinucleated giant cells, acute bronchopneumonia/bronchiolitis, and/or suppurative granulomas. *Streptococcus pneumoniae*, *Haemophilus influenzae*, *Staphylococcus aureus*, and *Pseudomonas* account for most cases of aspiration pneumonia. Infiltrate in the posterior upper lobe or apical lower lobe segments from recumbent aspiration, and basal lower lobe segments from upright or semi-recumbent aspiration are characteristic radiology findings. In the present case, there was interstitial pneumonia in areas surrounding the bronchi/bronchioles showing aspirated material in their lumina. The rest of the lungs showed eosinophilic edema fluid within the alveolar spaces bilateral. This case highlights the fact that aspiration can be masked by other respiratory pathologies, like pulmonary edema in this case. Aspiration of vegetable fibers was a finding on autopsy, which being so extensive could have been the single cause of death.

References

1. Pordeus ACB, Katz L, Soares MC, Maia SB, Amorim MMR. Acute pulmonary edema in an obstetric intensive care unit; A case series study. Medicine (Baltimore). 2018;97(28):e11508. https://doi.org/10.1097/MD.0000000000011508.
2. Mukhopadhyay S, Katzenstein A-LA. Pulmonary disease due to aspiration of food and other particulate matter: a clinicopathologic study of 59 cases diagnosed on biopsy or resection specimens. A J Surg Pathol. 2007;31(5):752–9. https://doi.org/10.1097/01.pas.0000213418.08009.f9.
3. Chakravarthy K, Swetha T, Nirmalan PK, Alagandala A, Sodumu N. Protocol-based management of acute pulmonary edema in pregnancy in a low-resource center. J Obstet Anaesth Crit Care. 2020;10:98–105.

Postpartum Febrile Illness: Recurrent Acute Rheumatic Fever

40

Ashutosh Goyal and Pradeep Vaideeswar

40.1 Clinical History

A 26-year-old female, with 30 weeks of gestation (gravida 4, parity 2, living 1, death 1, and abortion 1), was admitted with pain in her abdomen and progressive shortness of breath since 2 days. The patient had been diagnosed as a case of chronic RHD (severe MR, mild AR/TR, severe PH, and good biventricular function) in our tertiary-care institute and had been on regular follow-up and treatment for the past 5 years. She had been advised to have mitral valve replacement and tricuspid valve annuloplasty, but these options were refused by the patient and her relatives. She had been admitted to the same institute at 17 weeks' gestation with dyspnea and chest pain. The two-dimensional trans-thoracic echocardiography revealed severe MR, trivial AR, mild TR, and insignificant PH with good biventricular function (ejection fraction of 60%). She was advised to continue the pregnancy and was discharged after 4 days with digoxin/diuretic therapy and penicillin prophylaxis.

On examination during the current admission, the patient was in active labor. She was conscious with tachycardia (pulse rate of 128 per minute) and tachypnea (respiratory rate 48 per minute). The blood pressure was 130/90 mm Hg. There was bilateral pedal edema and raised JVP (10 cm of water). On auscultation, the patient had a pansystolic murmur, para-sternal heave, and palpable thrill. Obstetric examination revealed a uterus size of 32 weeks with a transverse lie (fetal head in the right hypochondriac region), a dilated cervix with 70% effacement, and blood stained liquor with blood clots. The fetal heart sounds were 150/min. In view of the transverse lie and abruptio placentae, a decision to perform a lower segment Cesarean section was taken. However post-surgery, the general condition was poor with fever (39 °C), tachycardia (pulse rate 150 per minute), raised JVP (>15 cm of water) and a deranged coagulation profile (platelet count of 100 x 10^9/L, prothrombin time of 59.2 s (control 13.2 s), international normalized ratio of 5.98, activated partial thromboplastin time 104 s (control 30.3 s), fibrinogen 91 mg/dL (200 to 400 mg/dL), fibrin degradation products >320 µg/mL (in pregnancy <20 µg/mL), and D-dimer 9.6 mg/L (last trimester of pregnancy <1.70 mg/L)). She succumbed after 23 h of admission.

A. Goyal
Seth GS Medical College & KEM Hospital, Mumbai, Maharashtra, India

P. Vaideeswar (✉)
Department of Pathology (Cardiovascular & Thoracic Division), Seth GS Medical College & KEM Hospital, Mumbai, Maharashtra, India

K. D. Jashnani (ed.), *Maternal Mortality - Lessons Learnt from Autopsy*,
https://doi.org/10.1007/978-981-19-3420-9_40

40.2 Autopsy Findings

The heart at autopsy was moderately enlarged (350 g). The apex was formed by both the ventricles. There was moderate enlargement of the right-sided chambers and left atrium, and mild enlargement of the left ventricle (Fig. 40.1). The great arterial relations were normal, but the pulmonary trunk and its branches were dilated with intimal thickening. There was moderate hypertrophy of both atria and marked hypertrophy of the right ventricle. The tricuspid annulus was dilated with moderate fusion of all the 3 commissures and mild thickening/rolling of the free margins of the valve leaflets. Few of the chordae tendineae attached to the anterior papillary muscle were thickened and fused. Both the commissures of the mitral valve (Fig. 40.2a) were moderately fused with moderate thickening and uprolling of the free margins, indicating the presence of MR. The chordae were moderately thickened but showed minimal fusion with preservation of the inter-chordal spaces (Fig. 40.2a). A jet lesion in the form of rugose endocardial irregularity was present in the posterior wall of the left atrium. The aortic valve also showed mild fusion and thickening of the commissures and cusps, respectively (Fig. 40.2b). The histopathology was a complete surprise. Both the left-sided valves, besides features of healed valvulitis, revealed microscopic fresh and organizing vegetations with Aschoff bodies, while all the chambers, particularly the left ventricle, showed interstitial granulomatous myocarditis with many Aschoff bodies (Fig. 40.2c, d), all of which indicated the recurrence of acute rheumatic fever. Other organ findings included chronic passive venous congestion of the lungs and liver and mediastinal tuberculous lymphadenitis. The uterus was corresponding to its postpartum state.

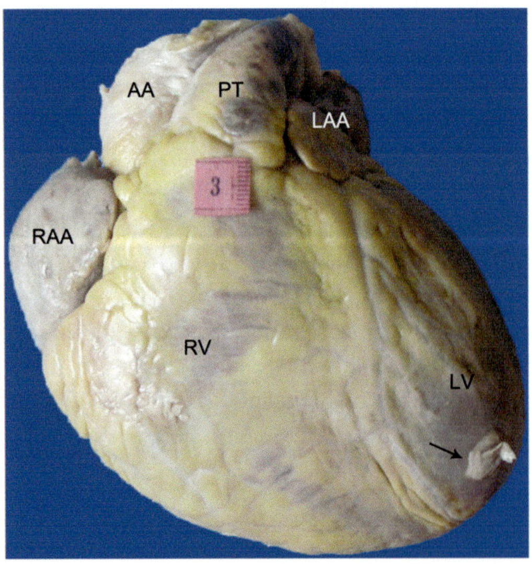

Fig. 40.1 Moderate cardiomegaly with moderate enlargement of the right-sided chambers. The pulmonary trunk PT is larger than aorta AA. Note a milk patch at the left ventricular LV apex (LAA, left atrial appendage; RAA, right atrial appendage; RV, right ventricle)

40.3 Final Cause of Death

Recurrent ARF.

40.4 Clinicopathologic Discussion

A rapid deterioration of the cardiovascular status after delivery had been noted in a patient with a long-standing rheumatic MR and bad obstetric history. The mortality was as a result of recurrent ARF. The case highlights the association of CVD with pregnancy, which is nowadays considered the main cause of maternal deaths. Such diseases arise *de-novo* in pregnancy, leading to direct causes of death, or there may be deterioration of the preexisting disorders (indirect causes of death) due to a number of changes in the cardiovascular functional physiology during gestation [1]. These include reduction in the peripheral vascular resistance, plasma volume expansion, increase in the heart rate, increased stroke volume and rise in the cardiac output [1, 2]. In addition, older maternal age and its frequent association with metabolic disorders add further burden to these physiological alterations [1, 2]. Hence such patients present with heart failure around 26 to 30 weeks of amenorrhea and during or after delivery, which are periods of maximum cardiovascular stress [1]. These adaptations and their accompanying symptomatology can mask the features of CVD with delayed diag-

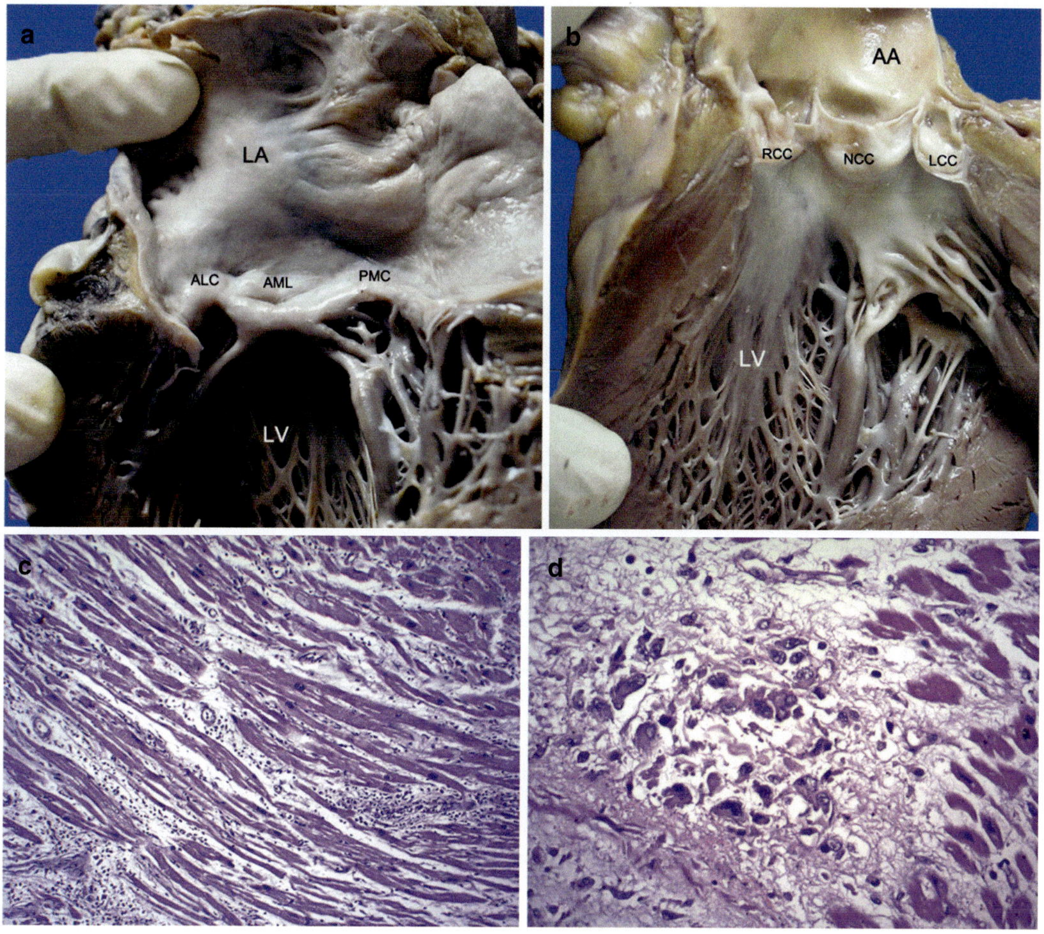

Fig. 40.2 (**a**) Opened out left ventricular LV inflow tract. Features of MR—valve leaflets are moderately thickened with thick margins. Commissures are mild fused. Mild chordal thickening with minimal fusion and shortening; (**b**) LV outflow tract showing minimal involvement of the aortic valve with mild fusion of the commissure between the coronary cusps (AA, ascending aorta; AML, anterior mitral leaflet; ALC, anterolateral commissure; LA, left atrium; LCC, left coronary cusp; NCC, noncoronary cusp; PMC, posteromedial commissure; RCC, right coronary cusp); (**c**) Patchy but prominent mononuclear cell infiltrate with focal interstitial aggregates (H&E × 200; (**d**) Proliferative phase of Aschoff body with Anitschkow cells and Aschoff's giant cells (H&E × 400)

nosis and at the same time can also unveil preexisting subclinical CVDs [1].

Hypertensive disorders are seen in 10% of pregnancies, while 1 to 4% of patients have a complicated gestational course accompanied by a growing spectrum of diverse CVDs. Though they appear infrequent, they are the commonest causes of mortality, especially due to corrected to uncorrected valvular or non-valvular CHDs. This may be the case in the developed countries [3, 4], but in developing and underdeveloped countries like India, RHD remains the leading cause of cardiac disorders in pregnancy, constituting about 69% of all cardiac cases [5]. Pregnancy is a hyperdynamic state and concurrent valvular heart disease can predispose the patients to pulmonary hypertension, pulmonary edema, heart failure, and arrhythmias, particularly after delivery when there is an auto-transfusion of blood from the utero-placental circulation and removal of compression from the inferior vena cava [5, 6]. The type of valvular deformity is the same as for the general population, where involvement of the left-sided valves and MS is found to be more common; moderate to severe stenosis has a higher risk of heart failure of 30 to 50%, respectively [5, 6]. Though it is said that regurgitant lesions are better tolerated during pregnancy, it is noted that moderate to severe MR also have a higher rate of heart failure of about 23% and require stringent surveillance [6]. In the case described, the patient had severe MR with mild AR/TR with the absence of significant PH, was well managed and advised to continue with her pregnancy. Though she had coagulation parameters that indicated DIC, the gross and histological features of DIC had been negative. Her sudden circulatory collapse could be explained on the basis of a recurrence of ARF [7] with verrucous endocarditis and granulomatous myocarditis. In this case, the recurrence and its severity can be explained on the basis of immunological modulations that occur in pregnancy [8].

References

1. Ramlakhan KP, Johnson MR, Roos-Hesselink JW. Pregnancy and cardiovascular disease. Nat Rev Cardiol. 2020;17(11):718–31.
2. Parsonage WA, Zentner D, Lust K, Kane SC, Sullivan EA. Heart disease and pregnancy: the need for a twenty-first century approach to care. Heart Lung Circ. 2021;30:45–51.
3. Salciccioli KB, Cotts TB. Pregnancy in women with adult congenital heart disease. Cardiol Clin. 2021;39:55–65.
4. Bortnick AE, Levine LD. Valvular heart disease in pregnancy. Clin Obstet Gynecol. 2021;63:910–22.
5. Khanna R, Chandra D, Yadav S, Sahu A, Singh N, Kumar S, et al. Maternal and fetal outcomes in pregnant females with rheumatic heart disease. Indian Heart J. 2021;73:185–9.
6. van Hagen IM, Thorne SA, Taha N, Youssef G, Elnagar A, Gabriel H, et al. Pregnancy outcomes in women with rheumatic mitral valve disease. Results from the registry of pregnancy and cardiac disease. Circulation. 2018;137:806–16.
7. Goyal A, Vaideeswar P, Daga P, Bhargav R. Acute rheumatic fever – a pathological analysis of clinically missed cases. Indian J Pathol Microbiol. 2021;64(4):651–4.
8. Morelli SS, Mandal M, Goldsmith LT, Kashani BN, Ponzio NM. The maternal immune system during pregnancy and its influence on fetal development. Res Rep Biol. 2015;6:171–89.

41 Common Atrioventricular Canal: A Fatality Due to a Commonality

Pradeep Vaideeswar and Balaji Baste

41.1 Clinical History

A 23-year-old primigravida had a normal, uneventful delivery after 36 weeks of gestation (male child, 2.98 kg). A week later, she developed fever and dizziness in the morning and was admitted for evaluation. The general condition was good with a pulse rate of 90 per minute and blood pressure of 110/70 mm Hg; systemic examinations had been normal. The uterus was well contracted and there was no discharge. The episiotomy wound was also healthy. The routine hematological and biochemical parameters were within normal limits. After 8 h of ward stay, she developed sudden respiratory distress while drinking carrot juice with the development of peripheral cyanosis; later she became unconscious. A diagnosis of aspiration was entertained and oral suctioning was done. She expired despite attempts at resuscitation.

P. Vaideeswar (✉)
Department of Pathology (Cardiovascular & Thoracic Division), Seth GS Medical College & KEM Hospital, Mumbai, Maharashtra, India

B. Baste
Department of Pathology, Seth GS Medical College & KEM Hospital, Mumbai, Maharashtra, India

41.2 Autopsy Findings

A complete autopsy was performed. On general examination, clubbing of the fingers and peripheral cyanosis on the lips and nails were noted. There was mild cardiomegaly (weight 230 g) with moderate enlargement and hypertrophy of the right-sided chambers. There was large 4.2 × 2.3 cm defect in the interatrial septum below the oval fossa with involvement of the crest of the interventricular septum (Fig. 41.1a). The septal aspect of the RAVV was largely devoid of chordae, dysplastic, rolled, shortened, and directly attached to the endocardium (Fig. 41.1a). The adjoining commissures were also poorly delineated. The pulmonary annulus was dilated; valve cusps were normal. The pulmonary trunk and its branches were dilated with the presence of intimal fatty streaks. The anterior leaflet of the LAVV was cleaved and dysplastic (Fig. 41.1b). Abnormal chordae had inserted into the left ventricular outflow tract, 2.3 cm below the aortic valve, producing narrowing in that region (Fig. 41.2a). The tracheobronchial tree showed some aspirated food material. The vasculature in both lungs appeared prominent (Fig. 41.2b). On histology, the lungs showed a range of changes in PH in the form of intimal fibrocellular thickening, medial hypertrophy, and several plexiform lesions (Fig. 41.3a, b).

K. D. Jashnani (ed.), *Maternal Mortality - Lessons Learnt from Autopsy*,
https://doi.org/10.1007/978-981-19-3420-9_41

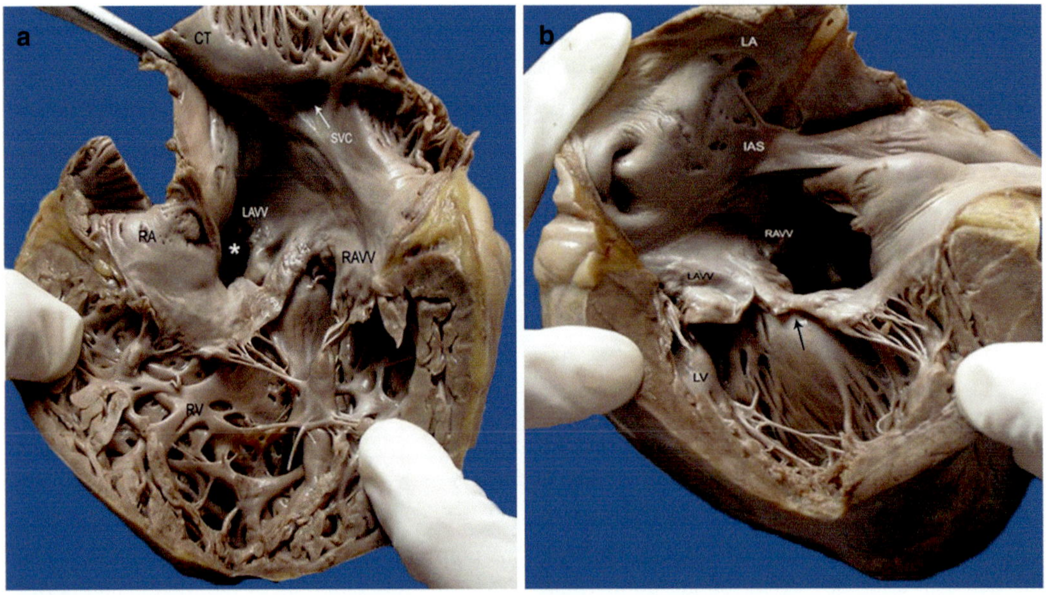

Fig. 41.1 (**a**) Opened out right ventricular RV inflow tract shows a large opening * below the fossa ovalis, which is covered by the right atrioventricular valvular RAVV tissue over its entire inferior margin. Note right ventricular RV hypertrophy; (**b**) Opened out left ventricular LV inflow tract showing the defect that abuts the left atrioventricular valvular LAVV annulus. Note a distinct cleft (arrow). The RAVV tissue can be seen from the left side (CT, crista terminalis; IAS, interatrial septum; LA, left atrium; RA, right atrium; SVC, superior vena cava)

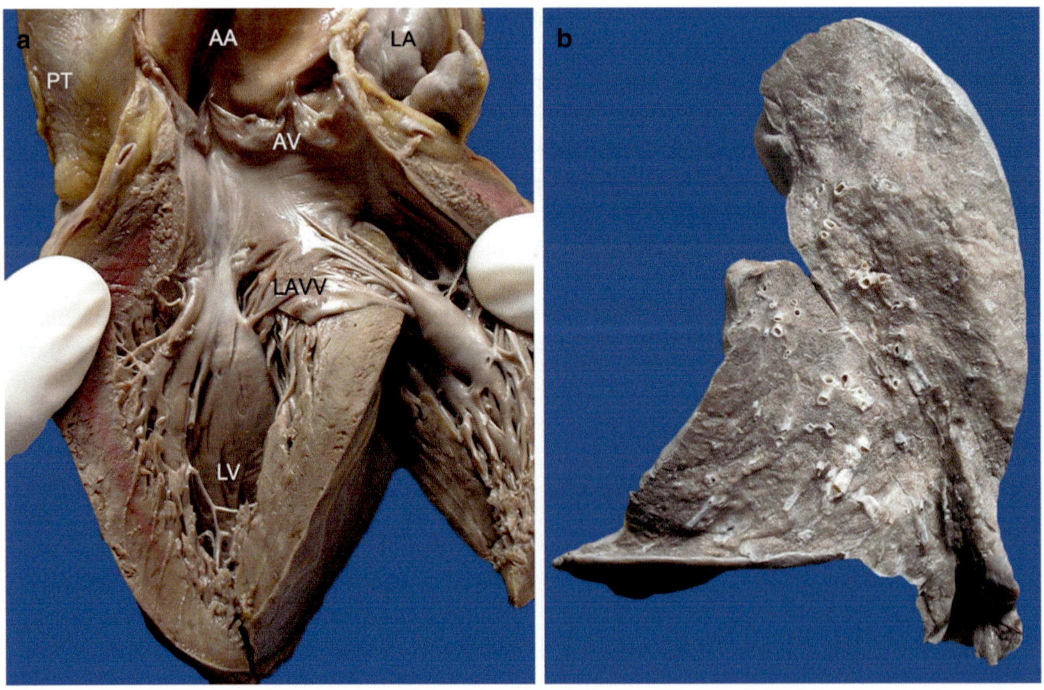

Fig. 41.2 (**a**) The left ventricular LV outflow tract is narrowed due to abnormal attachment of the chordae tendineae of the left atrioventricular valve LAAV (AA ascending aorta, AV aortic valve, LA left atrium, PT pulmonary trunk); (**b**) prominent vasculature seen over the cut surface of the left lung

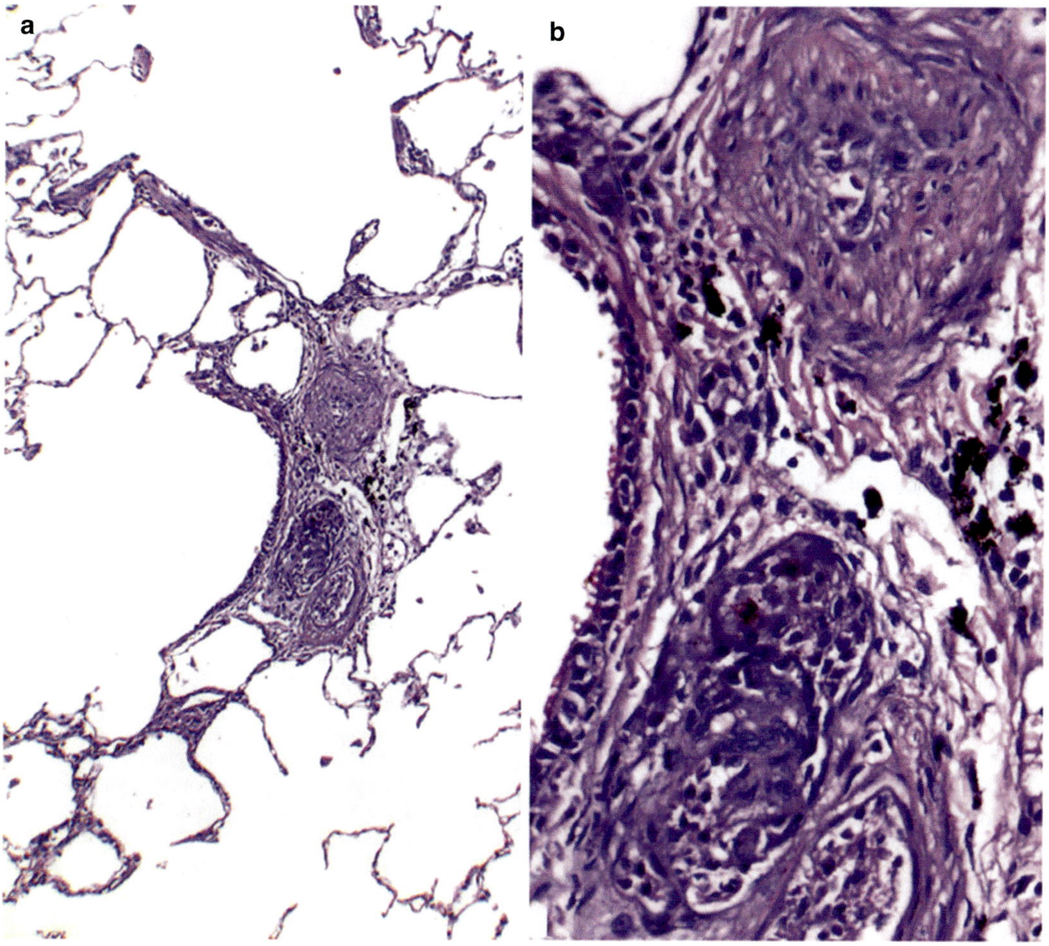

Fig. 41.3 (**a**) Thick-walled arteries seen in a clean background of alveolated parenchyma; (**b**) The artery on top shows marked medial hypertrophy, while the artery at the bottom shows the lumen to be replaced by multiple channels—plexiform lesion (H&E × 400)

41.3 Final Cause of Death

Partial AVSD with Eisenmengerization and right heart failure.

41.4 Clinicopathologic Discussion

An uncorrected CHD with significant left-to-right shunt and severe changes of PH were surprise findings at autopsy performed in the postpartum period in a young woman. Although pregnancy-induced hypertensive disorders are the commonest cardiovascular afflictions, rheumatic heart disease and its associated valvular deformities (see Chap. 1) are common in the middle and low-income countries. With improved methods of medical therapy, cardiological interventions, and palliative or corrective surgeries of CHDs, survival into adulthood is ensured, and a good number of such women would also conceive. Hence, in the developing/developed world, CHD represents an important subset of cardiovascular disease in pregnancy [1]. Since pregnancy is associated with certain physiological alterations in the cardiovascular system, pregnant women with CHD may develop adverse events (affecting the mother and the fetus) and hence these anomalies have been broadly classified into simple and complex defects [2]. Such risk stratification would help in the management of pregnancy, especially those with repairs or even counselling against pregnancy, particularly with complex anomalies [3, 4]. AVSD is considered a complex CHD, and ideally the pregnancy should have been discouraged. In this case, the lesion was undetected and unmasked during the postpartum state. It is to be noted that pregnancy can have symptoms similar to those of cardiac diseases.

The morphological hallmark of AVSD, also called endocardial cushion defect, AV canal defect, or common AV canal, is the presence of a common AV junction as compared to the separate right and left atrioventricular junctions in the normal heart. It accounts for 4 to 7% of all congenital cardiac anomalies and is commonly seen in women and individuals with Down's syndrome. [5]. The basic anatomical spectrum ranges from a single common AV valve or the presence of two valves within a common fibrous ring, constituting the complete or partial forms of AVSD, respectively. Apart from valvular malformations, this creates inter-atrial, AV or interventricular shunting, alterations in the ventricular geometry, and/or conduction defects [5]. Some uncorrected AVSD patients may reach child-bearing age in relatively good health, as was seen in our patient, but the level and degree of shunting decide the pregnancy outcome. There are only few reports of AVSDs during pregnancy in the recent past [6, 7].

The dimensions and location of the defect in this case indicate that there would have been a significant degree of left-to-right shunting. This is further substantiated by the histological features of pulmonary plexogenic lesions indicative of severe pulmonary hypertension. This coupled with pregnancy-induced changes (e.g., volume overload, increased cardiac output and decreased systemic vascular resistance) produces a reversal of shunt with the discharge of an increased volume of deoxygenated blood into the left-sided circulation. This leads to progressive hypoxemia and cardiac dysfunction, a scenario designated as the ES syndrome or Eisenmengerization [8]. The mortality of ES in pregnancy ranges from 26 to 40% and occurs in the last trimester, labor, or immediate postpartum period, the phases associated with acute, maximum, and potentially life-threatening hemodynamic changes. A similar chain of events would have occurred in our case, where rapid cardio-pulmonary decompensation led to sudden death, which was clinically misconstrued as being caused only by aspiration.

References

1. Salciccioli KB, Cotts TB. Pregnancy in women with adult congenital heart disease. Cardiol Clin. 2021;39:55–65.
2. Chan A, Wolfe DS, Zaidi AN. Pregnancy and congenital heart disease: a brief review of risk assessment and management. Clin Obstet Gynecol. 2020;63:836–51.
3. van Hagen IM, Roos-Hesselink JW. Pregnancy in congenital heart disease: risk prediction and counseling. Heart. 2021;106:1853–61.
4. Regitz-Zagrosek V, Roos-Hesselink JW, Bauersachs J, Blomström- Lundqvist C, Cífková R, De Bonis M, et al. 2018 ESC guidelines for the management of cardiovascular diseases during pregnancy. Eur Heart J. 2018;39:3165–241.
5. Taqatqa AS, Vettukattil JJ. Atrioventricular septal defects: pathology, imaging, and treatment options. Curr Cardiol Rep. 2021;23:93.
6. Chen X, Xiao B, Yang W, Chen Y, Zhang W, Zhu H. Complete endocardial cushion defects in pregnancy: a case report. J Med Case Rep. 2014;8:1–3.
7. Li Z, Sun H, Li J, Zhu Y. Management of leukemia and partial atrioventricular septal defect during pregnancy. Thorac Cardiovasc Surg Rep. 2021;10:e45–8.
8. Lopez BM, Malhame I, Davies LK, Gonzalez Velez JM, Marelli A, Rabai F. Eisenmenger syndrome in pregnancy: a management conundrum. J Cardiothorac Vasc Anesth. 2020;34:2813–22.

Choked Prosthetic Mitral Valve

42

Jabin Ullah, Pranita Zare, and Pradeep Vaideeswar

42.1 Clinical History

A 31-year-old pregnant woman (7 weeks' amenorrhea) presented with giddiness, dry cough, palpitation, and acute-onset dyspnea on exertion (New York Heart Association grade III) for the past 5 days. She was a known case of rheumatic MS, diagnosed at the age of 13 with previous balloon valvuloplasty (2002 and 2003) and mitral valve replacement (2018). She had stopped the penidure prophylaxis in 2018 and was currently on anticoagulants (warfarin), antiplatelet drugs, and calcium channel blockers. During an antenatal visit a week ago, she was diagnosed with gestational hypertension (blood pressure 186/100 mm Hg). The echocardiography performed showed no abnormality of the prosthetic mitral valve; the ejection fraction was 60%. She was switched from an oral anticoagulant to low-molecular-weight heparin. The course in the ward was uneventful and she was discharged after 4 days of admission.

On current admission, the general condition was fair with a pulse rate of 120 per minute and blood pressure of 90/50 mm Hg. Systemic examination revealed a clear chest with normal heart sounds and clicks of the mitral prosthesis. Routine investigations were within normal limits. Single intra-uterine gestational sac was seen on ultrasonography. Fetal cardiac activity was present and the crown-to-heel length was 20 mm (suggestive of 8 weeks of gestation). Fifteen hours after admission, the "click" at the mitral area was not heard; she had a sudden cardiac arrest and could not be revived.

42.2 Autopsy Findings

A complete autopsy was performed. The patient was averagely built and nourished. A healed sternotomy 10 cm scar was seen over the anterior chest wall. The heart appeared moderately enlarged in size and weighed 340 g. The epicardial surface was patchily opacified with adherent layers of pericardium (Fig. 42.1a) and sutures buried in the fibrous tissue were present over the superior vena cava, ascending aorta, and right atrium. There was moderate enlargement of the RV and mild enlargement of both atria as well as the LV. The main pulmonary artery was larger than the aorta; the branches were also dilated with intimal thickening. There was mild RV

J. Ullah
Department of Pathology, Seth GS Medical College & KEM Hospital, Mumbai, Maharashtra, India

P. Zare · P. Vaideeswar (✉)
Department of Pathology (Cardiovascular & Thoracic Division), Seth GS Medical College & KEM Hospital, Mumbai, Maharashtra, India

K. D. Jashnani (ed.), *Maternal Mortality - Lessons Learnt from Autopsy*,
https://doi.org/10.1007/978-981-19-3420-9_42

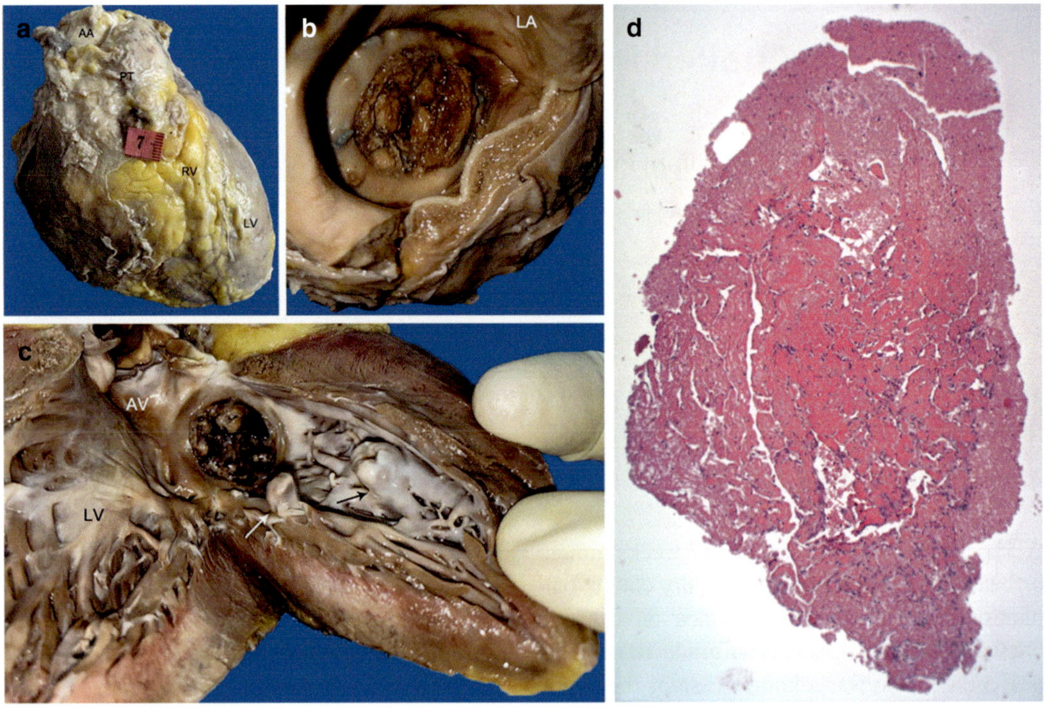

Fig. 42.1 (**a**) Moderate cardiomegaly. There is adherence of the pericardial layers over the right side of the heart. Note dilated pulmonary trunk PT. (**b**) The mitral prosthesis on the left atrial LA aspect is covered by reddish brown flattened thrombotic masses. (**c**) Similar material also obscures the prosthesis from the left ventricular LV aspect. Arrows point to the stumps of the papillary muscles (AA, ascending aorta; RV, right ventricle). (**d**) The thrombotic material was bland composed of fibrin and platelets (H&E × 100)

hypertrophy. The entire mitral valve had been excised (only the bases of papillary muscle were present) and had been replaced by a mechanical bi-leaflet disc valve. The prosthesis was completely obscured on its atrial (Fig. 42.1b) and ventricular (Fig. 42.1c) aspects by pale-brown, flattened to polypoidal thrombotic masses—PVT. On histology, the thrombi were composed of mainly fibrin and platelets and were bland (Fig. 42.1d). Small foci of ischemic scarring were seen in the LV. Fresh and healed infarcts restricted to the cortical region were seen in both kidneys. Changes in chronic passive venous congestion were seen in the lungs and liver.

42.3 Final Cause of Death

Prosthetic mitral valvular thrombosis.

42.4 Clinicopathologic Discussion

A young woman, with a past history of rheumatic MS and mechanical valve replacement, developed PVT in the first trimester of her pregnancy, despite anticoagulant therapy. RHD, a disease of poverty, continues to be rampant in this part of the world and manifests predominantly with left-sided valvular lesions, particularly MS [1]. Apart from the balloon valvotomy procedure and valve repairs, a well-established and definitive therapy is replacement of the diseased valve/s [2]. The prosthetic heart valves may be mechanical or biological (bioprostheses). The bioprosthetic valves typically do not require anticoagulation (unless there are other thromboembolic risk factors), but have a significantly high incidence of valve failure. This is an important concern for young women, who must consider the potential need for future additional valve surgery and plans for pregnancy. In these circumstances, the more durable mechanical valves are preferred (as in this case), but they require life-long anticoagulant therapy as they are inherently predisposed to the development of thrombosis with subsequent obstruction ("choked valve") and systemic embolism. Anticoagulation, if not adequately monitored, is associated with a bleeding tendency.

PVT has an estimated incidence of about 0.3 to 1.3% per patient year [2]. The risk of valve thrombosis and ensuing thromboembolic events depends upon the type of the mechanical valve and its location (most commonly in the mitral location) with other factors such as small valve size, implantation of multiple prosthetic valves, atrial fibrillation, and a previous history of thromboembolism [2]. Pregnancy presents a unique set of problems for women with such prostheses as gestation and puerperium are thrombophilic states, which enhance the chances of PVT. There are increased levels of the procoagulants, decreased levels of their inhibitors, and reduction in the rate of fibrinolysis [3], raising the risk of PVT up to 10%. The magnitude of risk for pregnant women with prosthetic valves in few large-scale studies [4–6] has shown that the maternal mortality rate ranged from 1.4 to 1.8% with mechanical valves, and the overall pregnancy loss rate was about 21%. When risk assessment is applied to pregnant women with CVD, our patient with mechanical valve would fall into the category of modified WHO class III [7] since she did not have severe pulmonary hypertension or left ventricular dysfunction. But it still indicates significantly increased risk of maternal mortality or severe morbidity [7]. Such patients would require expert counseling, regular cardiac and obstetric review and anticoagulation and its timely monitoring. Our patient had been on warfarin, the commonly used vitamin K antagonist. But since the drug can cross the placental barrier and is teratogenic, there was a switchover to low molecular weight heparin. It has been noted that such thrombotic episodes frequently occur in the first trimester during drug switchovers [8], as happened in the case presented. Additionally, there would also be increased heparin clearance by the kidneys during pregnancy and consequent sub-therapeutic levels. Unfortunately, despite normal dosage and levels, thrombotic episodes can occur in 4.4 to 8.7% of patients. Under these circumstances, medical therapy (a low-dose, slow infusion of fibrinolytic regimen) is preferred over surgery.

References

1. Watkins DA, Beaton AZ, Carapetis JR, Karthikeyan G, Mayosi BM, Wyber R, et al. Rheumatic heart disease worldwide. JACC scientific expert panel. J Am Coll Cardiol. 2018;72:1397–416.
2. Nishimura RA, Otto CM, Bonow RO, Carabello BA, Erwin JP 3rd, Fleisher LA, et al. 2017 AHA/ACC focused update of the 2014 AHA/ACC guideline for the management of patients with valvular heart disease: a report of the American College of Cardiology/American Heart Association task force on clinical practice guidelines. Circulation. 2017;135:e1159–95.
3. Economy KE, Valente AM. Mechanical heart valves in pregnancy: a sticky business. Circulation. 2015;132:79–81.
4. Steinberg ZL, Dominguez-Islas CP, Otto CM, Stout KK, Krieger EV. Maternal and fetal outcomes of anticoagulation in pregnant women with mechanical heart valves. J Am Coll Cardiol. 2017;69:2681–91.
5. Lawley CM, Lain SJ, Algert CS, Ford JB, Figtree GA, Roberts CL. Prosthetic heart valves in pregnancy, outcomes for women and their babies: a systematic review and meta-analysis. BJOG. 2015;122:1446–55.
6. Van Hagen IM, Roos-Hesselink JW, Ruys TP, Merz WM, Goland S, Gabriel H, et al. Pregnancy in women with a mechanical heart valve: data of the European Society of Cardiology Registry of pregnancy and cardiac disease (ROPAC). Circulation. 2015;132:132–42.
7. Regitz-Zagrosek V, Roos-Hesselink JW, Bauersachs J, Blomstrom-Lundgvist C, Cifkova R, De Bonis M, et al. 2018 ESC guidelines for the management of cardiovascular diseases during pregnancy. Eur Heart J. 2018;39:3165–241.
8. Romera AE, Sanchez JJ, Sierra JN, Paracuellos TS, Salguero FJV, Solanilla BR. Mitral valve thrombosis in term pregnancy: a case report and review of the literature. Taiwan J Obstet Gynecol. 2021;60:324–7.

Interstitial Lung Disease: Scarred, Stiff Lungs with Honeycombing

43

Kusum D. Jashnani, Lalita Yoganand Patil, and Sagar Punjabi

43.1 Clinical History

A 35-year-old female G3P2L2 with 6 months' amenorrhea was referred from a private hospital with c/o fever, cough, and breathlessness for the past 4–7 days.

O/E- P-80/minute, GC poor, BP 110/70 mm Hg, with SPO_2 100% on BMV at 15 L of O_2. She was conscious and oriented, bilateral creps were auscultated, P/A uterus 26 weeks, relaxed. P/V-Os multiparous, no show, no leak. She gave past H/o cough with breathlessness in her second pregnancy, details of which were not available.

Investigations during her hospital stay revealed T WBC count varying from 13,000 to 19,000/cumm. The platelet count was normal. Hb was 7.8 to 8.0 gm/dL; ESR was 77 to 102 mm/h. LFT, RFT, urine, and TFT all were WNL; HGT—110 g%, ferritin, d dimer was normal. HRCT was highly suspicious for COVID pneumonia with ARDS. However, the possibility of ILD couldn't be ruled out. CO-RADS 4. CT severity score: 23/25.

Treatment given at Nair—Inj Hydrocot, Inj Ceftriaxone, T Azee, Inj Pan 40, Inj Remdesivir, T Ivermectin, Inj Dexa, Inj Artesunate. Due to a drop in saturation, the patient was put on Bipap on day 9 of admission. The patient's condition deteriorated, she was intubated, and was declared dead next day, with a total hospital stay of 10 days. A complete autopsy was performed.

43.2 Autopsy Findings

Bilateral lungs weighing 560 g (right lung) and 480 g (left) were very firm in consistency throughout with a positive sink test. The pleura was thick, opaque, and fibrinous in places. The cut surface showed gray white areas of consolidation throughout. Many areas especially in the base showed tiny cystic spaces of size varying from 1 mm to 4 mm, filled with mucoid material; some were empty (Figs. 43.1 and 43.2). The heart weighed 330 g and showed right ventricular wall hypertrophy of over 1.2 cm (Fig. 43.6a). The uterus measuring 26 × 18 × 5 cm showed a male fetus weighing 920 g. The rest all organs were unremarkable.

Lungs showed varied changes of interstitial lung disease on histology, like areas of intraalveolar hemorrhage, intraalveolar edema, intraalveolar fibroblastic proliferation (fibroblastic foci), intraalveolar foamy macrophages, and neutrophils. Many alveoli showed the presence of an eosinophilic hyaline membrane along their septae, suggestive of ARDS. There was evidence of microscopic honey-

K. D. Jashnani (✉) · L. Y. Patil
Department of Pathology, Topiwala National Medical College and BYL Nair Charitable Hospital, Mumbai, Maharashtra, India

S. Punjabi
Department of Medicine, Topiwala National Medical College and BYL Nair Charitable Hospital, Mumbai, Maharashtra, India

K. D. Jashnani (ed.), *Maternal Mortality - Lessons Learnt from Autopsy*,
https://doi.org/10.1007/978-981-19-3420-9_43

combing consisting of irregular cysts of variable sizes and shapes lined by ciliated tall columnar epithelium, at places showing squamous metaplasia. Their lumina showed the presence of mucus and neutrophils. Interstitium was widened showing chronic inflammatory cells and fibrosis. There were scattered large areas of fibrosis in the lung parenchyma as well as in subpleural areas. The pleura was also fibrotically thickened and showed multiple congested dilated blood vessels. Many of the alveolar spaces showed type II pneumocyte hyperplasia (Figs. 43.3, 43.4 and 43.5). Uterine wall showed hypertrophied myometrial fibers with preischemic changes (Fig. 43.6b).

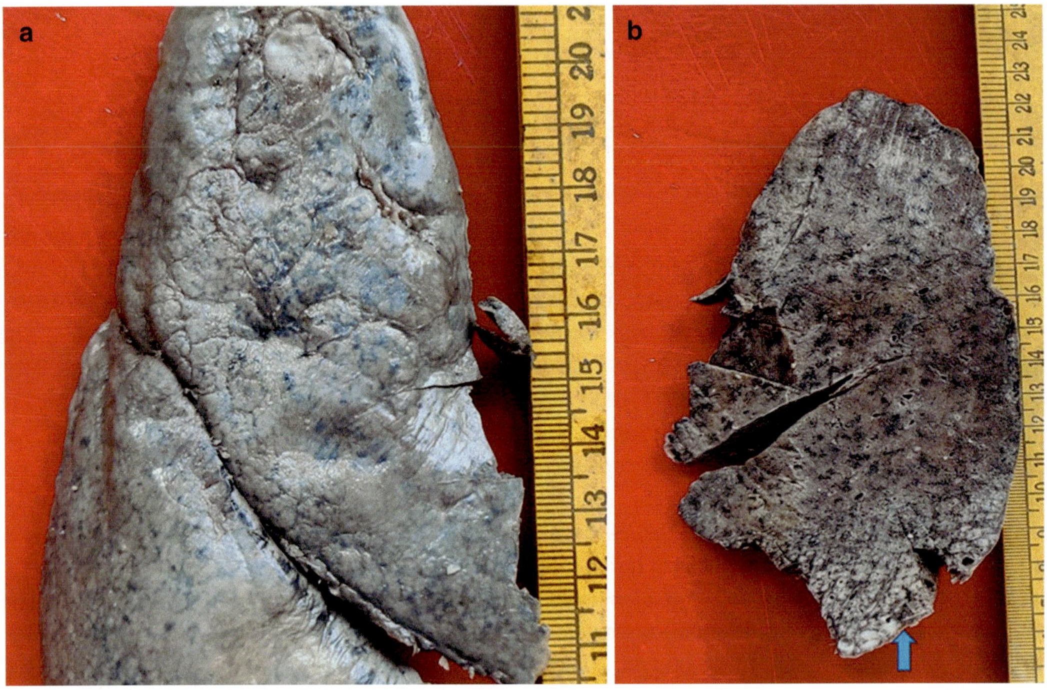

Fig. 43.1 Gross specimen of lung showing thick and opaque pleura, which is fibrinous at places (**a**). Cut surface of the lung shows gray white areas of consolidation throughout (**b**). The base shows multiple tiny cystic spaces of size varying from 1 mm to 4 mm, filled with mucoid material; some were empty (**b**—blue arrow)

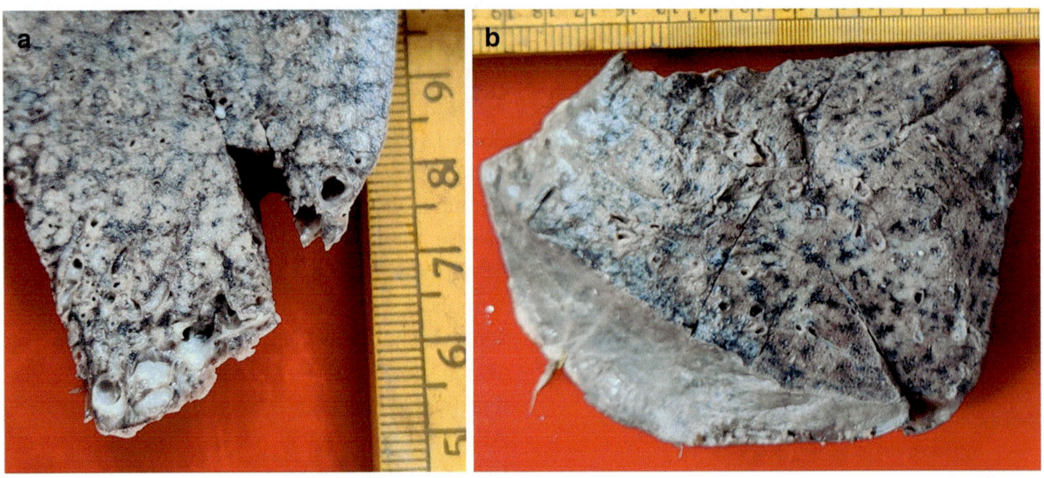

Fig. 43.2 Cut surface of the lung shows gray white areas of consolidation throughout (**b**). The base shows multiple tiny cystic spaces of varying sizes ranging from 1 mm to 4 mm, filled with mucoid material (**a**)

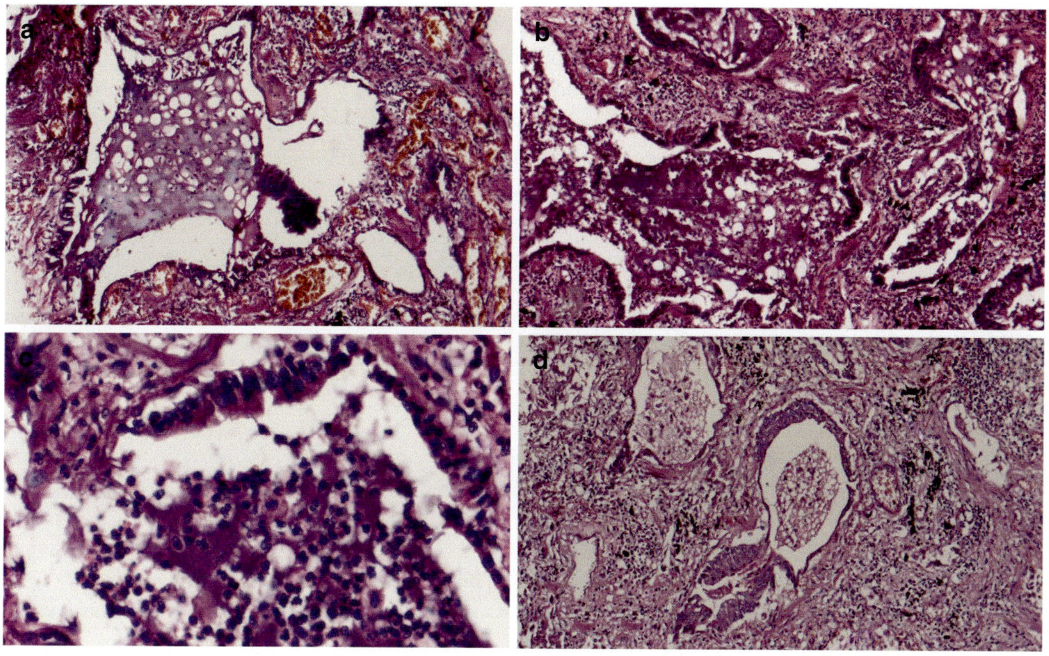

Fig. 43.3 Irregular cysts of variable sizes and shapes (**a**, **b**—H&E, 200×) lined by ciliated tall columnar epithelium (**c**—H&E, 400×), at places showing squamous metaplasia (**d**—H&E, 200×). Their lumina show the presence of mucus and neutrophils

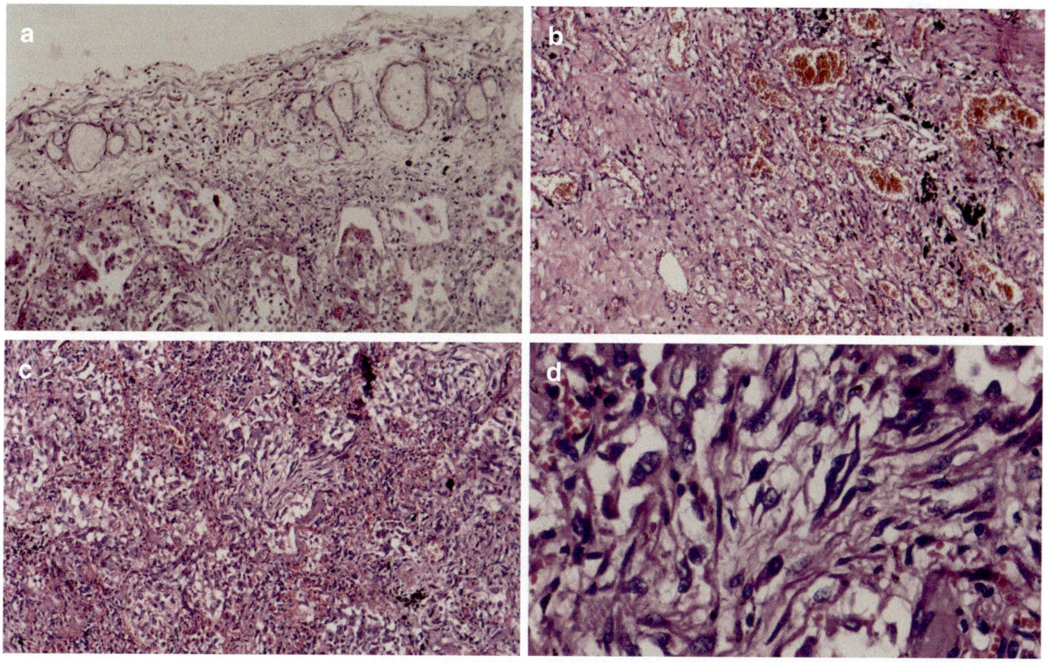

Fig. 43.4 The pleura is fibrotically thick, showing multiple congested dilated blood vessels and subpleural fibrosis (**a**—H&E, 200×). Area of fibrosis in the lung parenchyma (**b**—H&E, 200×). Intraalveolar fibroblastic proliferation-fibroblastic foci (**c**, **d** H&E, 200×, 400×)

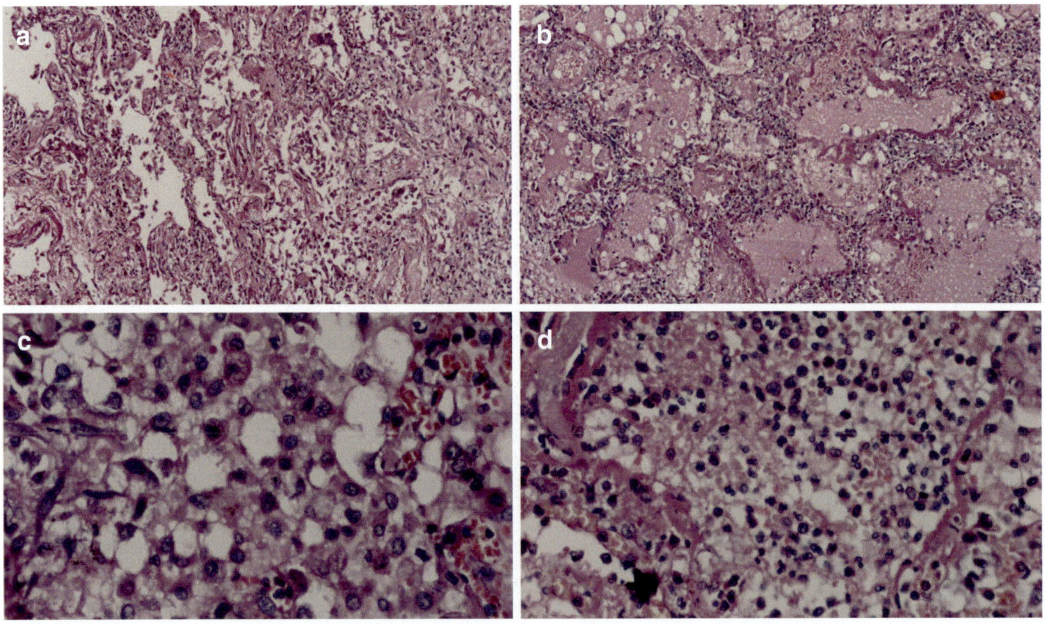

Fig. 43.5 Intraalveolar fibroblastic foci (**a**—H&E, 200×), Eosinophilic hyaline membrane along alveolar septal walls (**b**—H&E, 200×), Intraalveolar foamy macrophages (**c**—H&E, 400×), Intraalveolar neutrophils (**d**—H&E, 400×)

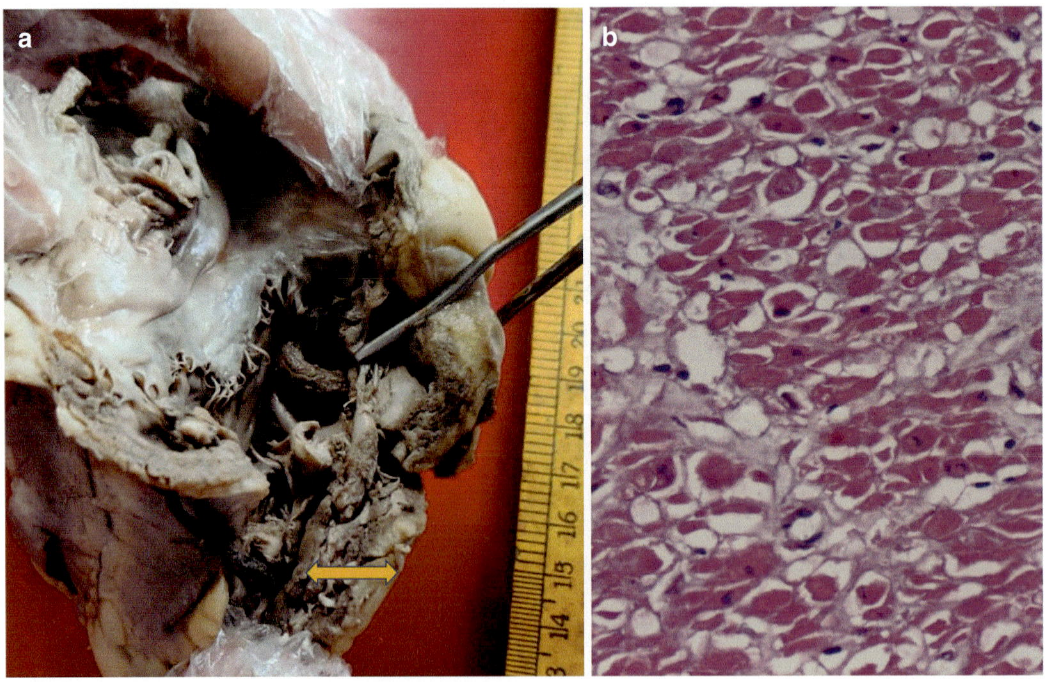

Fig. 43.6 Gross specimen of the heart showing thick right ventricular wall (**a**—yellow arrow). Uterine wall showing hypertrophied myometrial fibers with preischemic changes (**b**—H&E, 200×)

43.3 Final Cause of Death

Cor pulmonale in a case of interstitial lung disease.

43.4 Clinicopathologic Discussion

Interstitial lung disease (ILD) is another term for pulmonary fibrosis, which means "scarring" and "inflammation" of the interstitium. Fibrosis results from epithelial cell dysfunction and myofibroblast dysfunction. Both immune and stromal mechanisms may be contributing to fibrosis progression. Breathlessness is the main clinical complaint in ILD, often accompanied by cough.

Types of ILD include:

- ILD related to autoimmune diseases.
- ILD caused by inhalation of coal dust, asbestos, and tobacco smoke.
- Genetic ILD.
- Idiopathic ILD.

Idiopathic or genetic ILD cannot be prevented, but it is possible to prevent some types with known causes by wearing a respirator around harmful substances, by quitting smoking and taking immunizations for flu and pneumonia to help protect the lungs. There is no cure for ILD as scarring cannot be reversed. Treatment in the form of steroids, pirfenidone, and nintedanib can help slow the progression of the disease. People with mild ILD are stable and can function normally without treatment. People with severe forms of ILD will need regular therapy for the rest of their lives. Pulmonary rehabilitation (physical exercise and breathing techniques) can improve lung efficiency and help people lead somewhat satisfying lives. Lung transplantation may be an option of last resort for people with severe ILD, which can otherwise lead to a series of life-threatening complications like pulmonary hypertension, right-sided heart failure (cor pulmonale) and respiratory failure.

HRCT of the chest provides invaluable information in the form of four patterns of diffuse parenchymal lung disease: (1) ground glass opacity and consolidation, (2) reticulation with parenchymal distortion (fibrosis), (3) nodules, and (4) mosaic patterns and cysts.

In cases of antemortem diagnosis, Surgical Lung Biopsy (SLB) is considered the gold standard in the histologic diagnosis of ILD. However, SLBs carry significant morbidity and mortality. Transbronchial forceps biopsy (TBBX) can diagnose diseases with centrilobular distribution, such as sarcoidosis, berylliosis, and hypersensitivity pneumonitis; it however cannot be used for the diagnosis of UIP/IPF. Cryobiopsy is one more method for obtaining lung tissue fragments (>1 cm) for the diagnosis of interstitial lung disease. However, it may not always be easy to diagnose ILD on biopsies, owing to its varied patterns in different areas, as this feature is very well seen in the index case. Only the cases with unusual clinical presentations and HRCT findings that are not classic for UIP/IPF end up meeting criteria for histopathologic confirmation [1].

As early as 2009, Leslie KO [2] offered six histopathological patterns of ILD:

Pattern 1: Acute lung injury characterized by interstitial edema, intra-alveolar fibrin, reactive type 2 cells, DAD in the form of hyaline membranes, necrosis, and alveolar eosinophils.

Pattern 2: Fibrosis—dense collagen deposition in the lung parenchyma, with some degree of irreversible alteration of lung architecture. Cystic spaces seen are referred to as "microscopic honeycombing" in histopathology. Temporal heterogeneity is characterized by zones of normal lung tissue adjacent to zones of microscopic honeycombing with intervening fibroblastic foci as seen in UIP. Honeycomb lung represents end-stage pulmonary fibrosis. Interstitial fibrosis, subpleural fibrosis, honeycombing only, peribronchiolar fibrosis, and pleuritis are other types of this pattern.

Pattern 3: Interstitial chronic inflammatory infiltrates (lymphocytes and plasma cells) with and without granulomas.

Pattern 4: Alveolar filling with cells or non-cellular material- neutrophils, macrophages, blood and siderophages, eosinophilic material (PAP), OP, etc. The OP pattern is characterized by the presence of intraluminal tufts of plump fibroblasts within terminal bronchioles, alveolar ducts, and alveoli, also known as COP.

Pattern 5: Nodules—single or multiple. These can be neoplastic, nodular ILD, miliary infections, granulomatous disease, pneumoconiosis, etc.

Pattern 6: Minimal changes in pathology in patients with clinical evidence of ILD, which needs review of the clinical and HRCT findings.

As per the latest 2018 ATS/ERS/JRS/ALAT guidelines for the histopathologic diagnosis of idiopathic pulmonary fibrosis [3] are as follows:

1. UIP-dense fibrosis with architectural distortion (destructive scarring/honeycombing)
   (a) Subpleural/paraseptal/patchy lung fibrosis
   (b) Fibroblast foci
2. Probable UIP—Some histologic features from column 1 are present but preclude a definite diagnosis of UIP/IPF
   AND
   (a) No features of an alternative diagnosis
   OR
   (b) Honeycombing only.
3. Indeterminant for UIP: Fibrosis with or without architectural distortion, with other features suggesting an alternative diagnosis.
4. Alternative diagnosis: Features of other histologic patterns of IIPs (e.g., absence of FF or loose fibrosis) or other diseases (e.g., hypersensitivity pneumonitis, Langerhans cell histiocytosis, sarcoidosis, LAM).

The present patient had past history of similar complaints of breathlessness and cough during her last delivery 4 years back, the details of which were not available. This tells us that it would have been the same ILD present for the past many years with progression, leading to her death now. We should remember here that our tertiary care hospital provides services to low socioeconomic group of patients. So, it is not a surprise that it was not diagnosed earlier as ILD. It was not difficult to diagnose ILD now as we had access to autopsy specimens of bilateral lungs.

References

1. Kebbe TA. Review Article Interstitial lung disease: the diagnostic role of bronchoscopy. J Thorac Dis. 2017;9(10):S996–S1010. https://doi.org/10.21037/jtd.2017.06.39.
2. Leslie KO. My approach to interstitial lung disease using clinical, radiological and histopathological patterns. J Clin Pathol. 2009;62:387–401.
3. Smith ML. The histologic diagnosis of usual interstitial pneumonia of idiopathic pulmonary fibrosis. Where we are and where we need to go. Mod Pathol. 2022;35(Suppl 1):8–14. https://doi.org/10.1038/s41379-021-00889-5.

Diffuse Alveolar Damage in COVID-19 Infection

44

Kusum D. Jashnani, Lalita Yoganand Patil, and Giselle Dsilva

44.1 Clinical History

A 29-year-old female with 3 months of pregnancy was transferred to our tertiary care hospital with complaints of (c/o) breathlessness grade IV for 4 days and mild grade fever. O/E-Afebrile, P-117/min, BP-120/66 mm Hg, SPO2–85% on mechanical ventilation, RR-26/min conscious oriented, RS – B/L crepitations.

There was h/o admission in another hospital since the last 21 days with a RAT (COVID) positive test with c/o breathlessness, fever, and generalized weakness. She was conscious, oriented and had bilateral crepitations on auscultation. She received treatment for COVID pneumonia with sepsis. Limited information about her investigations done outside were available to us. These were CRP of 7.5 mg/L on day 1 of her outside admission, which increased to 320 mg/L on day 18th. D dimer on day 1 was 778 μg/mL. LFT and RFT were within normal limits. She was a known case of DM, HTN, and hypothyroidism for 6–7 months, noncompliant with treatment, and not registered anywhere for ANC. The patient's condition was deteriorating, so she was intubated, mechanical ventilation was started, and she was transferred to our hospital with a negative RT-PCR test, done 4 days back. HGT was 226 mg/dL with an ECG showing sinus tachycardia on admission in our hospital. GC continued to be poor, and she was declared dead within 8 h of admission. A complete autopsy was performed.

K. D. Jashnani (✉) · L. Y. Patil
Department of Pathology, Topiwala National Medical College & BYL Nair Charitable Hospital, Mumbai, Maharashtra, India

G. Dsilva
Department of Medicine, Topiwala National Medical College and BYL Nair Charitable Hospital, Mumbai, Maharashtra, India

44.2 Autopsy Findings

Bilateral lungs weighed 520 g each; they were very firm in consistency, with rounded borders, completely gray white and consolidated. Two well-defined areas of necrosis, 4 × 3 × 4 and 2 × 1 × 2 cm in size were seen, suggestive of abscess (Fig. 44.1). Bilateral lungs on histopathology showed features of diffuse alveolar damage classic of COVID infection. There was evidence of intraalveolar hemorrhage, neutrophils, edema fluid, fibrin and macrophages. Eosinophilic hyaline membranes along the alveolar septae, fibrin thrombi in small- and medium-sized blood vessels, and occasional tiny foci of fibrosis were also seen (Figs. 44.2, 44.3, 44.4). Additional findings of well-defined abscess consisting of destruction of lung parenchyma with the presence of dense neutrophilic collection were seen as well as few multinucleated cells—probably type 2 pneumocytes (Fig. 44.5d) as already described in the COVID literature.

K. D. Jashnani (ed.), *Maternal Mortality - Lessons Learnt from Autopsy*,
https://doi.org/10.1007/978-981-19-3420-9_44

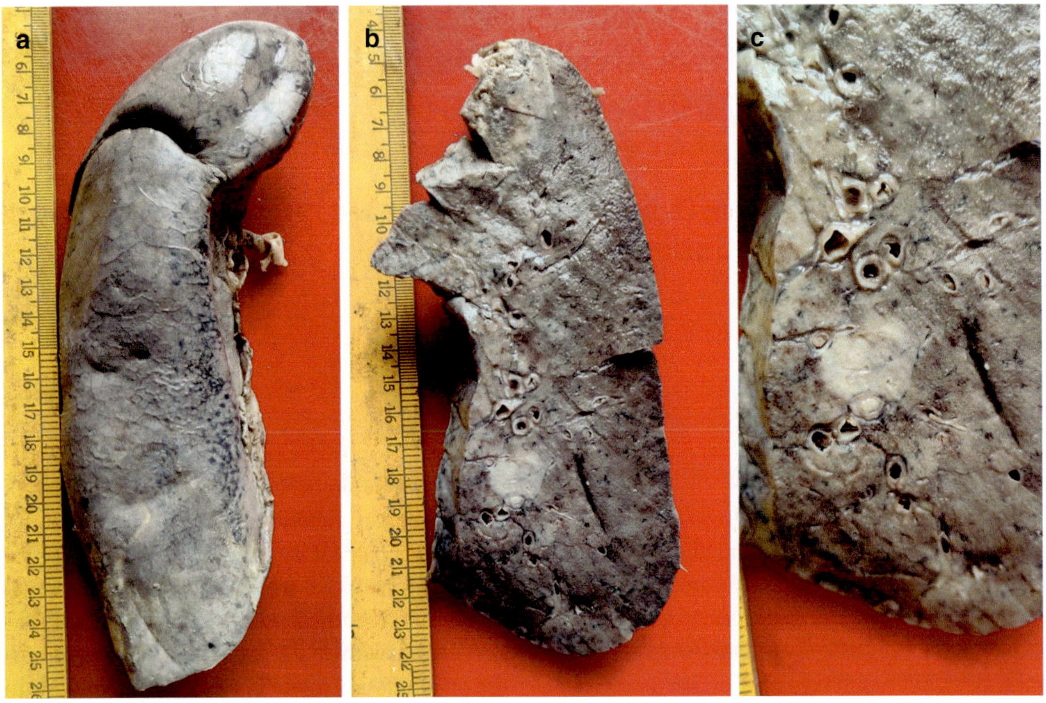

Fig. 44.1 Gross specimen of lung showing thick opaque pleura with rounded borders on external surface (**a**). It was firm in consistency with gray-white areas all throughout and a well-defined area of 2 × 1 × 2 cm of abscess seen in the lower part on the cut surface (**b**, **c**)

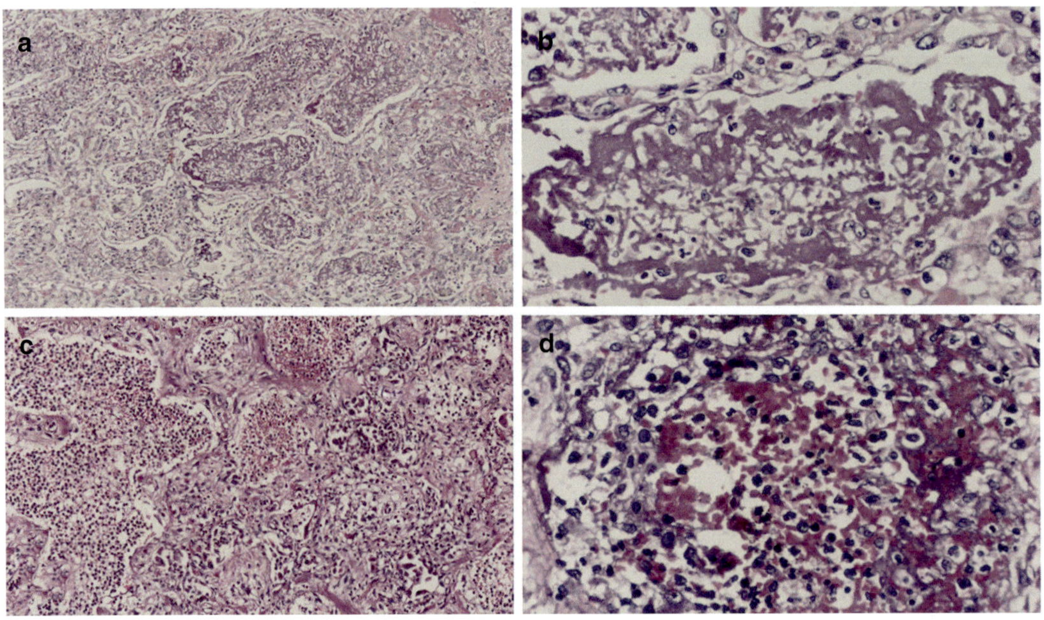

Fig. 44.2 Histopathologic examination of the lung showing the presence of fibrin within the alveolar spaces (H&E, 200×—**a**, H&E, 400×—**b**). Intraalveolar presence of a mixture of neutrophils, RBCs, and little fibrin (H&E, 200×—**c**, H&E, 400×—**d**)

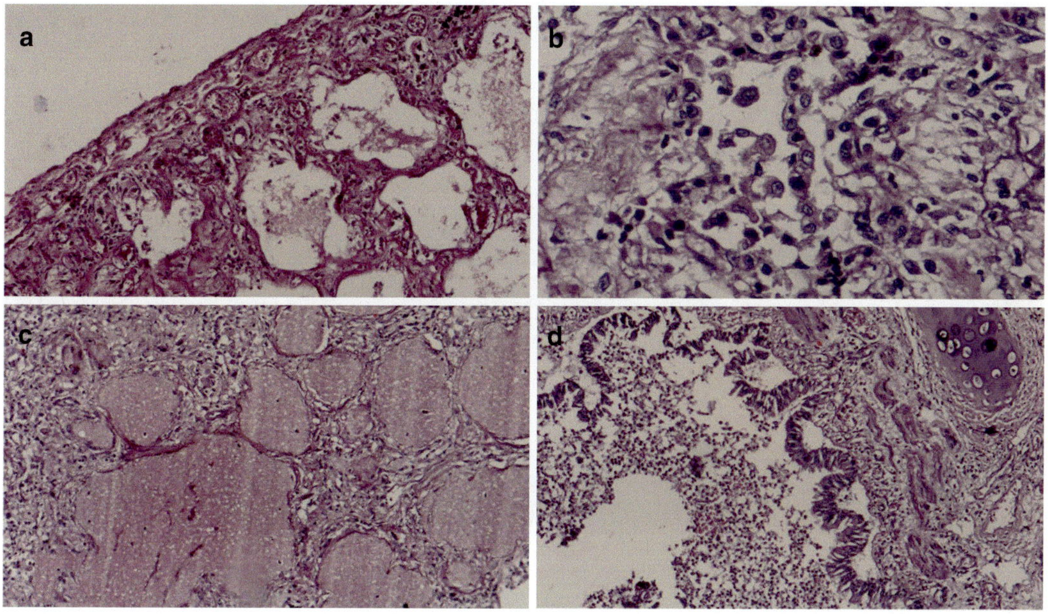

Fig. 44.3 Histopathologic examination of the lung showing pleural fibrous thickening, Type 2 pneumocyte hyperplasia (H&E, 200×—**a**, H&E, 400×—**b**). There is the presence of vacuolated edema fluid within the alveolar spaces and bronchial lumina neutrophils (H&E, 200×—**c**, H&E, 400×—**d**)

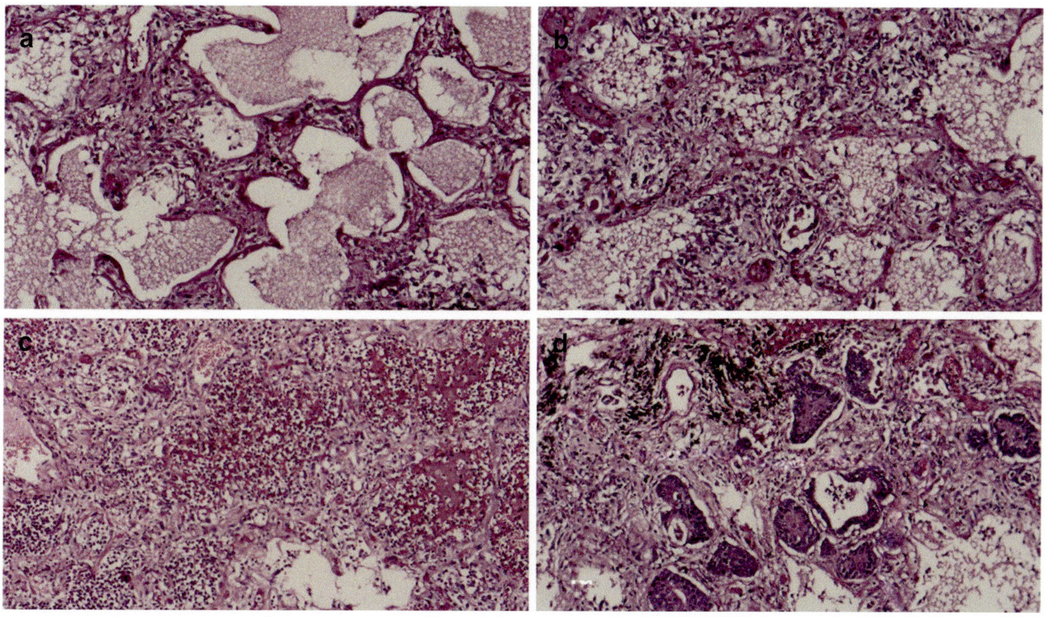

Fig. 44.4 Histopathologic examination of the lung showing eosinophilic hyaline membranes along the alveolar septae (H&E, 200×—**a**), areas of severe acute lung injury (diffuse alveolar damage) in the *acute* exudative stage. (H&E, 200×—**b**, H&E, 200×—**c**) and foci of squamous metaplasia (H&E, 200×—**d**)

The spleen weighing 210 g was enlarged and showed 2 large infarcts 7 × 5 × 5 cm and 3 × 4 × 3 cm. Microscopy confirmed the infarction with the presence of thrombi in few small- and medium-sized arteries (Fig. 44.5). The liver weighing 1.8 kg appeared pale yellow. The uterus

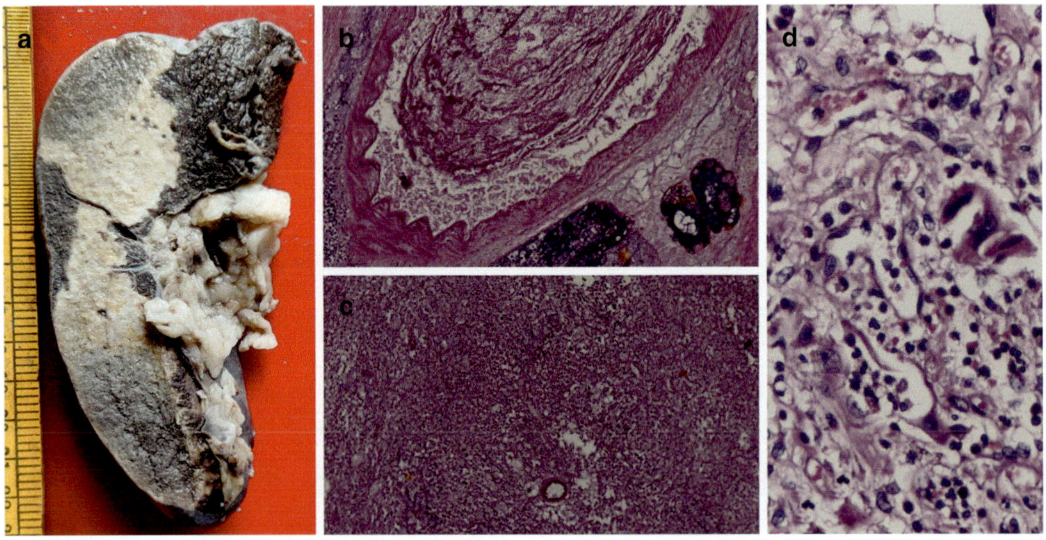

Fig. 44.5 Gross specimen of a slice of the spleen showing large wedge-shaped gray-white infarcts (**a**). Histopathologic examination of spleen showing a thrombus in a medium-sized artery, coagulation necrosis of splenic parenchyma (H&E, 400×—**b**, H&E, 200×—**c**), enlarged multinucleated atypical type 2 pneumocytes (H&E, 200×—**d**)

weighing 400 g showed a fetus weighing 150 g. The rest of the organs were unremarkable on gross as well as microscopy.

44.3 Final Cause of Death

Diffuse alveolar damage with ARDS in a pregnant woman with Covid-19 infection.

44.4 Clinicopathologic Discussion

SARS-CoV-2, the etiologic agent of COVID-19, initially identified in the Hubei province of China in December 2019, was a global pandemic declared by the World Health Organization in March 2020, with substantial mortality due to acute respiratory distress syndrome [1, 2]. This novel virus was identified as a cause of pneumonia [1]. Radiologic findings in the form of ground glass opacities with progression to consolidation with CT score risk and CORAD's score have been used to identify COVID pneumonia till now. The pathology of this progression consists of DAD at different stages and vascular and thrombosis-induced injury. SARS-CoV-2 being a coronavirus utilizes angiotensin converting enzyme 2 (ACE2) as a source of cellular entry. The combination of ACE2 and transmembrane protease serine 2 (TMPRSS2) allows for viral entry into the cells of the nasopharynx and large upper airway, as well into the alveolar AT2 cells, as all these cells express ACE2. This explains the patterns of lung injury both in the upper airways and in the distal alveolar lung tissue [3]. Patients develop coagulation system abnormalities, particularly elevated D-dimer levels, which predispose patients to thrombotic disease. Pro-inflammatory cytokines such as interleukin-6 (IL-6) are also elevated, similar to those seen in sepsis-induced ARDS in general [4].

Diffuse alveolar damage (DAD) has been primarily reported in autopsy studies of the lungs in COVID-19 to date. Congested and edematous lungs with patchy or diffuse involvement as consolidation, along with increased weight of each lung, are seen on gross examination. Macroscopic nodularity represents patches of acute lung injury rather than organizing pneumonia. Diffuse alveolar damage (DAD) describes a sequence of events following severe acute lung injury caused by any one of a variety of insults. Clinically, DAD is characterized by respiratory distress and diffuse pulmonary infiltrates. Although DAD may be considered as the pathological feature of ARDS, not all patients with ARDS have DAD and not all patients with DAD have ARDS. Patients with clinical definition of ARDS and having DAD appear to have worse outcomes than patients with ARDS but without DAD [5, 6].

Microscopic evaluation of the lungs has shown hyaline membranes (with both short and longer duration of disease) and type 2 pneumocyte (AT2 cell) hyperplasia as frequent findings. Interstitial fibroblastic proliferation with fibromyxoid stroma, organizing pneumonia, squamous metaplasia, and alveolar wall acute inflammation have been less frequently noticed. AT2 cell hyperplasia and interstitial fibroblastic proliferation were seen in deceased with longer duration of illness, so also organizing pneumonia and squamous metaplasia. Large vessel thrombi were seen in patients with longer disease duration. Microthrombi containing fibrin and platelets, sometimes admixed with inflammatory cells, were detected in small arteries (<1.0 mm) and in alveolar capillaries [6, 7].

Atypical, enlarged, and sometimes multinucleated pneumocytes with basophilic intracytoplasmic inclusions have been seen [7]. Immunohistochemistry, in situ hybridization, or EM has not been done to confirm these as viral inclusions. Alveolar wall injury with neutrophils with capillary proliferation and necrosis has been seen in a subset of cases, suggesting an endotheliitis [7]. Though vascular thrombi, both fibrin and platelet types, are reported as a component of DAD, they are more frequently seen in COVID-19 infection. This can be explained by direct viral infection of endothelial cells, hypercoagulable state, or systemic immune reaction and be a key aspect of COVID-19 disease pathogenesis. The current patient's lungs showed all the features of DAD, as described in the literature of COVID-19 patients, which also explains her clinical presentation of breathlessness and fever.

References

1. Zhu N, Zhang D, Wang W, Li X, Yang B, Song J, et al. A novel coronavirus from patients with pneumonia in China, 2019. N Engl J Med. 2020;382:727–33.
2. Cucinotta D, Vanelli M. WHO declares COVID-19 a pandemic. Acta Biomed. 2020;91:157–60.
3. Lukassen S, Chua RL, Trefzer T, Kahn NC, Schneider MA, Muley T, et al. SARS-CoV-2 receptor ACE2 and TMPRSS2 are primarily expressed in bronchial transient secretory cells. EMBO J. 2020;39:e105114.
4. Bikdeli B, Madhavan MV, Jimenez D, Chuich T, Dreyfus I, Driggin E, et al. COVID-19 and thrombotic or thromboembolic disease: implications for prevention, antithrombotic therapy, and follow-up. J Am Coll Cardiol. 2020;75:2950–73.
5. Barton LM, Duval EJ, Stroberg E, Ghosh S, Mukhopadhyay S. COVID-19 Autopsies, Oklahoma, USA. Am J Clin Pathol. 2020;153:725–33.
6. Bosmuller H, Traxler S, Bitzer M, Haberle H, Raiser W, Nann D, et al. The evolution of pulmonary pathology in fatal COVID-19 disease: an autopsy study with clinical correlation. Virchows Arch. 2020;477:349–57.
7. Borczuk AC, Salvatore SP, Seshan SV, et al. COVID-19 pulmonary pathology: a multi-institutional autopsy cohort from Italy and new York City. Mod Pathol. 2020;33:2156–68. https://doi.org/10.1038/s41379-020-00661-1.

Takayasu Arteritis: Third Trimester Tragedy

45

Pradeep Vaideeswar

45.1 Clinical History

The body of a 29-year-old woman was referred to our institute for a medicolegal autopsy. She was in her third trimester of pregnancy when she developed sudden unconsciousness with frothing at the mouth and bleeding from her nostrils after a bout of vomiting. During her past antenatal visits, she was diagnosed to have hypothyroidism, while an ultrasound had revealed a small contracted right kidney with compensatory hypertrophy of the left kidney. Other details, including her routine parameters and investigations were not available.

45.2 Autopsy Findings

The heart was markedly enlarged in size (410 g) with marked enlargement (Fig. 45.1a) and moderate concentric hypertrophy of the LV. The great arteries had a normal relationship. The pulmonary trunk (Fig. 45.1a) and its branches were also dilated with thickening of the wall and a tree-bark appearance of the intima at places. The ascending (Fig. 45.1a), transverse and the entire descending aortic segments (Fig. 45.1b) showed an aneurysmal dilatation with thickening of their walls and extensive atherosclerosis with calcification and ulceration. Aneurysmal out-pouching was also seen in the anterolateral aspect of the dilated ascending aorta. The right coronary artery was dominant, and all the arteries were widely patent with normal thickness of their walls. The RBCA (Fig. 45.2a, b) showed the presence of fresh occlusive thrombus right at its origin, extending for its entire length of 2 cm with circumferential thickening of its wall and atherosclerotic calcification. The available lengths of the RCCA, RSA, LCCA, and LSA also had similar appearances (Fig. 45.2a, b), but devoid of thrombi. The aortic annulus was dilated. All the 3 cusps had rounded and everted margins with the presence of bird's nest-like jet lesion in the subaortic region. This indicated the possibility of long-standing aortic regurgitation. The intrapulmonary arteries were also rigid and dilated; parenchyma was normal.

The entire aorta and its branches had an almost similar appearance. Apart from intimal atherosclerotic plaques with complications (Figs. 45.3, 45.4a, b), significant changes were seen in the media and adventitia. There was multifocal destruction of the media with fibrosis, vascularisation and clusters of mononuclear cells. At places, there was a frank granulomatous reaction (Fig. 45.4c, d). There was extensive adventitial and peri-adventitial fibrosis, inflammation, and endarteritis obliterans (Fig. 45.4e). A similar appearance was noted in the extrapulmonary

P. Vaideeswar (✉)
Department of Pathology (Cardiovascular & Thoracic Division), Seth GS Medical College & KEM Hospital, Mumbai, Maharashtra, India

K. D. Jashnani (ed.), *Maternal Mortality - Lessons Learnt from Autopsy*,
https://doi.org/10.1007/978-981-19-3420-9_45

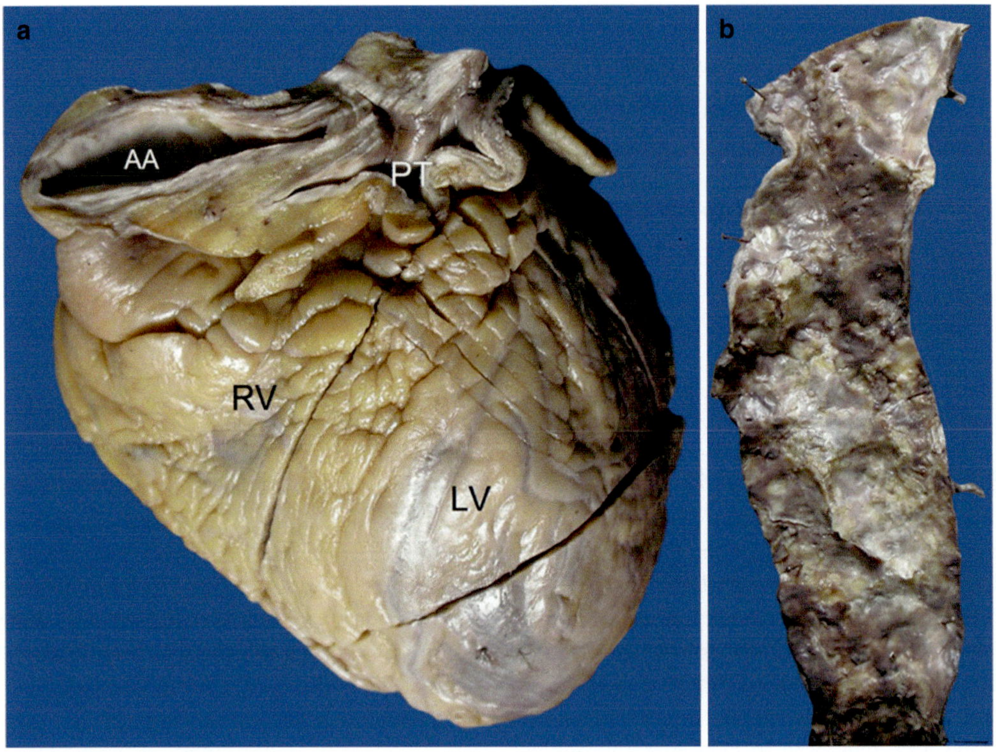

Fig. 45.1 (**a**) Marked cardiomegaly with rounding of the apex. Note the enlargement of the LV and dilatation of the AA and PT. The walls of the arteries are thickened (RV, right ventricle); (**b**) Dilated descending aorta with severe complicated atherosclerosis

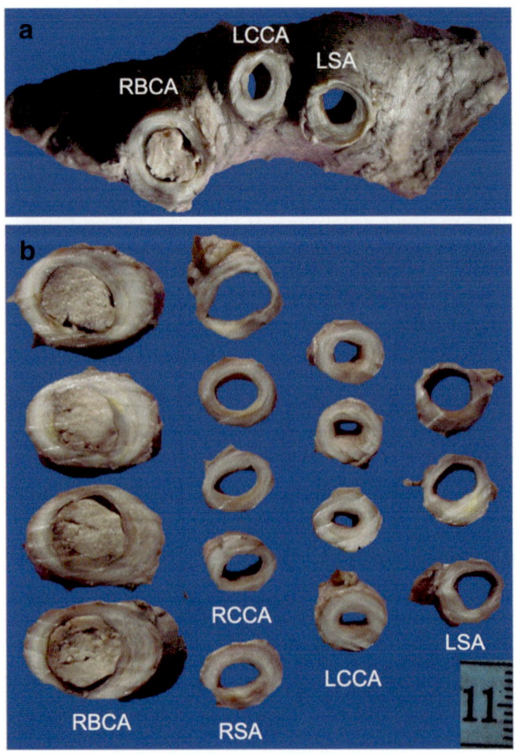

Fig. 45.2 (**a**) End-on view of the arch arteries showing thickening of their walls and occlusive fresh friable thrombus in the RBCA; (**b**) Serial cross-sections of the arch arteries showing similar features. The occlusive thrombus was present along the entire length of the RBCA

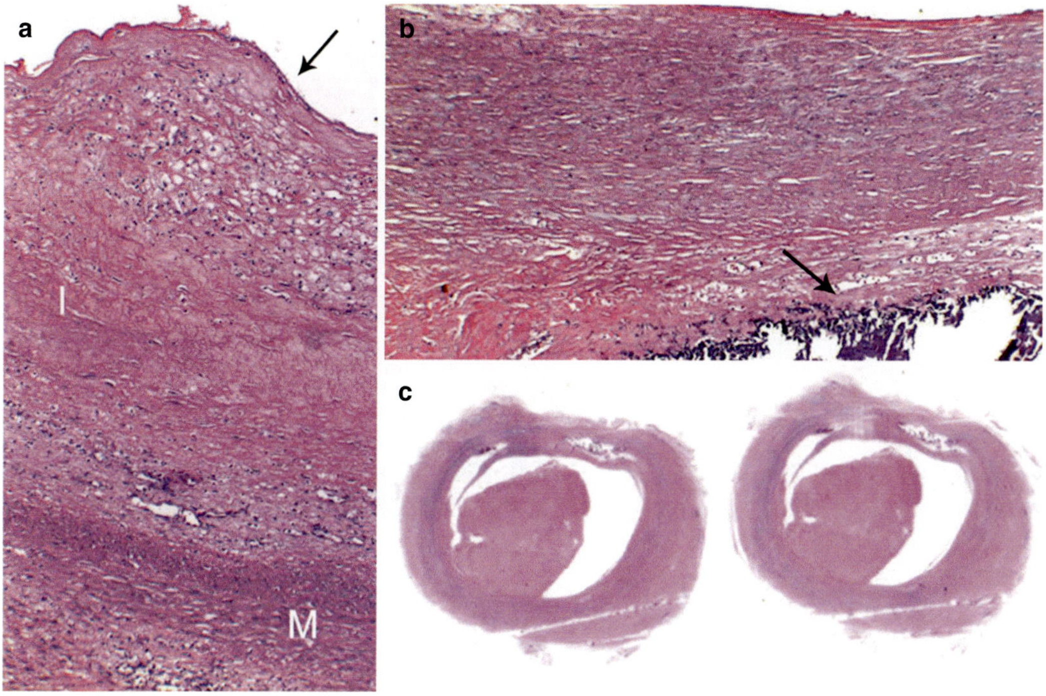

Fig. 45.3 (**a**) Intimal atheroma composed of foam cells (H&E × 200); (**b**) Intimal fibrous plaque with basal calcification (arrow, H&E × 200); (**c**) Scanned section of RBCA with thick wall and luminal thrombus (I intima, M media)

arteries. The intrapulmonary branches showed present intimal fibro-cellular thickening and sprinkling of inflammatory cells. A diagnosis of TA was made. The right kidney was small and contracted (6 × 3 × 1 cm), while the left measured 13 × 5 × 3 cm. No abnormalities were noted in the uterus, placenta, or fetus. No obvious infarcts or ischemic changes were seen in the brain. The thyroid showed lymphocytic thyroiditis. Other organs were normal.

45.3 Final Cause of Death

Diffuse TA with thrombotic occlusion of RBCA.

45.4 Clinicopathologic Discussion

Well-established primary vasculitic process was encountered as a surprise finding at autopsy in a case of maternal mortality. These vasculitic syndromes are a heterogeneous group of disorders that have varied demographic characteristics, etio-pathogenetic mechanisms, inflammatory responses, clinical manifestations, and natural histories. The commonality is inflammation of the vessel walls, and vasculitides are mainly classified on the basis of their vascular calibers [1]. In the illustrated case, there was LVV with dominant involvement of the large vessels (aorta and its branches), best exemplified by TA [2]. Moreover, TA affects women of reproductive age (second and third decades of life), and hence it remains the most common type of LVV diagnosed or identified before or during pregnancy [3].

TA has a worldwide distribution with a prevalence of 1.2 to 2.6 per 100,000 individuals per year, but a higher degree of occurrence in the Southeast Asian and Indian subcontinents with a male-to-female ratio of 1:8 [2]. Though the etio-pathogenesis is not exactly known, there is presumably a complex interaction between genetic/immunological factors and infectious agents (particularly tuberculosis) [4]. This ultimately sets in an autoimmune

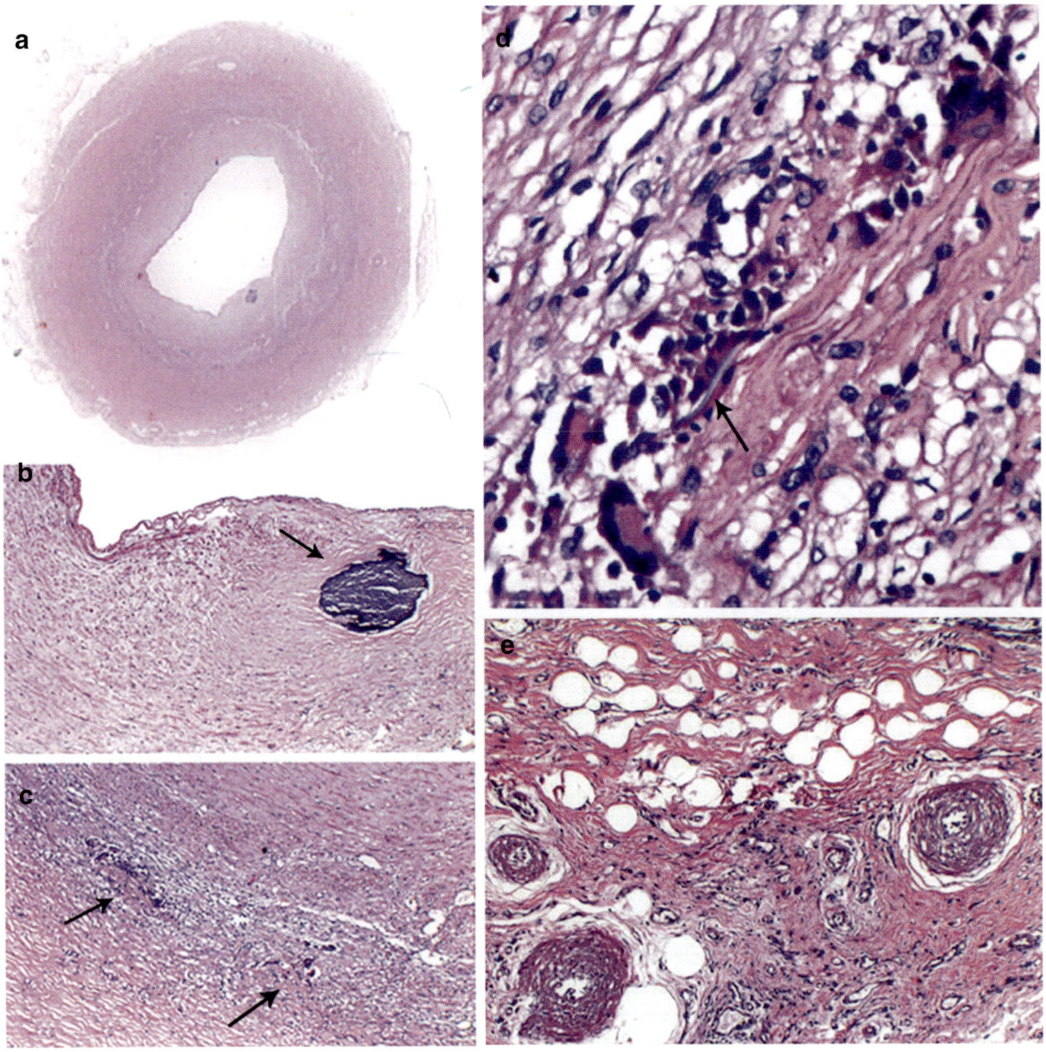

Fig. 45.4 (**a**) Scanned section of LCCA; (**b**) Intimal thickening with calcification (arrow, H&E × 200); (**c**) Granulomatous inflammation (arrows) at the medio-adventitial junction (H&E × 200); (**d**) Giant cell ingesting the elastic fiber—"elastophagia" (H&E × 400); (**e**) End-arteritis obliterans in the thickened adventitia (H&E × 200)

granulomatous panarteritis of the aorta and other large arteries. Depending on the anatomical patterns, TA is categorized as Type I—aortic arch and its branches; Type IIa—ascending aorta, arch and its branches; Type IIb—ascending aorta, arch, its branches and descending thoracic aorta; Type III—thoracic aorta and abdominal aorta; Type IV—abdominal aorta; and Type V—entire aorta [5]. Involvement of coronary arteries is labeled C (+) and involvement of pulmonary arteries is denoted as P (+) [5]. The inflammation has active, healing, and chronic inflammatory phases, culminating in stenosis, obliteration, or dilatation of the affected arteries [2, 5]. Most commonly in the Indian subcontinent, there is frequent affection of the thoracoabdominal aorta and renal arteries, constituting 'middle aortic syndrome'. Involvement of the entire aorta (Type V) and the pulmonary arteries [P (+)] and telescoped inflammatory phases were noted in our case; the aorta was slightly dilated and its branches exhibited stenosis of their lumens.

In the early stages of the disease (pre-pulseless and vasculitic phases), the patients present with constitutional symptoms without or with angiodynia, i.e., tenderness or pain over the vessels. Organ specific features related to vascular stenosis/occlusion are seen in the late stage of TA. Since there is a wide spectrum of manifestations, specific diagnostic criteria (Ishikawa diagnostic criteria or American College of Rheumatology classification criteria) have been outlined to identify these patients [2, 5]. Most patients, in general, present with hypertension, blood pressure differences between the upper and lower limbs, bruits, claudication, and pulselessness. This patient was not clinically diagnosed as a case of TA. Severe hypertension, preeclampsia, and eclampsia are the most common obstetric complications in patients with TA, and the prevalence is said to be around 40% as compared to 8% in patients without the disease [6–8]. Other complications include intrauterine growth retardation, pre-term delivery, or even fetal loss [6–8]. Unfortunately, no details were available in this case during autopsy. In addition, the adaptive changes in the cardiovascular system and modifications in the levels of both hormones and cytokines during pregnancy may increase the disease activity [6–8]. This predisposes the pregnant woman with TA to the development of hypertensive complications, cardiac failure, aortic regurgitation, aortic dissection, renal insufficiency, and stroke. In our case, despite the presence of secondary atherosclerosis, few arterial walls showed the presence of active granulomatous inflammation and the presence of occlusive thrombus in major branches. Hence it is imperative to control the hypertension and disease activity to minimize adverse maternal and fetal outcomes. TA should remain an important differential diagnosis in patients with gestational hypertension.

References

1. Jennette JC, Falk RJ, Bacon PA, Basu N, Cid MC, Ferrario F, et al. 2012 revised international Chapel Hill consensus conference nomenclature of vasculitides. Arthritis Rheum. 2013;65:1–11.
2. Vaideeswar P, Deshpande JR. Pathology of Takayasu's arteritis: a brief review. Ann Ped Cardiol. 2013;6:52–8.
3. Machen L, Clowse MEB. Vasculitis and pregnancy. Rheum Dis Clin N Am. 2017;43:239–47.
4. Hrisrova D, Marchev S. Takayasu arteritis – a systematic review. Acta Medica Bulgarica. 2019;46:56–64.
5. Hata A, Noda M, Moriwaki R, Numano F. Angiographic findings in Takayasu arteritis: new classification. Int J Cardiol. 1996;54:S155–63.
6. Comarmond C, Mirault T, Biard L, Nizard J, Lambert M, Wechsler B, et al. Takayasu arteritis and pregnancy. Arthritis. Rheumatol. 2015;67:3262–9.
7. Comarmond C, Saadoun D, Nizard J, Cacoub P. Pregnancy issues in Takayasu arteritis. Semin Arthritis Rheum. 2020;50:911–4.
8. Ross C, D'Souza R, Pagnoux C. Pregnancy outcomes in systemic vasculitides. Curr Rheumatol Rep. 2020;22:63.

Abbreviations

2-D	Two-dimensional
3-D	Three-dimensional
AA	Ascending aorta
ACE2	Angiotensin converting enzyme 2
ACOG	American College of Obstetrics and Gynaecology
ADAMTS13	A disintegrin and metalloproteinase with a thrombospondin Type 1 motif, member 13
AFB	Acid fast bacilli
AFE	Amniotic fluid embolism
AFI	Acute febrile illness
AFI	Amniotic fluid index
AFLP	Acute fatty liver of pregnancy
AKI	Acute kidney injury
ALAT	Latin American Thoracic Society
ALF	Acute liver failure
AMH	Anti-Mullerian hormone
ANA	Antinuclear antibody
ANC	Antenatal care
ANC	Antenatal clinic
AP	Acute pancreatitis
APC gene	Adenomatous polyposis coli gene
APLA	Antiphospholipid antibodies
APS	Antiphospholipid syndrome
aPTT	Activated partial thromboplastin time
ATT	Antituberculous treatment
AR	Aortic regurgitation
ARDS	Acute respiratory distress syndrome
ARF	Acute renal failure
ARF	Acute rheumatic fever
ARVD/C	Arrhythmogenic right ventricular dysplasia/cardiomyopathy
AT-1AA	Angiotensin type 1 receptor autoantibody
AT2	Type 2 pneumocyte
ATS	American Thoracic Society
AV	Atrioventricular
AVM	Arteriovenous malformation
AVSD	Atrioventricular septal defect
B/L	Bilateral
BiPAP	Bilevel positive airway pressure
BP	Blood pressure
BUN	Blood urea nitrogen
Ca	Calcium
CBC	Complete blood count
CCF	Congestive cardiac failure
CHD	Congenital heart disease
CIAB	Cried immediately after birth
CKD	Chronic kidney disease
cm	Centimetre
c/o	Complaints of
COP	Cryptogenic organizing pneumonia
CO-RADS	COVID-19 Reporting and Data System
COVID	Coronavirus disease

K. D. Jashnani (ed.), *Maternal Mortality - Lessons Learnt from Autopsy*,
https://doi.org/10.1007/978-981-19-3420-9

CPAP	Continuous positive airway pressure
CPC	Chronic passive congestion
CPR	Cardiopulmonary resuscitation
Cr	Creatinine
CRP	C-reactive protein
CRRT	Continuous renal replacement therapy
CSF	Cerebrospinal fluid
CT	Computed tomography
CVD	Cardiovascular disease
CVS	Cardiovascular system
CVST	Cerebral venous sinus thrombosis
D & C	Dilatation and curettage
D & E	Dilatation and evacuation
DAD	Diffuse alveolar damage
DC	Differential count
DCM	Dilated cardiomyopathy
DCT/ICT	Direct/indirect Coombs test
DIC	Disseminated intravascular coagulation
DM	Diabetes mellitus
DNA	Deoxyribonucleic acid
DOE	Dyspnea on exertion
DPS	Deep painful stimuli
dsDNA	double-stranded deoxyribonucleic acid
E	Eosinophils
ECF	Extracellular fluid
ECG	Electrocardiogram
EMB	Endomyocardial biopsy
ERS	European Respiratory Society
ES	Eisenmenger syndrome
ESR	Erythrocyte sedimentation rate
ET-1	Endothelin 1
FDP	Fibrin degradation products
FF	Fibroblast foci
FFP	Fresh frozen plasma
FHF	Fulminant hepatic failure
FHS	Fetal heart sounds
FLF	Fulminant liver failure
FNAC	Fine-needle aspiration cytology
fNSIP	Fibrotic nonspecific interstitial pneumonia
FTND	Full-term normal delivery
g	Grams
G/P/L	Gravida/parity/live
G/P/L/A	Gravida/parity/live/abortion
G/P/L/D	Gravida/parity/live/death
GBM	Glomerular basement membrane
GC	General condition
GCM	Giant cell myocarditis
GCS	Glasgow Coma Scale
GFR	Glomerular filtration rate
GMS	Grocott-Gomori's methenamine silver
GN	Glomerulonephritis
GTCS	Generalized tonic clonic convulsions
H&E	Hematoxylin and eosin
h/o	History of
HAV	Hepatitis A virus
Hb	Hemoglobin
Hb A	Hemoglobin A
Hb F	Fetal hemoglobin
HbS	Sickle hemoglobin
HBsAg	Hepatitis B surface antigen
HCM	Hypertrophic cardiomyopathy
HCV	Hepatitis C virus
HELLP	Hemolysis, elevated liver enzymes, low platelet count
HEV	Hepatitis E virus
Hg	Mercury
HGT	Hemo glucose test
HIV	Human immunodeficiency virus
HIV 1	Human immunodeficiency virus-1
HRCT	High resonance computed tomography
HSV	*Herpes simplex* virus
HTLV	Human T-lymphotrophic virus
HTN	Hypertension
HUS	Hemolytic uremic syndrome
ICH	Intracranial hemorrhage
ICU	Intensive care unit
IgG	Immunoglobulin G
IgM	Immunoglobulin M
IL	Interleukins
ILD	Interstitial lung disease
Inj	Injection
IPF	Idiopathic pulmonary fibrosis

ISN/RPS	International Society of Nephrology/Renal Pathology Society
IT	Intermediate trophoblast
ITP	Immune thrombocytopenic purpura
IUCD	Intrauterine contraceptive device
IUFD	Intrauterine fetal death/demise
IUGR	Intrauterine growth retardation
JRS	Japanese Respiratory Society
JVP	Jugular venous pressure
K	Potassium
kg	Kilogram
L	Lymphocytes
L/min	Liters/minute
LAM	Lymphangioleiomyomatosis
LAVV	Left atrioventricular valve
LCCA	Left common carotid artery
LDH	Lactate dehydrogenase
LFT	Liver function test
LMP	Last menstrual period
LN	Lupus nephritis
LRTI	Lower respiratory tract infection
LSA	Left subclavian artery
LSCS	Lower segment cesarean section
LV	Left ventricle
LVH	Left ventricular hypertrophy
LVV	Large-vessel vasculitis
M	Monocytes
MI	Myocardial Infarction
MICU	Medical intensive care unit
MODS	Multiple organ dysfunction syndrome
MR	Mitral regurgitation
MRI	Magnetic resonance imaging
MRI/MRV	Magnetic resonance imaging/magnetic resonance venography
MS	Mitral stenosis
MTP	Medical termination of pregnancy
NCC	Neurocysticercosis
NICU	Neonatal intensive care unit
NIV	Noninvasive ventilation
NO	Nitric oxide
Nucleated RBC	Nucleated red blood cell
NYHA	New York Heart Association
O/E	On examination
O_2	Oxygen
OP	Organizing pneumonia
OPD	Outpatient department
P	Polymorphs
P	Pulse
P/A	Per abdomen
P/V	Per vaginum
PAP	Pulmonary alveolar proteinosis
PAS	Periodic acid Schiff
PH	Pulmonary hypertension
PHC	Primary health center
PIGF	Placental growth factor
PIH	Pregnancy-induced hypertension
PND	Paroxysmal nocturnal dyspnea
PP	Post-partum
PPCM	Peripartum cardiomyopathy
PPH	Postpartum hemorrhage
PRBCs	Parasitized red blood cells
PS	Peripheral smear
PT	Prothrombin time
PT	Pulmonary trunk
PT/INR	Prothrombin time/international normalized ratio
PTAH	Phosphotungstic acid hematoxylin
PVT	Prosthetic valve thrombosis
RAT	Rapid antigen test
RAVV	Right atrioventricular valve
RBBB	Right bundle-branch block
RBCs	Red blood cells
RBC/HPF	Red blood cells/high power field
RBCA	Right brachiocephalic artery
RCCA	Right common carotid artery
RCN	Renal cortical necrosis
RDP	Random donor platelets
RFT	Renal function test
RHD	Rheumatic heart disease
RHP	Rudimentary horn pregnancy
RMAT	Rapid malaria antigen test
RNP	Ribonucleoprotein

RPGN	Rapidly progressive glomerulonephritis
RPOC	Retained products of conception
RR	Respiratory rate
RS	Respiratory system
RSA	Right subclavian artery
RV	Right ventricle
SARS-CoV-2	Severe acute respiratory syndrome coronavirus 2
sFlt1	Soluble fms like tyrosine kinase 1
SGOT (AST)	Serum glutamic oxaloacetic transaminase (aspartate aminotransferase)
SGPT (ALT)	Serum glutamic pyruvic transaminase (alanine aminotransferase)
SLE	Systemic lupus erythematosus
SLIUF	Single live intrauterine fetus
Sm	Smith
SOB	Shortness of breath
SPO_2	Peripheral capillary oxygen saturation
spp.	Species
SSA	Sjogren syndrome-related antigen A
SSS	Superior sagittal sinus
T	Tablet
TB	Tuberculosis
TBLB	Transbronchial lung biopsy
TFT	Thyroid function test
TIBC	Total iron binding capacity
TLC	Total leucocyte count
TMPRSS2	Transmembrane protease serine 2
TNF	Tumor necrosis factor
TR	Tricuspid regurgitation
TTP	Thrombotic thrombocytopenic purpura
TWBC	Total white blood cell
UIP	Usual interstitial pneumonia
USG	Ultrasonography
UTI	Urinary tract infection
UVA	Uterine vascular anomalies
VEGF	Vascular endothelial growth factor
VTE	Venous thromboembolism
vWF	von Willebrand factor
WBC	White blood cells
WHO	World Health Organization
WNL	Within normal limits
ZN	Ziehl-Neelsen

MIX
Papier aus verantwortungsvollen Quellen
Paper from responsible sources
FSC® C105338

If you have any concerns about our products,
you can contact us on
ProductSafety@springernature.com

In case Publisher is established outside the EU,
the EU authorized representative is:
Springer Nature Customer Service Center GmbH
Europaplatz 3, 69115 Heidelberg, Germany

Printed by Libri Plureos GmbH
in Hamburg, Germany